Introduction to Drug Metabolism

INTRODUCTION TO DRUG METABOLISM

Second edition

G. GORDON GIBSON, PhD
Professor of Molecular Toxicology
School of Biological Sciences
University of Surrey

and

PAUL SKETT, Fil.dr.
Senior Lecturer in Pharmacology
University of Glasgow

BLACKIE ACADEMIC & PROFESSIONAL
An Imprint of Chapman & Hall
London · Glasgow · New York · Tokyo · Melbourne · Madras

Published by
Blackie Academic & Professional, an imprint of Chapman & Hall,
Wester Cleddens Road, Bishopbriggs, Glasgow G64 2NZ

Chapman & Hall, 2–6 Boundary Row, London SE1 8HN, UK

Blackie Academic & Professional, Wester Cleddens Road, Bishopbriggs, Glasgow G64 2NZ, UK

Chapman & Hall Inc., One Penn Plaza, 41st Floor, New York NY10119, USA

Chapman & Hall Japan, Thomson Publishing Japan, Hirakawacho Nemoto Building, 6F, 1-7-11 Hirakawa-cho, Chiyoda-ku, Tokyo 102, Japan

DA Book (Aust.) Pty Ltd., 648 Whitehorse Road, Mitcham 3132, Victoria, Australia

Chapman & Hall India, R. Seshadri, 32 Second Main Road, CIT East, Madras 600 035, India

First edition 1986
Second edition 1994

© 1994 Chapman & Hall

Typeset in 10/12 pt Times New Roman by ICON Graphic Services, Exeter
Printed in Great Britain by Page Bros, Norwich, Norfolk

ISBN 0 7514 0042 4

A catalogue record for this book is available from the British Library

Library of Congress Catalog Card Number: 93-73495

Printed on acid-free text paper, manufactured in accordance with ANSI/NISO Z39.48-1992 and ANSI/NISO Z39.48-1984 (Permanence of Paper).

Preface to second edition

It is now eight years since the publication of the first edition of *Introduction to Drug Metabolism* and much has changed in the world of drug biotransformation. The routes of metabolism are still relevant but much new information is available about the enzymology of the reactions (including a completely new method of naming many of the enzyme isoforms), the control mechanisms and methods of studying drug metabolism. We felt, therefore, that it was time to update the text to incorporate these new ideas.

The textbook is intended to be a primer in drug metabolism for advanced undergraduate classes in science, medicine, dentistry and pharmacy, and for postgraduate students new to the area of drug metabolism. It is also useful as a source book of methods for undergraduate experiments in drug metabolism.

The layout and content of the text is little changed from the first edition, as this was well received and we do not believe in tampering with something that is working. We intended to show the routes of metabolism first (chapter 1) and then further describe the enzymology of the reactions (chapter 2), followed by the important phenomena of induction and inhibition (chapter 3). The lessons learned in the first three chapters are used to illustrate how factors can affect drug metabolism (chapters 4 and 5) and the pharmacological, toxicological and clinical significance of drug metabolism (chapters 6 and 7). Chapter 8 is the methods section for a menu of drug metabolism related practicals.

The expertise of the two authors is complementary, with one based on biochemistry and toxicology and the other on pharmacology and medicine. This is reflected in the balanced approach to the subject in this text. There is no other textbook at this level on drug metabolism – students have recourse only to more advanced texts, monographs and review articles. Many of these are given as a further reading list at the end of each chapter.

We are indebted to our many colleagues and former students for comments on the first edition which have helped to make the second edition, we believe, better. In particular, we would like to thank Dr Tachio Aimoto, Setsunan University, and Dr L. Chasseaud for the great amount of effort put into searching out errors in the first edition. Also we acknowledge the help of the staff at Blackie Academic & Professional during preparation of the second edition. Again, all comments on this edition will be welcome.

G.G.G.
P.S.

Contents

1 Pathways of drug metabolism

1.1 Introduction

The routes by which drugs may be metabolised or biotransformed are many and varied and include the chemical reactions of oxidation, reduction, hydrolysis, hydration, conjugation and condensation. It is important that these pathways are studied as the route of metabolism of a drug can determine whether it shows any pharmacological or toxicological activity. Drug metabolism is normally divided into two phases, phase I (or functionalisation reactions) and phase II (or conjugative reactions). The chemical reactions normally associated with phase I and phase II drug metabolism are given in Table 1.1.

Table 1.1 Reactions classed as phase I or phase II metabolism

Phase I	Phase II
Oxidation	Glucuronidation/glucosidation
Reduction	Sulfation
Hydrolysis	Methylation
Hydration	Acetylation
Dethioacetylation	Amino acid conjugation
Isomerisation	Glutathione conjugation
	Fatty acid conjugation
	Condensation

The reactions of phase I are thought to act as a preparation of the drug for the phase II reactions, i.e. phase I 'functionalises' the drug by producing or uncovering a chemically reactive group on which the phase II reactions can occur. Thus, the phase II reactions are usually the true 'detoxification' pathways and give products that account for the bulk of the inactive, excreted products of a drug. Many of the reactions of both phase I and phase II are capable of being performed on the same compound and, thus, there is a possibility of interaction of the various metabolic routes in terms of competing reactions for the same substrate.

This chapter will examine the different types of reactions involved in drug metabolism using the phase I and II classification as a basis. Examples of each type of reaction will be given and, where possible, these will be actual reactions of drug substrates rather than model substrates. This will show the pharmacological, toxicological and clinical relevance of the reactions. Attention will be drawn to competing reactions for the same substrate where appropriate.

There is a close relationship between the biotransformation of drugs and the normal biochemical processes occurring in the body and many of the enzymes involved in drug metabolism are, in fact, principally involved in the metabolism of endogenous compounds and only metabolise drugs because they closely resemble the natural compound. A separate section of the chapter will be devoted to the metabolism of endogenous compounds by 'drug metabolising' enzymes.

In the limited space available, it is only possible to give a flavour of the range of reactions involved in drug biotransformation. It would be impossible to list every reaction undergone by every drug and inevitably there will be omissions. Information regarding specific drugs will be found in specialist publications. A list of further reading material will be found at the end of the chapter from which further information on specific pathways can be obtained.

1.2 Phase I metabolism

Phase I metabolism includes oxidation, reduction, hydrolysis and hydration reactions as well as other rarer miscellaneous reactions. The reactions will be discussed in terms of reaction type and, with respect to oxidation, site of enzyme – the classification of phase I reactions can be found in Table 1.2. Oxidation performed by the microsomal mixed-function oxidase system (cytochrome P450-dependent) is considered separately because of its importance and the diversity of reactions performed by this enzyme system.

Table 1.2 Sub-classification of phase I reactions

Oxidation involving cytochrome P450
Oxidation – others
Reduction
Hydrolysis
Hydration
Isomerisation
Miscellaneous

1.2.1 Oxidations involving the microsomal mixed-function oxidase (cytochrome P450)

The mixed-function oxidase system found in microsomes (endoplasmic reticulum) of many cells (notably those of liver, kidney, lung and intestine) performs many different functionalisation reactions (summarised in Table 1.3). All of the above reactions require the presence of molecular oxygen and NADPH as well as the complete mixed-function oxidase system (cytochrome P450, NADPH–cytochrome P450 reductase and lipid). All reactions involve the initial insertion of a single oxygen atom into the drug molecule. A subsequent rearrangement and/or decomposition of this product may occur leading to the final products seen. The mechanism of insertion of this single oxygen atom is discussed at length in chapter 2. An example of each reaction is given below.

Table 1.3 Reactions performed by the microsomal mixed-function oxidase system

Reaction	Substrate
Aromatic hydroxylation	Lignocaine
Aliphatic hydroxylation	Pentobarbitone
Epoxidation	Benzo[a]pyrene
N-Dealkylation	Diazepam
O-Dealkylation	Codeine
S-Dealkylation	6-Methylthiopurine
Oxidative deamination	Amphetamine
N-Oxidation	3-Methylpyridine
	2-Acetylaminofluorene
S-Oxidation	Chlorpromazine
Phosphothionate oxidation	Parathion
Dehalogenation	Halothane
Alcohol oxidation	Ethanol

(a) *Aromatic hydroxylation.* This is a very common reaction for drugs and xenobiotics containing an aromatic ring. In this example (Figure 1.1) the local anaesthetic and antidysrhythmic drug, lignocaine, is converted to its 3-hydroxy derivative.

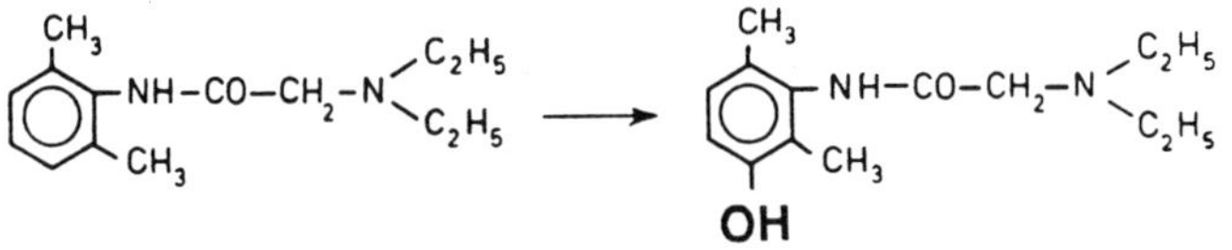

Figure 1.1 The 3-hydroxylation of lignocaine.

(b) *Aliphatic hydroxylation.* Another very common reaction, e.g. pentobarbitone hydroxylated in the pentyl side chain (Figure 1.2).

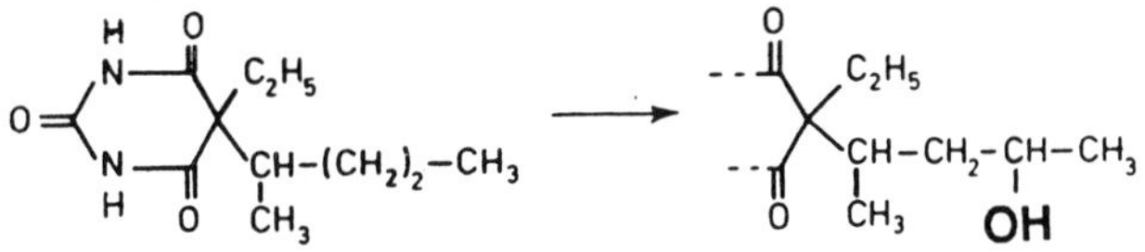

Figure 1.2 The side-chain hydroxylation of pentobarbitone.

(c) *Epoxidation.* Epoxides are normally unstable intermediates but may be stable enough to be isolated from polycyclic compounds (e.g. the precarcinogenic polycyclic hydrocarbons). Epoxides are substrates of epoxide hydratase (discussed later) forming dihydrodiols but they may also spontaneously

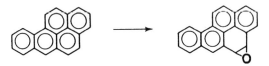

Figure 1.3 The formation of benzo[a]pyrene-4,5-epoxide.

decompose to form hydroxylated products. It has been suggested that epoxide formation is the first step in aromatic hydroxylation. Figure 1.3 shows the epoxidation of benzo[a]pyrene to its 4,5-epoxide.

(d) *Dealkylation.* This reaction occurs very readily with drugs containing a secondary or tertiary amine, an alkoxy group or an alkyl substituted thiol. The alkyl group is lost as the corresponding aldehyde. The reactions are often referred to as *N*-, *O*- or *S*-dealkylations depending on type of atom the alkyl group is attached to. In the example of *N*-demethylation in Figure 1.4, diazepam is converted to *N*-desmethyldiazepam with the loss of methanal. The reaction is considered to occur in two steps, the first being hydroxylation of the methyl group on the nitrogen, and the second a decomposition of this intermediate (see Figure 1.5).

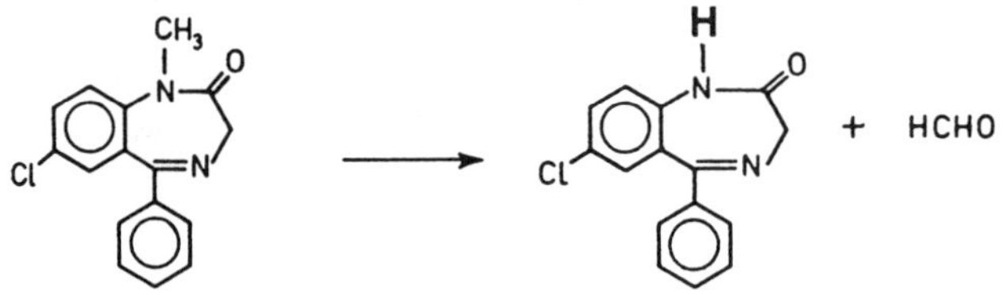

Figure 1.4 The *N*-demethylation of diazepam.

Unstable intermediate

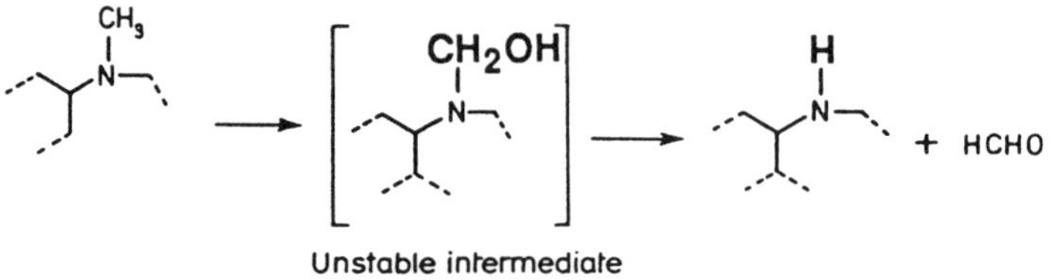

Figure 1.5 The mechanism of *N*-demethylation of diazepam.

Figure 1.6 shows the *O*-demethylation of codeine to yield morphine. The reaction proceeds via a hydroxy intermediate as in *N*-dealkylation.

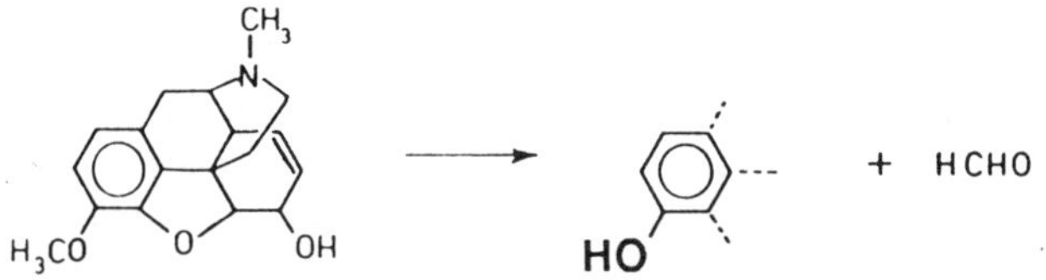

Figure 1.6 The *O*-demethylation of codeine.

Various *S*-methyl compounds can be *S*-demethylated by hepatic microsomes but a soluble factor appears to be necessary as well. This reaction may not, therefore, be a true microsomal one. The *S*-demethylation of *S*-methylthiopurine is illustrated in Figure 1.7.

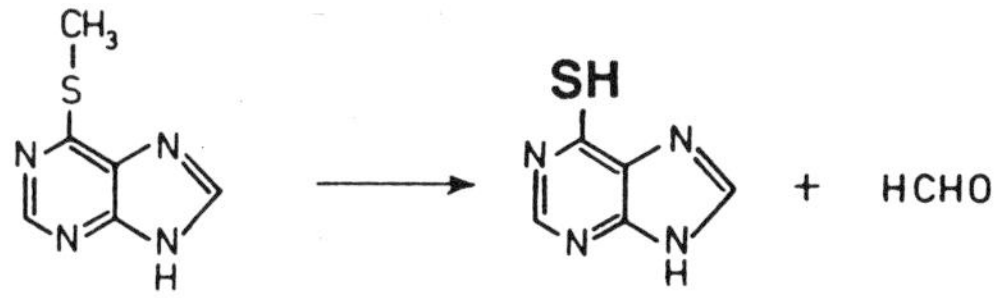

Figure 1.7 The *S*-demethylation of *S*-methylthiopurine.

(e) *Oxidative deamination*. Amines containing the structure $-CH(CH_3)-NH_2$ are metabolised by the microsomal mixed-function oxidase system to release ammonium ions and leave the corresponding ketone. This is a different substrate specificity to the other enzyme-metabolising amines, namely monoamine oxidase (MAO – see later) and the two enzymes do not compete for the same substrates. Figure 1.8 shows the deamination of amphetamine. The ketone formed in this case is phenylmethylketone. As with dealkylation, oxidative deamination involves an intermediate hydroxylation step (Figure 1.9) with subsequent decomposition to yield the final products.

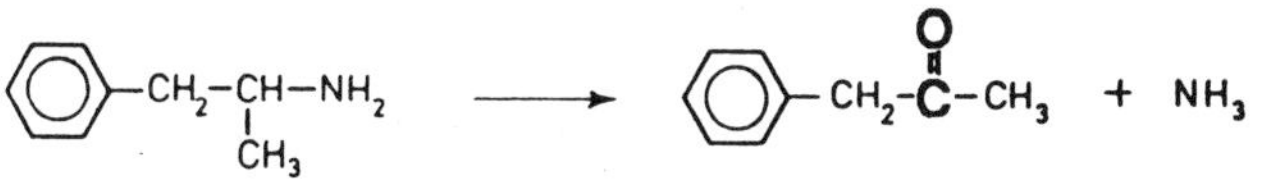

Figure 1.8 The oxidative deamination of amphetamine.

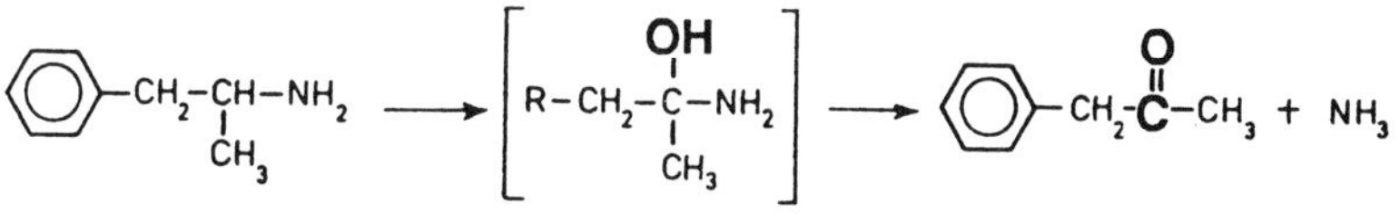

Figure 1.9 The mechanism of oxidative deamination of amphetamine.

(f) N-*oxidation*. Hepatic microsomes in the presence of oxygen and NADPH can form *N*-oxides. These oxidation products may be formed by the mixed-function oxidase system or by separate flavoprotein *N*-oxidases (see later). The enzyme involved in *N*-oxidation depends on the substrate under study. Many different chemical groups can be *N*-oxidised including amines, amides, imines, hydrazines and heterocyclic compounds. In Figure 1.10 the *N*-oxidation of 3-methylpyridine (a cytochrome P450-dependent reaction) is illustrated.

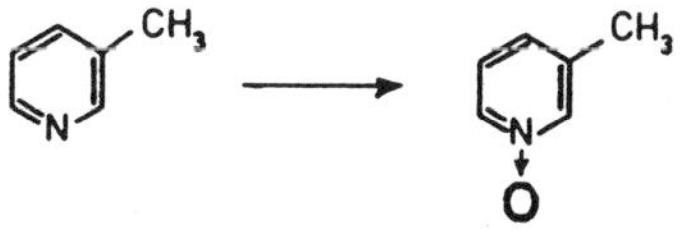

Figure 1.10 The *N*-oxidation of 3-methylpyridine.

N-oxidation may manifest itself as the formation of a hydroxylamine as in the metabolism of 2-acetylaminofluorene (2-AAF) (Figure 1.11). This is of interest as the hydroxylamine of 2-AAF is thought to be a proximate carcinogen giving the toxicity of 2-AAF.

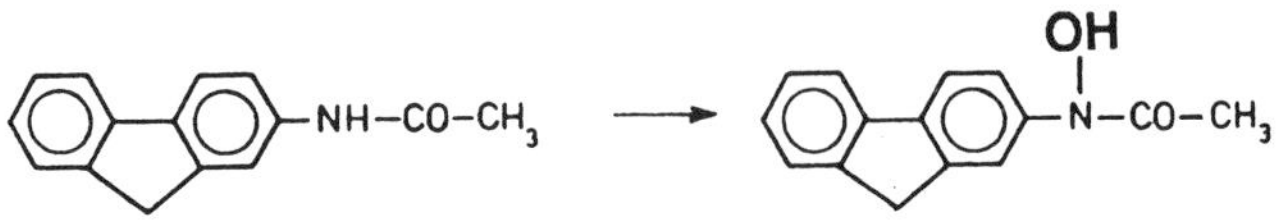

Figure 1.11 The *N*-hydroxylation of 2-acetylaminofluorene.

(g) S-*oxidation*. Phenothiazines can be converted to their *S*-oxides by the microsomal mixed-function oxidase system. As an example the *S*-oxidation of chlorpromazine is shown in Figure 1.12.

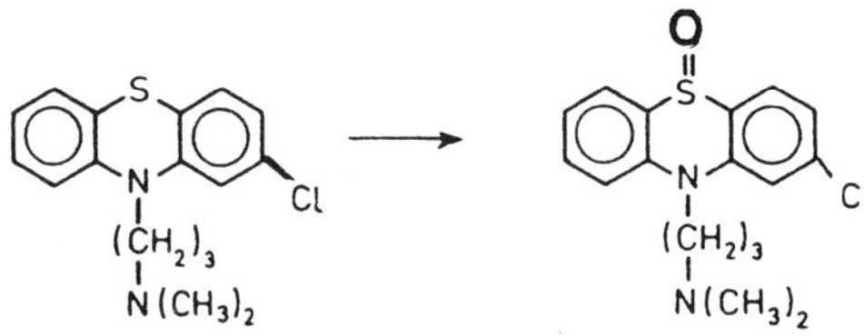

Figure 1.12 The *S*-oxidation of chlorpromazine.

(h) *Phosphothionate oxidation*. The replacement of a phosphothionate sulfur atom with oxygen is a reaction common to the phosphothionate insecticides, e.g. parathion (Figure 1.13). The product paraoxon is a potent anticholinesterase.

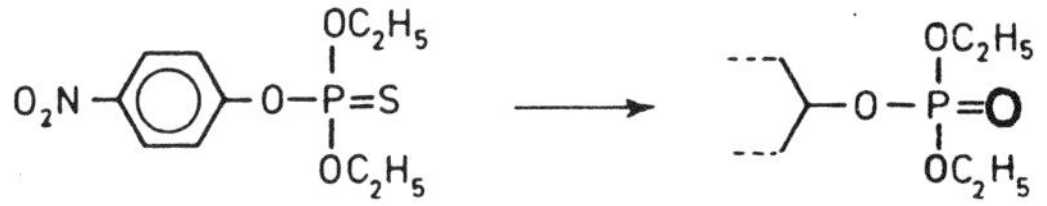

Figure 1.13 The oxidation of parathion.

(i) *Dehalogenation*. The halogenated general anaesthetics, e.g. halothane, undergo oxidative dechlorination and debromination to yield the corresponding alcohol or acid (Figure 1.14).

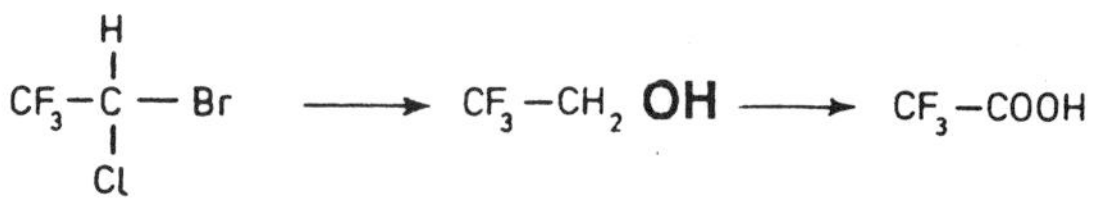

Figure 1.14 The oxidative dehalogenation of halothane.

One apparently unusual oxidation reaction performed by the mixed-function oxidase system is the conversion of ethanol to ethanal (Figure 1.15). In this case the microsomal ethanol-oxidising system appears to dehydrogenate ethanol, as does alcohol dehydrogenase (see below). This may still be a hydroxylation reaction, however, as illustrated in Figure 1.15 but other mechanisms have also been proposed.

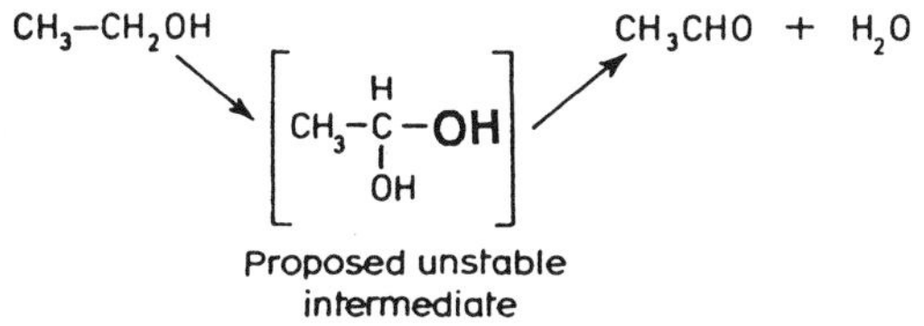

$$CH_3-CH_2OH \quad \left[CH_3-\overset{\overset{\displaystyle H}{|}}{\underset{\underset{\displaystyle OH}{|}}{C}}-OH \right] \quad CH_3CHO \; + \; H_2O$$

Proposed unstable
intermediate

Figure 1.15 The oxidation of ethanol.

The microsomal mixed-function oxidase system can, thus, catalyse a large range of oxidation reactions on a variety of substrates (Table 1.3). There is another mixed-function oxidase found in the mitochondria which is more selective in its substrates and is mainly involved in endogenous steroid metabolism (see section 1.5).

1.2.2 Oxidation other than the microsomal mixed-function oxidase

A number of enzymes in the body not related to mixed-function oxidase can oxidise drugs. These are listed in Table 1.4. Most of these enzymes are primarily involved in endogenous compound metabolism and will be dealt with in section 1.5. A number, however, are more intimately involved in drug metabolism and are discussed below.

Table 1.4 Oxidative enzymes other than
mixed-function oxidase

Alcohol dehydrogenase
Aldehyde dehydrogenase
Xanthine oxidase
Amine oxidases
Aromatases
Alkylhydrazine oxidase

(a) *Alcohol dehydrogenase.* This enzyme catalyses the oxidation of many alcohols to the corresponding aldehyde and is localised in the soluble fraction of liver, kidney and lung cells. Unlike the microsomal ethanol-oxidising system mentioned above, this enzyme uses NAD^+ as co-factor (Figure 1.16) and is a true dehydrogenase (the MEOS is an oxidase).

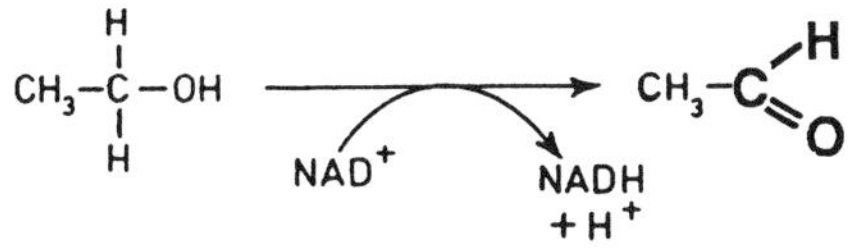

$$CH_3-\overset{\overset{\displaystyle H}{|}}{\underset{\underset{\displaystyle H}{|}}{C}}-OH \xrightarrow[\underset{NAD^+}{}]{\quad\quad\quad} \overset{\displaystyle NADH}{\underset{+H^+}{}} CH_3-C\overset{\displaystyle H}{\underset{\displaystyle O}{\lessgtr}}$$

Figure 1.16 The oxidation of ethanol by alcohol dehydrogenase.

In naive animals the cytochrome P450-mediated oxidation of ethanol is thought to be of minor importance but following induction by ethanol, the microsomal oxidation of ethanol increases dramatically and may account for

80% of ethanol clearance in certain cases. In non-induced situations, alcohol dehydrogenase is the major metaboliser of ethanol.

(b) *Aldehyde oxidation.* Aldehydes can be oxidised by a variety of enzymes involved in intermediary metabolism, e.g. aldehyde dehydrogenase, aldehyde oxidase and xanthine oxidase (the latter two being soluble metalloflavoproteins). The product of the reaction is the corresponding carboxylic acid (Figure 1.17).

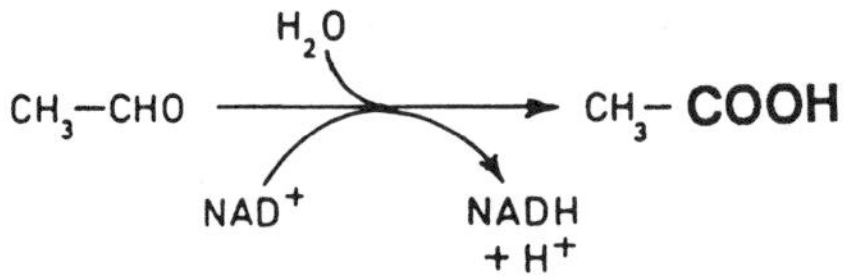

Figure 1.17 The oxidation of acetaldehyde.

(c) *Xanthine oxidase.* This enzyme will metabolise the xanthine-containing drugs, e.g. caffeine, theophylline and theobromine, and the purine analogues, to the corresponding uric acid derivative (Figure 1.18).

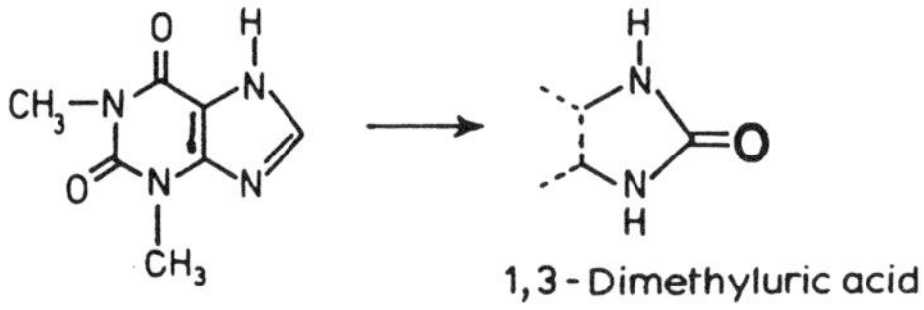

1,3 - Dimethyluric acid

Figure 1.18 The oxidation of theophylline.

(d) *Amine oxidases.* This group of enzymes can be subdivided into monoamine oxidases (responsible for the metabolism of endogenous catecholamines), diamine oxidases (deaminating endogenous diamines, e.g. histamine) and the flavoprotein N-oxidases and N-hydroxylases (which have been discussed above).

Monoamine oxidase metabolises dietary exogenous amines, e.g. tyramine (found in cheese, etc.) to the corresponding aldehyde (cf. oxidative deamination by the mixed-function oxidase) and is found in mitochondria, at nerve endings and in the liver. The enzyme does not metabolise the amphetamine class of drugs that are metabolised by the mixed-function oxidase.

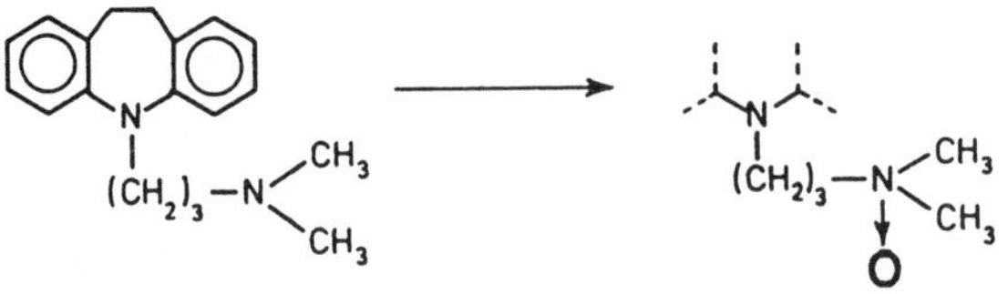

Figure 1.19 The N-oxidation of imipramine.

Diamine oxidase is primarily involved with endogenous metabolism and is of little relevance here, whereas the N-oxidases are of importance in the metabolism of drugs, e.g. imipramine (Figure 1.19). These enzymes are found in liver microsomes. They appear to require NADPH and molecular oxygen, but are not mixed-function oxidases – they are flavoproteins.

(e) *Aromatases.* Xenobiotics containing a cyclohexanecarboxylic acid group can be converted to the corresponding benzoic acid by a liver and kidney mitochondrial enzyme. The enzyme requires the co-enzyme A derivative of the acid as substrate, and oxygen and FAD as co-factors (Figure 1.20).

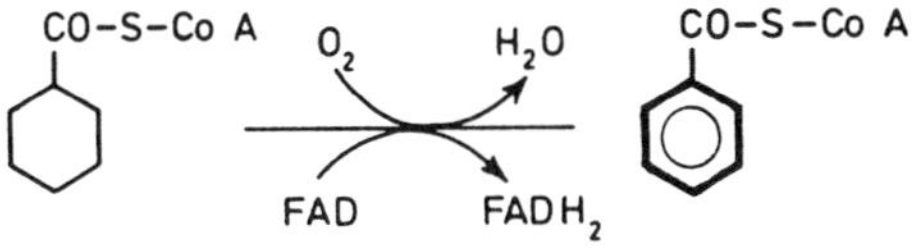

Figure 1.20 The aromatisation of cyclohexanecarboxylic acid CoA.

(f) *Alkylhydrazine oxidase.* Carbidopa can be converted to 2-methyl-3', 4'-dihydroxyphenylpropionic acid (Figure 1.21) by oxidation of the nitrogen function and subsequent rearrangement and decomposition of the intermediate. The exact mechanism is not known.

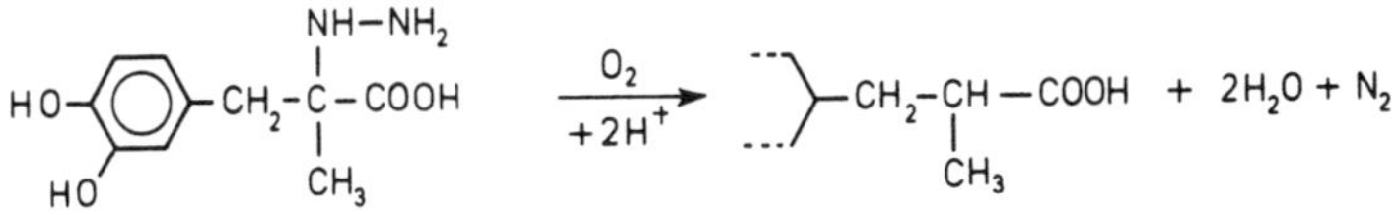

Figure 1.21 The oxidation of carbidopa.

1.2.3 Reductive metabolism

A number of reductive reactions can be catalysed by hepatic microsomes. These reactions require NADPH but are generally inhibited by oxygen, unlike the mixed function oxidase reactions that require oxygen. A list of the types of compounds undergoing reduction is given in Table 1.5.

Table 1.5 Compounds undergoing reduction by hepatic microsomes

Azo-compounds
Nitro-compounds
Epoxides
Heterocyclic ring compounds
Halogenated hydrocarbons

Azo- and nitro-reduction can be catalysed by cytochrome P450 (but can also be catalysed by NADPH–cytochrome c (P450) reductase) and can involve substrates such as prontosil red (forming sulfanilamide) and chloramphenicol (Figure 1.22). The former reaction led to the discovery of the sulfonamides. The

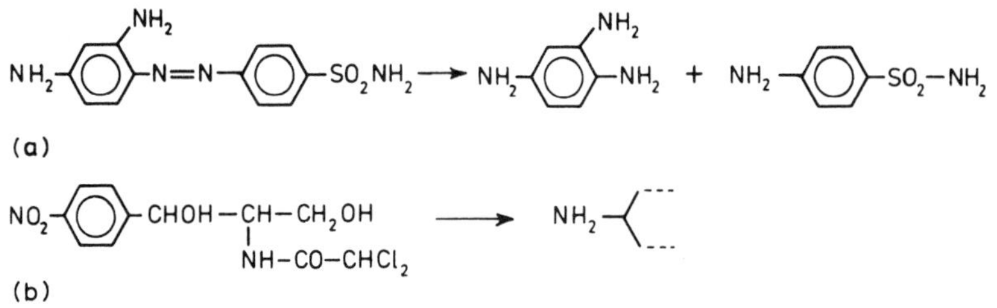

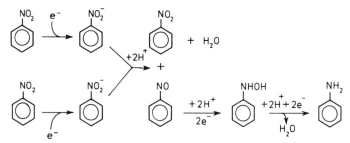

(a)

(b)

Figure 1.22 Reduction of (a) prontosil red and (b) chloramphenicol.

Figure 1.23 Stepwise reduction of aromatic nitro-group.

latter reaction is thought to occur in a stepwise fashion as is seen in the reduction of nitrobenzene (Figure 1.23).

Epoxides can be converted back to the parent hydrocarbon, e.g. benzo[*a*]anthracene-8,9-epoxide whereas some heterocyclic compounds can be ring cleaved by reduction (Figure 1.24). The products of the latter reaction are unstable and break down further to yield rearrangement and hydrolysis products.

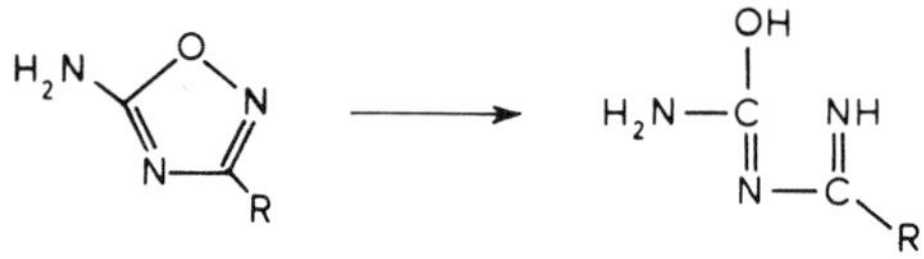

Figure 1.24 Ring cleavage of oxadiazoles.

Fluorocarbons of the halothane type can be defluorinated by liver microsomes in anaerobic conditions (cf. oxidative dehalogenation of halothane) as shown in Figure 1.25.

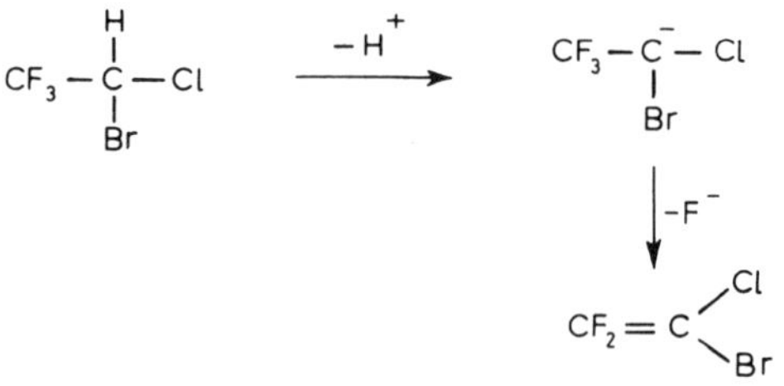

Figure 1.25 Reductive defluorination of halothane.

1.2.4 Hydrolysis

Esters, amides, hydrazides and carbamates can readily be hydrolysed by various enzymes.

(a) *Ester hydrolysis*. The hydrolysis of esters can take place in the plasma (non-specific acetylcholinesterases, pseudocholinesterases and other esterases) or in the liver (specific esterases for particular groups of compounds). Procaine is metabolised by the plasma esterase (Figure 1.26) whereas pethidine (meperidine) is only metabolised by the liver esterase.

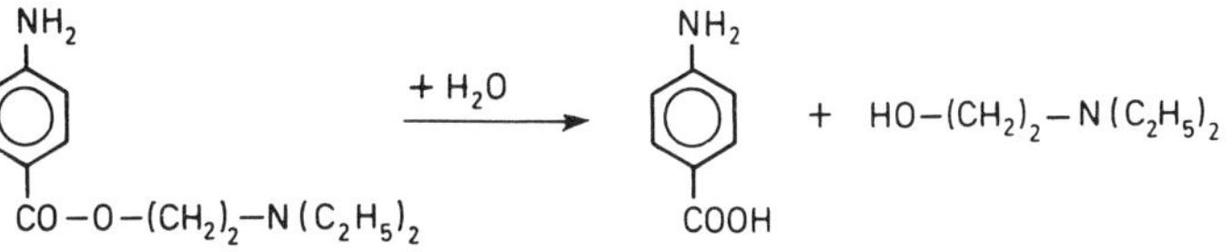

Figure 1.26 Hydrolysis of procaine

(b) *Amide hydrolysis*. Amides may be hydrolysed by the plasma esterases (which are so non-specific that they will also hydrolyse amides although more slowly than the corresponding esters) but are more likely to be hydrolysed by the liver amidases. Ethylglycylxylidide, the *N*-deethylated phase I product of lignocaine, is hydrolysed by the liver microsomal fraction to yield xylidine and ethylglycine (Figure 1.27).

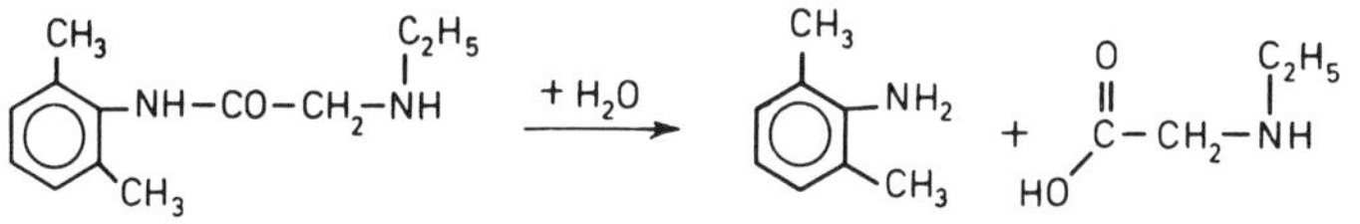

Figure 1.27 Hydrolysis of monoethylglycylxylidide.

(c) *Hydrazide and carbamate hydrolysis*. Less common functional groups in drugs can also be hydrolysed such as the hydrazide group in isoniazid (Figure 1.28) or the carbamate group in the previously used hypnotic, hedonal.

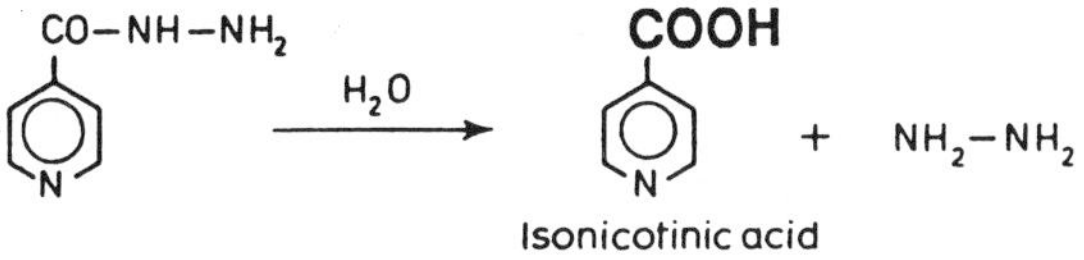

Isonicotinic acid

Figure 1.28 Hydrolysis of isoniazid.

The hydrolysis of proteins and peptides by enzymes can also be mentioned here but these enzymes are mainly found in gut secretions and are little involved in drug metabolism except in the further metabolism of glutathione conjugates (discussed later) and in the metabolism of peptide/protein drugs taken orally.

1.2.5 Hydration

Hydration can be regarded as a specialised form of hydrolysis where water is added to the compound without causing the compound to dissociate. Epoxides are particularly prone to hydration by the enzyme, epoxide hydratase, yielding the dihydrodiol. This enzyme is also called epoxide hydrase or hydrolase. The precarcinogenic polycyclic hydrocarbon epoxides in particular undergo this reaction (e.g. benzo[a]pyrene 4,5-epoxide (Figure 1.29)). The reaction forms a *trans*-diol.

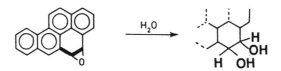

Figure 1.29 Hydration of benzo[a]pyrene-4,5-epoxide.

1.2.6 Other phase I reactions

Many other reactions which cannot be classified into the groups mentioned above have been proposed as possible routes of metabolism for specific drugs. A list of some of these reactions is given in Table 1.6. Further details of these reactions can be found in the reading list at the end of the chapter.

Table 1.6 Other reactions involved in drug metabolism

Reaction	Compound
Ring cyclisation	Proguanil
N-Carboxylation	Tocainide
Dimerisation	N-OH-2-Acetylaminofluorene
Transamidation	Propiram
Isomerisation	α-Methylfluorene-2-acetic acid
Decarboxylation	L-Dopa
Dethioacetylation	Spironolactone

1.2.7 Summary of phase I metabolism

As can be seen from the above, virtually every possible chemical reaction that a compound can undergo can be catalysed by the drug-metabolising enzyme systems. In most cases the final product contains a chemically reactive functional group, such as –OH, –NH$_2$, –SH, –COOH, etc. and, thus, as we shall see below, is in the correct chemical state to be acted upon by the phase II or conjugative enzymes. Indeed it is recognised that the main function of phase I metabolism is to prepare the compound for phase II metabolism and not to prepare the drug for excretion. Phase II is usually the true 'detoxification' of drugs and gives products that are generally water-soluble and easily excreted.

It will also be appreciated that many drugs can undergo a number of the reactions listed: indeed some drugs can pass along many of the routes of metabolism described above. The importance of a particular pathway varies with many factors (most of which are described in chapters 4 and 5) and it is obviously very difficult to predict the metabolism of a drug from the data given above. Computer-based expert systems for the prediction of routes of drug metabolism are available and are becoming more accurate as data is added into them but it is still not possible to fully predict the metabolism of a particular compound from its structure.

1.3 Phase II metabolism

The phase II or conjugation reactions are listed in Table 1.7. It is seen that they involve a diverse group of enzymes, generally leading to a water-soluble product which can be excreted in bile or urine.

1.3.1 Conjugation with sugars

The major route of sugar conjugation is glucuronidation (conjugation with α-D-glucuronic acid) although conjugation with glucose, xylose and ribose are also possible.

Table 1.7 Conjugation reactions

Reaction	Enzyme	Functional group
Glucuronidation	UDP–Glucuronyltransferase	–OH –COOH –NH$_2$ –SH
Glycosidation	UDP–Glycosyltransferase	–OH –COOH –SH
Sulfation	Sulfotransferase	–NH$_2$ –SO$_2$NH$_2$ –OH
Methylation	Methyltransferase	–OH –NH$_2$
Acetylation	Acetyltransferase	–NH$_2$ –SO$_2$NH$_2$ –OH
Amino acid conjugation		–COOH
Glutathione conjugation	Glutathione-S-transferase	Epoxide Organic halide
Fatty acid conjugation		–OH
Condensation		Various

(a) *Glucuronidation.* Glucuronidation is the most widespread of the conjugation reactions probably due to the relative abundance of the cofactor for the reaction, UDP–glucuronic acid. UDP–glucuronic acid, being part of intermediary metabolism and closely related to glycogen synthesis, is found in all tissues of the body (Figure 1.30). The enzymes involved are located in the cytosol. UDP–glucuronic acid can be considered as an energy-rich intermediate for the transfer of the glucuronic acid moiety.

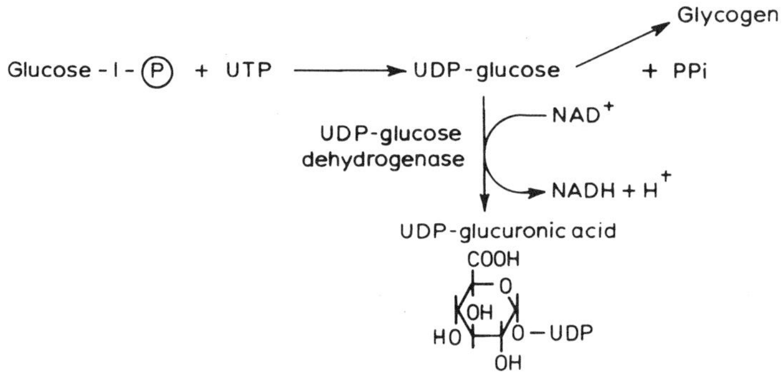

Figure 1.30 Synthesis of UDP–glucuronic acid.

Glucuronide formation is quantitatively the most important form of conjugation for drugs and endogenous compounds (for a discussion of this latter point, see the section on endogenous compound metabolism) and can occur with alcohols, phenols, hydroxylamines, carboxylic acids, amines, sulfonamides and thiols.

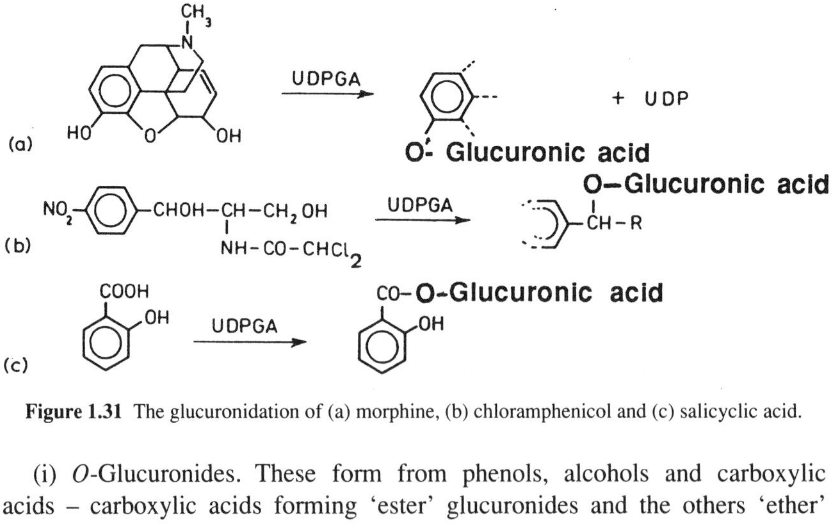

Figure 1.31 The glucuronidation of (a) morphine, (b) chloramphenicol and (c) salicyclic acid.

(i) *O*-Glucuronides. These form from phenols, alcohols and carboxylic acids – carboxylic acids forming 'ester' glucuronides and the others 'ether' glucuronides. Examples of each of these are shown in Figure 1.31. The reaction is the same in each case requiring the microsomal enzyme, UDP–glucuronosyl-transferase. It is interesting to note that inversion takes place during the reaction with the α-glucuronic acid forming a β-glucuronide. The O-glucuronides are often excreted in bile and thus released into the gut where they can be broken down to the parent compound by β-glucuronidase and possibly reabsorbed. This is the basis of the 'enterohepatic circulation' of drugs discussed in more detail in chapter 7.

(ii) *N-glucuronides.* N-glucuronides form from amines (mainly aromatic), amides and sulfonamides. It has also been suggested that tertiary amines can form glucuronides giving quaternary nitrogen conjugates. N-glucuronides may form spontaneously, i.e. without the presence of enzyme. Figure 1.32 shows some examples of N-glucuronide formation.

N.B. Double glucuronide on amine and sulfonamide

(a)

(b)

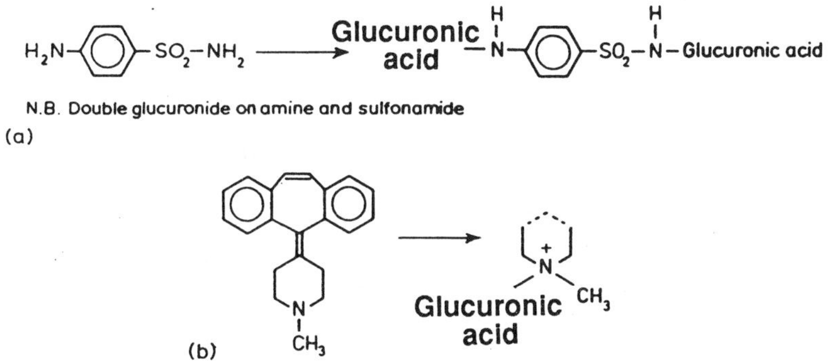

Figure 1.32 The glucuronidation of (a) sulfanilamide and (b) cyproheptidine.

(iii) *S-glucuronides.* Thiol groups can react with UDPGA in the presence of UDP–glucuronosyltransferase to yield S-glucuronides. An example of this is given in Figure 1.33 with antabuse as substrate.

Direct attachment of glucuronic acid to the carbon skeleton of drugs has also been reported (i.e. C-glucuronidation).

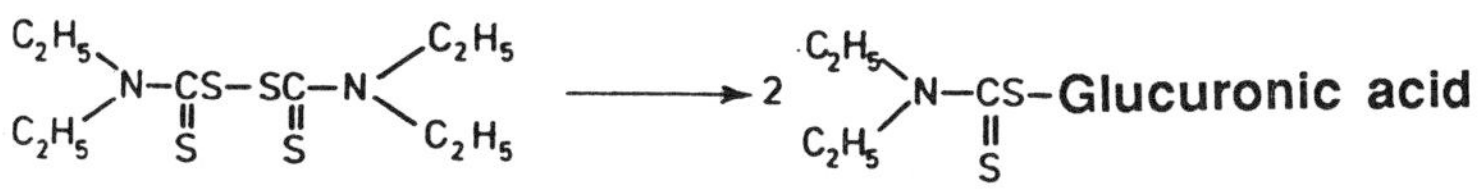

Figure 1.33 The glucuronidation of antabuse.

(b) *Other sugars.* In most species conjugation with glucuronic acid is by far the most important sugar conjugation but in insects conjugation with glucose is more prevalent. The reaction is exactly analogous to glucuronide formation but UDP–glucose is used instead of UDPGA and glucosides are formed. Similar O-,

N- and *S*-glucosides can be formed. Such reactions are also of importance in plants and have been found in mammals to a limited extent.

In certain circumstances UDP–xylose or UDP–ribose can be used giving the corresponding xyloside or riboside. *N*-ribosides seem to be the most common and may form non-enzymically but *O*-xylosides of bilirubin have been found and require a microsomal transferase for formation. An example of a *N*-riboside formation is shown in Figure 1.34.

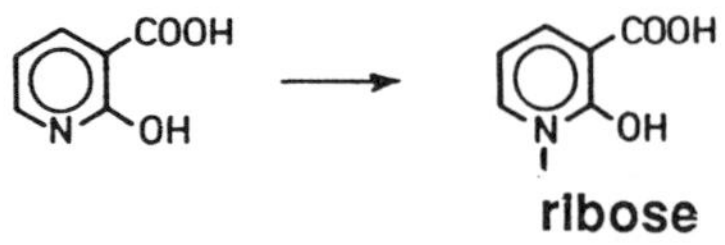

Figure 1.34 The *N*-ribosylation of 2-hydroxynicotinic acid.

1.3.2 Sulfation

Sulfation is a major conjugation pathway for phenols but can also occur for alcohols, amines and, to a lesser extent, thiols. As with sugar conjugation an energy-rich donor is required – in this case 3'-phosphoadenosine-5'-phosphosulfate (PAPS) (Figure 1.35). PAPS is produced by a two-stage reaction from ATP and sulfate as illustrated in Figure 1.36. These reactions occur in the cytosol.

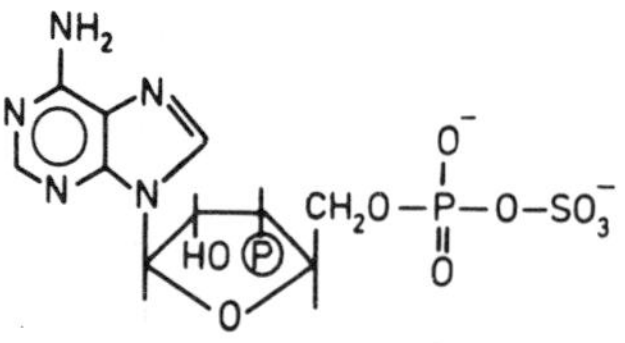

Figure 1.35 The structure of PAPS.

$$SO_4^{2-} + ATP \xrightarrow{\text{ATP-sulfurylase}} \text{Adenosine-5'-phosphosulfate (APS)} + PPi$$

$$APS + ATP \xrightarrow{\text{APS-kinase}} \text{3'-Phosphoadenosine-5'-phosphosulfate (PAPS)} + ADP$$

Figure 1.36 The formation of PAPS.

Sulfation occurs by interaction of the drug and PAPS in the presence of the cytosolic enzyme, sulfotransferase. Various isoenzymes have been described named after their preferred substrates – a list of these is given in Table 1.8.

The phenol, alcohol and arylamine sulfotransferases are fairly non-specific and will metabolise a wide range of drugs and xenobiotics but the steroid sulfotransferases are specific for a single steroid or a number of steroids of a particular type. For example oestrone sulfotransferase will sulfate oestrone and,

Table 1.8 Sulfotransferases and their substrates

Isoenzyme	Substrate	Site
Phenol sulfotransferase	Isoprenaline	Liver Kidney Gut
Alcohol sulfotransferase	Dimetranidazole	Liver
Steroid sulfotransferase	Oestrone	Liver
Arylamine sulfotransferase	Paracetamol	Liver

to a lesser extent, other oestrogens while testosterone is sulfated by another sulfotransferase. Some examples of sulfate conjugation are shown in Figure 1.37.

As is seen most drugs and endogenous compounds that can be glucuronidated can also be sulfated and this leads to the possibility of competition for the substrate between the two pathways. In general, sulfate conjugation predominates at low substrate concentration and glucuronide conjugation at high concentration due to the kinetics of the two reactions and the limited supply of PAPS in the cell compared to UDPGA.

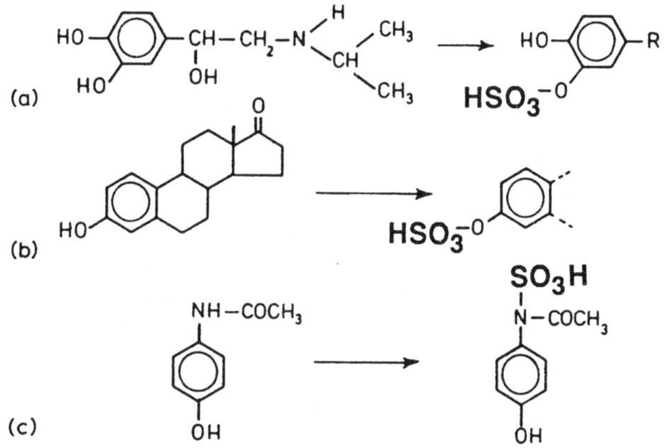

Figure 1.37 Sulfate conjugation of (a) isoprenaline, and (b) oestrone and (c) paracetamol.

1.3.3 Methylation

Methylation reactions are mainly involved with endogenous compound metabolism but some drugs may be methylated by non-specific methyltransferases found in the lung, and by the physiological methyltransferases. A list of the methyltransferases and their substrates is given in Table 1.9.

The co-factor, S-adenosylmethionine (SAM), is required to form methyl conjugates and is produced from L-methionine and ATP under the influence of the enzyme, L-methionine adenosyltransferase (Figure 1.38). SAM can also be considered as a high-energy intermediate (cf. UDPGA and PAPS above).

Table 1.9 The methyltransferases

Enzyme	Substrate	Site
Phenylethanolamine *N*-methyltransferase	Noradrenaline	Adrenals
Non-specific *N*-methyltransferase	Various (desmethylimipramine)	Lung
Imidazole *N*-methyltransferase	Histamine	Liver
Catechol *O*-methyltransferase	Catechols	Liver Kidney Skin Nerve tissue
Hydroxyindole *O*-methyltransferase	*N*-Acetylserotonin	Pineal gland
S-Methyltransferase	Thiols	Liver Kidney Lung

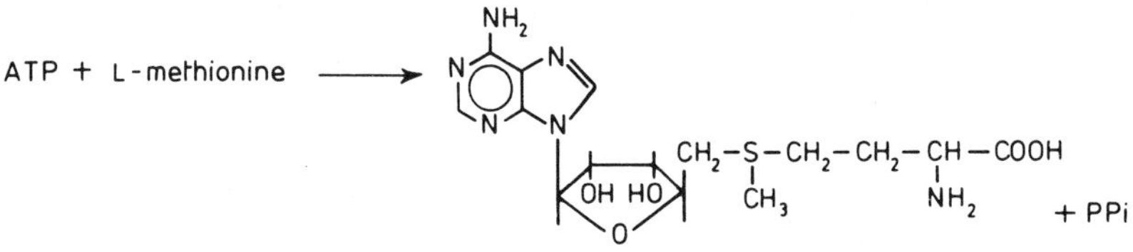

Figure 1.38 The formation of *S*-adenosylmethionine.

The non-specific *N*-methyltransferase found in the lung can reverse the *N*-demethylation reactions of phase I metabolism (see Figure 1.39) but most of the other methyltransferases are specific for endogenous compounds (see section 1.5) except the *S*-methyltransferase that is found in the microsomal fraction and which will methylate many thiols (see Figure 1.40) such as thiouracil. In general, unlike other conjugation reactions, methylation leads to a less polar product and thus hinders excretion of the drug.

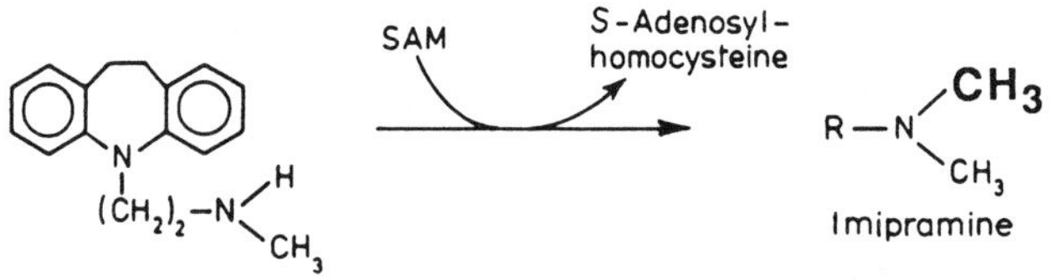

Figure 1.39 The *N*-methylation of desmethylimipramine.

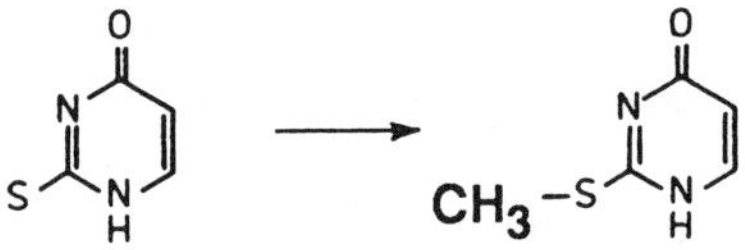

Figure 1.40 The *S*-methylation of thiouracil.

1.3.4 Acetylation

Acetylation reactions are common for aromatic amines and sulfonamides and require the co-factor, acetyl-CoA, which may be obtained from the glycolysis pathway or via direct interaction of acetate and coenzyme A (Figure 1.41). Acetylation takes place mainly in the liver and, interestingly, is found in the Kupffer cells and not in the more usual location of the hepatocytes. Acetylation can also take place in the reticuloendothelial cells of the spleen, lung and gut, and the enzyme is referred to as *N*-acetyltransferase. Some examples of acetylation are shown in Figure 1.42.

$$CH_3-COO^- \quad + \quad CoASH \quad \xrightarrow{\text{CoA-S-acetyltransferase}} \quad CH_3-Co-S-CoA$$

Figure 1.41 The formation of acetyl-CoA.

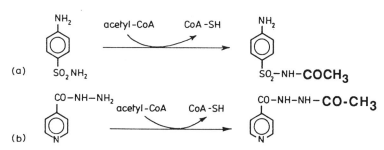

Figure 1.42 The *N*-acetylation of (a) sulfanilamide and (b) isoniazid.

Sulfanilamide can also be acetylated on the amine nitrogen to give a diacetylated product. The acetyl-sulfonamides are of particular interest as they are appreciably less soluble in water than the parent drug and the renal toxicity of the earlier sulfonamides has been attributed to precipitation of these conjugates in the kidney.

1.3.5 Amino acid conjugation

Exogenous carboxylic acids, in common with acetate noted above, can form CoA derivatives in the body and can then react with endogenous amines, such as amino acids to form conjugates. Amino acid conjugation is, thus, a special form of *N*-acylation, where the drug and not the endogenous co-factor is activated. The usual amino acids involved are glycine, glutamine, ornithine, arginine and taurine. The generalised reaction is given in Figure 1.43. This pathway was implicated in the first described production of a drug metabolite by Keller in 1842 when hippuric acid was found as a urinary excretion product of benzoic acid (Figure 1.44). The particular amino acid used is related to the intermediary metabolism of the species under study such that ureotelic animals (those excreting urea) tend to use glycine while uricotelic species (those excreting uric acid) use predominantly ornithine.

$$R-COOH + ATP \longrightarrow R-CO-AMP + PPi$$

$$R-CO-AMP + CoASH \longrightarrow R-CO-S-CoA + AMP$$

$$R-CO-S-CoA + R'-NH_2 \longrightarrow R-CO-NH-R' + CoASH$$

Figure 1.43 The amino acid conjugation of carboxylic acids.

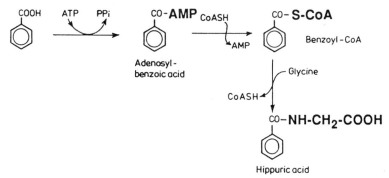

Figure 1.44 The glycine conjugation of benzoic acid.

1.3.6 Glutathione conjugation

Glutathione is recognised as a protective compound within the body for the removal of potentially toxic electrophilic compounds. Many drugs either are, or can be metabolised by phase I reactions to, strong electrophiles, and these can react with glutathione to form (in general) non-toxic conjugates. The list of compounds conjugated to glutathione includes epoxides, haloalkanes, nitroalkanes, alkenes, and aromatic halo-and nitro-compounds. Examples of these are given in Figure 1.45. The enzymes catalysing the reactions above are the glutathione-*S*-

Table 1.10 The isoenzymes of glutathione-*S*-transferases

Old name	New name	Substrate
L2	1–1	4-Nitrophenyl acetate
BL	1–2	Mixture of L2 and B2
B2	2–2	Ethacrynic acid
A2	3–3	1,2-Dichloro-4-nitrobenzene
AC	3–4	Mixture of A2 and C2
P	3–6	
C2	4–4	*trans*-4-phenyl-3-buten-2-one
S	4–6	
E	5–5	
M	6–6	
P	7–7	
K	8–8	

Taken from Mannervik and Danielson (1988).

transferases which are located in the cytosol of liver, kidney, gut and other tissues. At least six isoenzymes are known with differing substrate specificity as shown in Table 1.10. The glutathione conjugates may be excreted directly in urine, or more usually bile, but more often further metabolism of the conjugate takes place as illustrated in Figure 1.46.

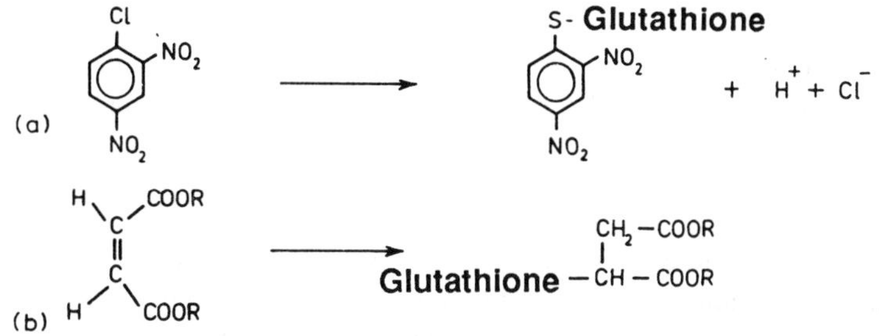

Figure 1.45 Glutathione conjugation of (a) 2,4-dinitro-1-chlorobenzene and (b) esters of maleic acid.

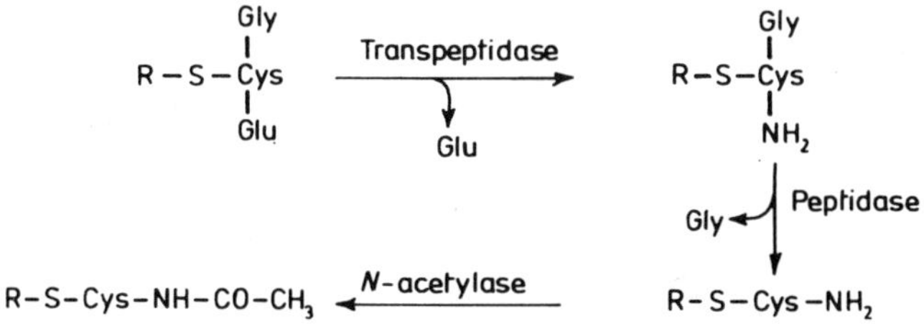

Figure 1.46 The further metabolism of a glutathione conjugate.

The tripeptide glutathione (Gly–Cys–Glu), once attached to the acceptor molecule, can be attacked by a glutamyltranspeptidase, which removes the glutamate, and a peptidase, which removes the glycine to yield the cysteine conjugate of the xenobiotic. These enzymes are found in the liver and kidney cytosol. N-Acetylation of the cysteine conjugate can then occur via the normal N-acetylation pathway described above to yield the N-acetylcysteine conjugate or mercapturic acid. The glycylcysteine and cysteine conjugates and the

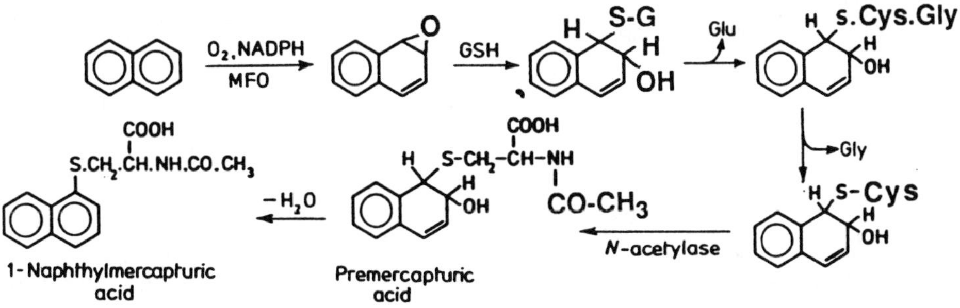

Figure 1.47 The phase I and II metabolism of naphthalene.

mercapturic acids are all found as excretion products depending on the substrate and species under study. One example of this complete process is found for the metabolism of naphthalene (Figure 1.47).

As well as being broken down by this process, sulfur-containing conjugates secreted in bile can also be further metabolised by an enzyme in the gut called C–S lyase (or cysteine conjugate β-lyase). This idea has been further expanded when dealing with certain sulfur-containing compounds or compounds that form sulfur-containing conjugates, such as 2-acetamido-4(chloromethyl)-thiazole, caffeine and propachlor. In these cases the methylthio derivates found as excretion products have been postulated to arise as shown in Figure 1.48. The breakdown of the glutathione conjugate is performed by a C–S lyase in the intestinal microflora transferring the –SH group from glutathione to the substrate, where subsequent *S*-methylation and reabsorption take place. The *S*-methylated compound is oxidised in the liver to a methylthio derivative and then excreted. The series of reactions for the anti-inflammatory drug, 2-acetamido-4-chloromethyl-thiazole is shown in Figure 1.49.

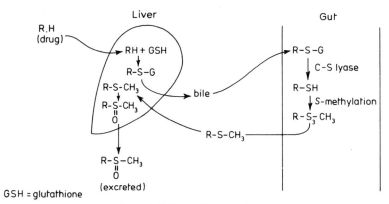

Figure 1.48 Phase III metabolism.

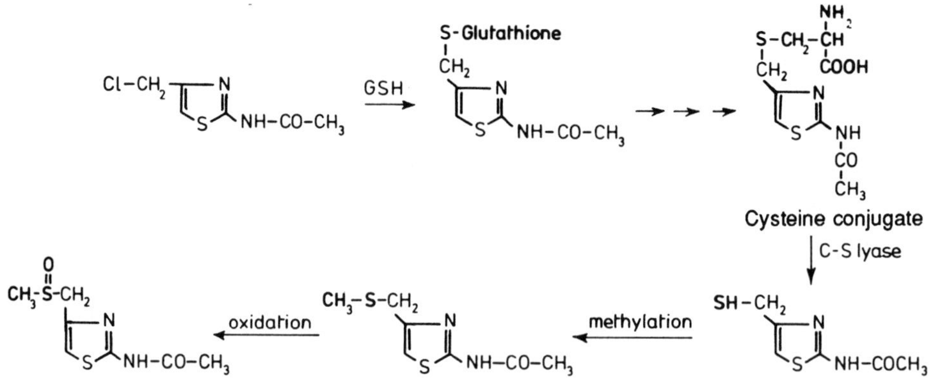

Figure 1.49 The metabolism of 2-acetomido-4-chloromethylthiazole.

1.3.7 Fatty acid and cholesteryl ester conjugation

Fatty acid conjugation has been shown to occur for 11-hydroxy-Δ^9-tetrahydro-cannabinol. The fatty acids involved are stearic and palmitic acid (Figure 1.50). The microsomal fraction from liver catalyses this reaction. Little is known, however, of the mechanism or whether other compounds can be conjugated in this way. Drugs containing carboxylic acid groups can also be esterified as part of a mixed triglyceride with a fatty acid or as a cholesteryl ester.

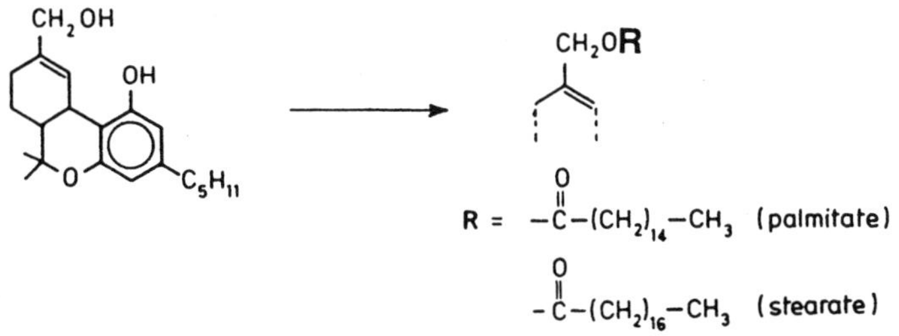

$$R = -\overset{O}{\underset{\|}{C}}-(CH_2)_{14}-CH_3 \quad (palmitate)$$

$$-\overset{O}{\underset{\|}{C}}-(CH_2)_{16}-CH_3 \quad (stearate)$$

Figure 1.50 The conjugation of 11-hydroxy-Δ^9-THC to palmitic and stearic acids.

1.3.8 Condensation reactions

These reactions may not be enzymatic but purely chemical (cf. *N*-glucuronide formation) and have been found for amines and aldehydes. One example is the condensation of dopamine and its own metabolite, 3,4-dihydroxyphenylethanal to yield the alkaloid, tetrahydropapaveroline, which is a potent dopamine antagonist (Figure 1.51).

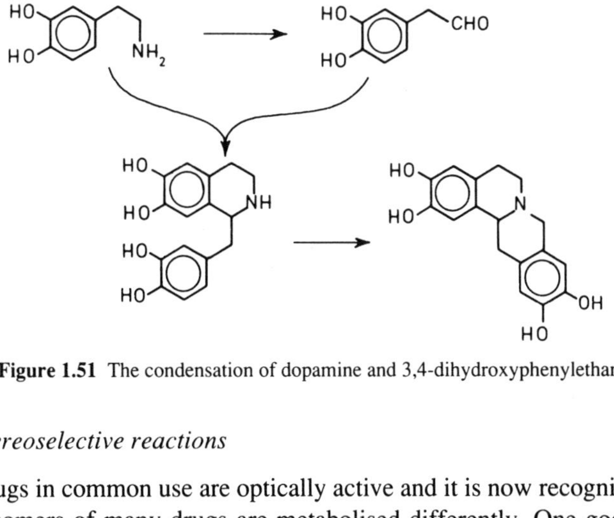

Figure 1.51 The condensation of dopamine and 3,4-dihydroxyphenylethanal.

1.3.9 Stereoselective reactions

Many drugs in common use are optically active and it is now recognised that the optical isomers of many drugs are metabolised differently. One good example of this is the metabolism of warfarin, which exists as *R*- and *S*-isomers with *S*-warfarin disappearing from plasma at a faster rate than the *R*-isomer. The metabolic routes for optical isomers tends to be the same but the rate of metabolism often differs. Further examples of this and the relationship to pharmacological activity, induction and toxicity will be found in chapters 3 and 6.

1.3.10 Summary of phase II metabolism

The above brief description of phase II reactions shows the range of possible products of metabolism which have in common the requirement for some form of energy-rich or 'activated' intermediate whether it be an activated co-factor (e.g. UDPGA, PAPS, SAM, acetyl-coenzyme A) or activated drug. In the main, phase II metabolites are more water-soluble (cf. *N*-methylation) and conjugation reactions are regarded as preparing the drug for excretion by one pathway or another.

1.4 Summary

In the preceding pages the various reactions that drugs can undergo have been described and the relative importance of the reactions discussed. It will be seen that very many different reactions can be found depending on the drug under study. A book of this type cannot claim to cover all of these reactions but it is hoped, however, that this chapter has given some insight into the complexity of drug metabolism and the interactions of the complementary, sequential and competing pathways.

The final section of this chapter deals with the interrelationship of drug and endogenous compound metabolism in an attempt to indicate where the overlap between the two may occur and how this may lead to interactions between drugs and endogenous metabolism.

1.5 Endogenous metabolism related to drug metabolism

The enzymes discussed above, the 'drug-metabolising' enzymes, are a diverse group performing a range of different reactions. As well as biotransforming many drugs, the majority of the enzymes also metabolise endogenous compounds and it has been suggested that the true function of these enzymes is in endogenous metabolism, and that it is purely fortuitous that they also metabolise drugs and other xenobiotics. The greater affinity for the 'natural' substrate in many cases would seem to support this idea but this evidence is not conclusive. It is, however, accepted that the same enzymes metabolise exogenous and endogenous compounds in many cases.

In this section we will look at endogenous metabolism catalysed by the 'drug-metabolising' enzymes discussed above. The section will be split into phase I and II reactions.

1.5.1 Phase I

(a) *Mixed-function oxidase.* Phase I metabolism is dominated by the mixed-function oxidase system and this is known to be involved in the metabolism of steroid hormones, thyroid hormones, fatty acids and prostaglandins and derivatives. The metabolism of steroids is intimately linked to that of drugs as can be seen from the common developmental patterns and physiological control. Indeed, steroid biosynthesis is dependent on cytochrome P450 at many stages. This may be of the microsomal or the mitochondrial type of mixed-function oxidase (see chapter 2) depending on the reaction being studied. The importance of this enzyme is best illustrated by looking at the biosynthesis of steroids from cholesterol.

The rate-limiting step in steroid biosynthesis is the conversion of cholesterol to pregnenolone and this is a multi-stage reaction referred to as side-chain cleavage (Figure 1.52). A specific form of cytochrome P450 has been isolated from the mitochondria of steroid-producing tissues that performs the above reaction. It is seen that the first two steps are simple aliphatic hydroxylations and require NADPH and molecular oxygen as co-factors (cf. drug metabolism).

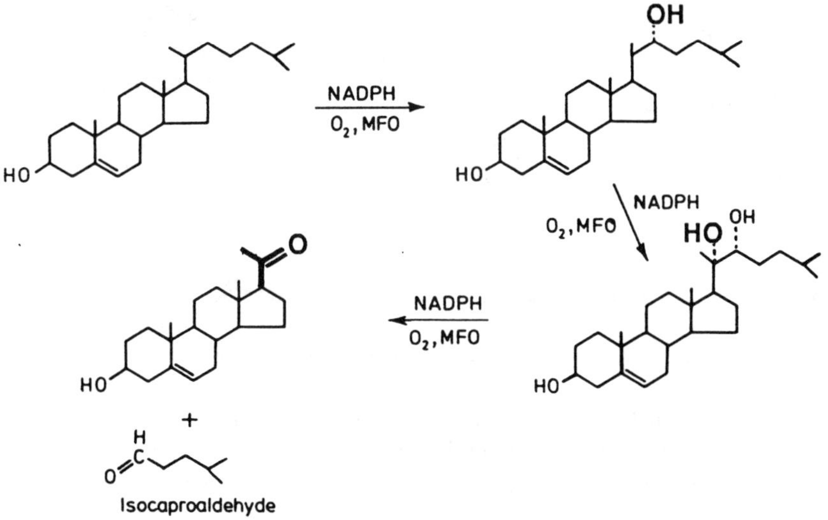

Isocaproaldehyde

Figure 1.52 The conversion of cholesterol to pregnenolone.

The further metabolism of pregnenolone also involves the mixed-function oxidase at many stages (Figure 1.53) some of which take place in the microsomal fraction and some in the mitochondria. Most of the reactions are found

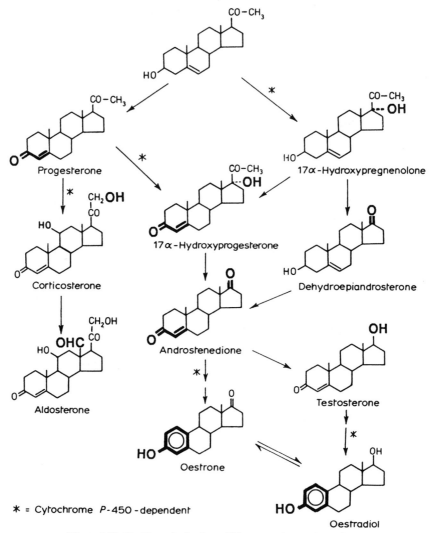

Figure 1.53 The biosynthesis of steroid hormones from pregnenolone.

predominantly in the steroid-synthesising tissues but may also be seen else-where. Thus we have cholesterol side-chain cleavage, 11β-, 17α-, and 21-hydroxylations and aromatisation of androgens all dependent on cytochrome P450.

The breakdown of steroids by the liver and other tissues is also, to a great extent, dependent on the mixed-function oxidase system. All steroids are hydroxylated in various positions by this enzyme and, in most cases, the metabolites are less active. One such example is androst-4-ene-3,17-dione (the precursor of the male sex hormone, testosterone) which is hydroxylated in

the 6β-, 7α- and 16α positions preferentially (Figure 1.54). The enzymes in this
case are located in the microsomal fraction of the liver and are exactly the same
enzymes that metabolise drugs. Other steroids are hydroxylated in different
positions by the same enzymes.

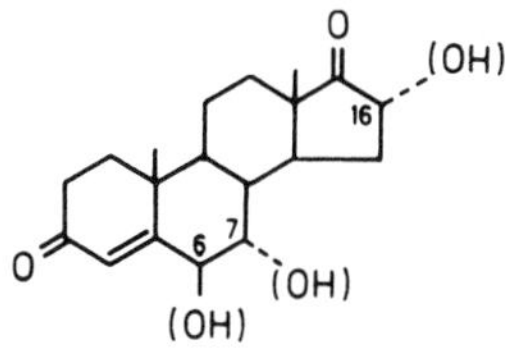

Figure 1.54 The hydroxylation of androst-4-ene-3,17-dione.

A somewhat different scheme is seen for vitamin D (Figure 1.55). After ring
opening by UV light of 7-dehydrocholesterol to yield vitamin D_3, the vitamin is
converted to its active form by 25-hydroxylation in the liver and subsequent
1-hydroxylation by the kidney mitochondria. Both of the hydroxylations are
catalysed by mixed-function oxidases.

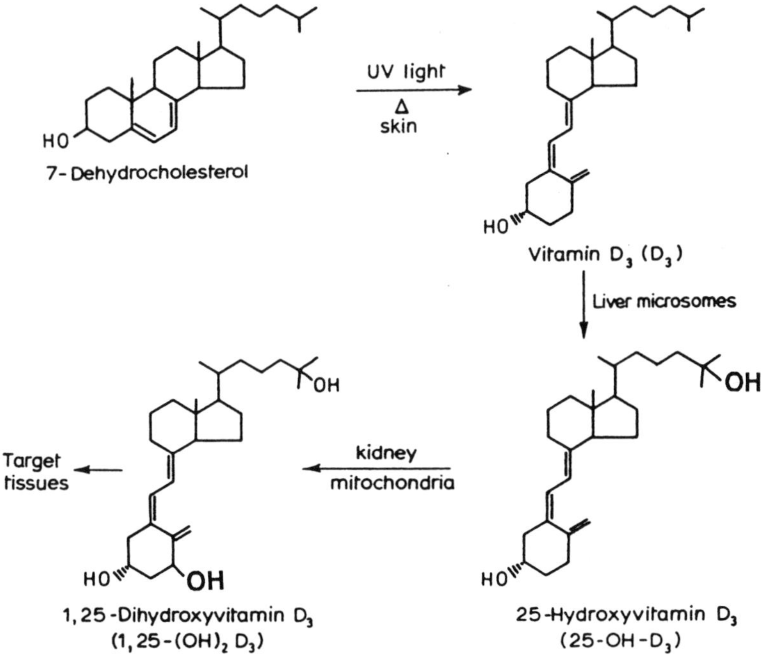

Figure 1.55 The activation of vitamin D_3.

The mixed-function oxidase system also metabolises thyroid hormones by
de-iodination (a mechanism for saving the body's store of iodine) and fatty
acids. Fatty acids are metabolised by hydroxylation in the ω- and (ω-1)-positions

and can also be converted to the epoxide and thus to the dihydroxyacid (Figure 1.56). It has been postulated that the biosynthesis of prostaglandins is also related to the mixed-function oxidase system in requiring cytochrome P450. The prostaglandin synthetase enzyme is closely related to the mixed-function oxidase (Figure 1.57). The breakdown of prostaglandins by hydroxylation is also a cytochrome P450-dependent process.

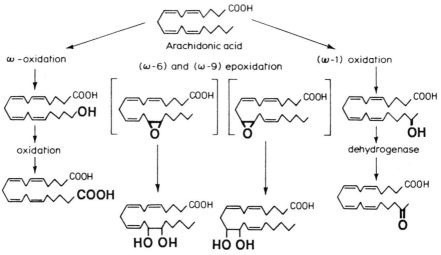

Figure 1.56 The oxidation of fatty acids.

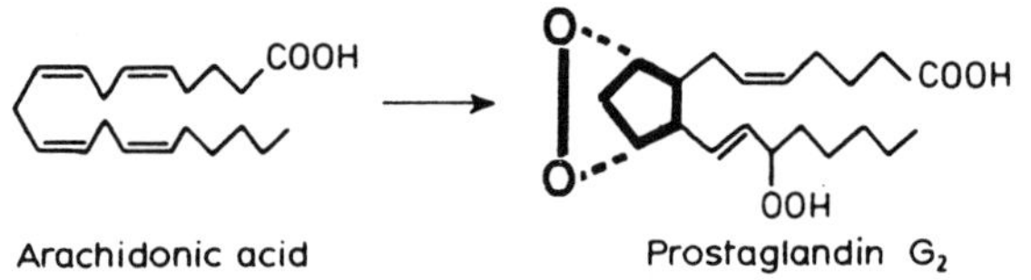

Figure 1.57 The prostaglandin synthetase reaction.

(b) *Other oxidations*. Other oxidation reactions, which are not cytochrome P450-dependent but are related to drug metabolism, occur with endogenous compounds. The hydroxysteroid oxidoreductases for instance are able to oxidise alcohols to ketones but their physiological function is in steroid metabolism (Figure 1.58).

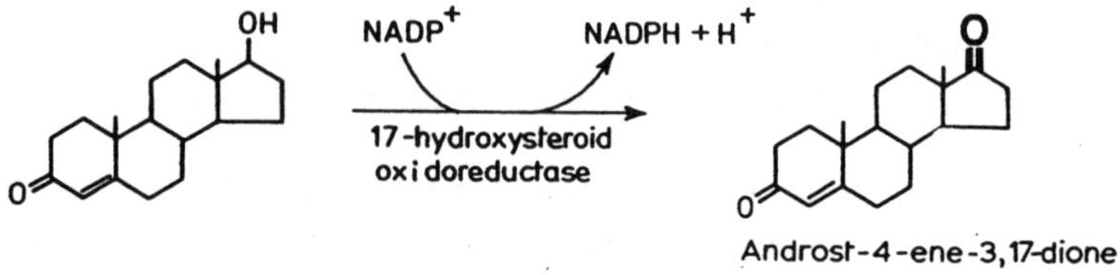

Figure 1.58 The oxidation of testosterone.

The monoamine oxidase is primarily an enzyme to break down endogenous neurotransmitters, e.g. noradrenaline (Figure 1.59), but it can also metabolise exogenous amines of similar structure (cf. drug metabolism, earlier in this chapter) whereas diamine oxidase deaminates the endogenous amines, histamine, putrescine and cadaverine.

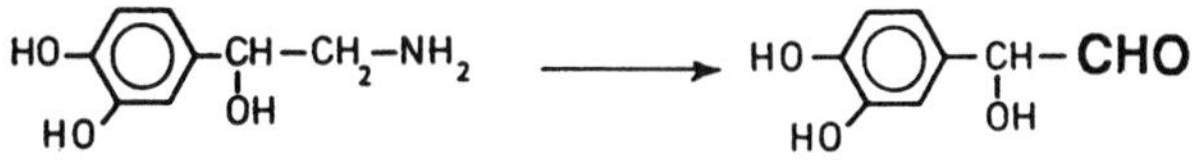

Figure 1.59 The oxidation of noradrenaline.

The xanthine oxidases are primarily related to breakdown of endogenous purines to uric acid via xanthine (Figure 1.60).

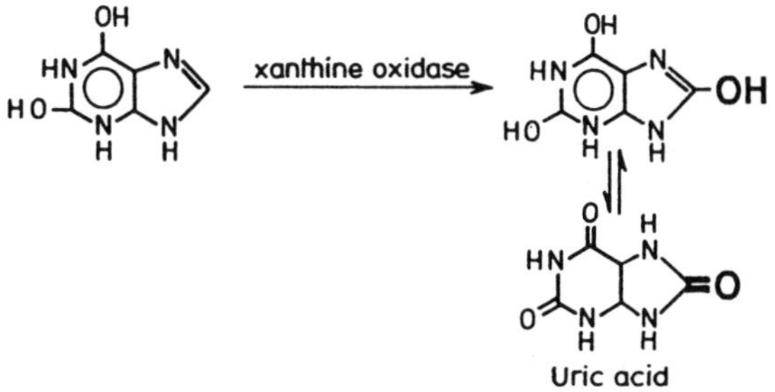

Uric acid

Figure 1.60 The oxidation of xanthine.

(c) *Other phase I reactions.* Of the other phase I reactions noted above, hydrolysis is the one which shows most overlap between endogenous and exogenous metabolism. The plasma esterases are closely related to acetylcholinesterase, the enzyme which inactivates acetylcholine (Figure 1.61). Certain reduction reactions are also seen in the metabolism of endogenous compounds such as the conversion of 4-androstene-3, 17-dione to testosterone (see Figure 1.53) and to 5α-androstane-3, 17-dione (Figure 1.62) but the relationship of these reactions

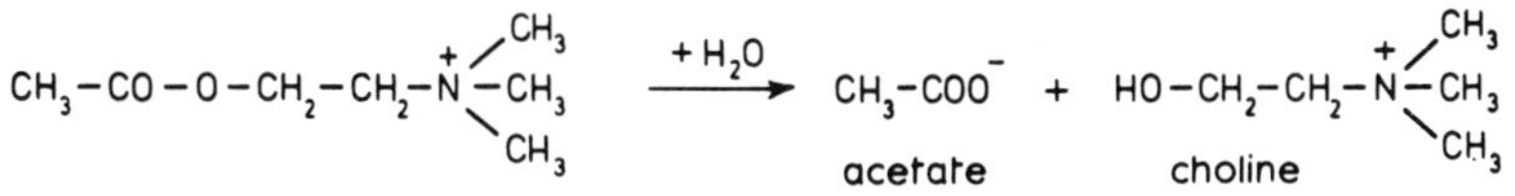

Figure 1.61 The hydrolysis of acetylcholine.

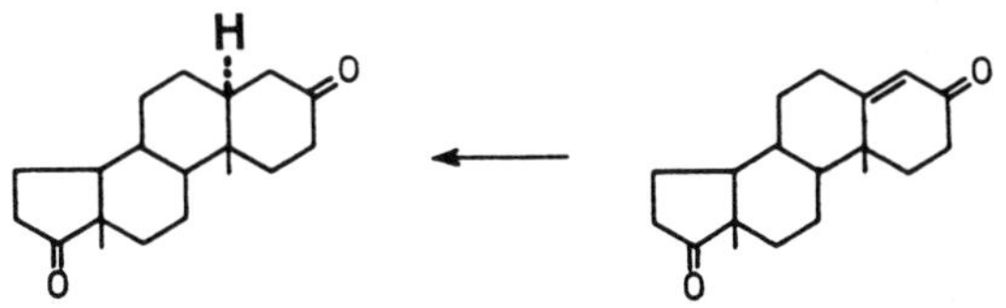

Figure 1.62 The 5α-reduction of androst-4-ene-3,17-dione.

Table 1.11 Endogenous metabolism by phase I enzymes

Enzyme	Endogenous substrates
Mixed-function oxidase	Steroids
	Sterols
	Thyroid hormones
	Fatty acids
	Prostaglandins
	Vitamin D
	Leukotrienes
Monoamine oxidase	Monoamine neurotransmitters
Diamine oxidase	Histamine
	Putrescine
	Cadaverine
Xanthine oxidase	Xanthine
Hydroxysteroid oxidoreductase	Steroids
Acetylcholinesterase	Acetylcholine
Reductases	Steroids

to reduction of drug substrates is unclear. A summary of phase I reactions related to endogenous metabolism is given in Table 1.11.

1.5.2 Phase II

(a) *Glucuronidation*. Glucuronidation is a common pathway of metabolism for many endogenous compounds including steroid hormones, catecholamines, bilirubin and thyroxine. As with glucuronidation of drugs, this process is a preparation for excretion of the compound. Many steroids are excreted as glucuronides into the bile and thus in the faeces. The excretion of bilirubin is dependent on glucuronide formation, and the liver contains a specific form of UDP–glucuronosyltransferase for bilirubin. An example of steroid glucuronide formation is shown in Figure 1.63.

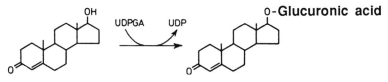

Figure 1.63 The formation of testosterone 17-glucuronide.

(b) *Sulfation*. Sulfate formation is involved in the biosynthesis of steroids and heparin, each of which have specific sulfotransferases and do not interfere to any great extent with drug metabolism.

(c) *Methylation*. Methylation is predominantly a reaction involving endogenous compounds although certain exogenous compounds may also be metabolised (see above). The methyltransferases are listed in Table 1.9 and include phenylethanolamine N-methyltransferase (PNMT) which converts noradrenaline to adrenaline in the adrenal gland, imidazole N-methyltransferase (IMT) which inactivates histamine in the liver, catechol O-methyltransferase (COMT) which inactivates catecholamines mainly in nerve cells and liver, and hydroxy-indole-O-methyltransferase (HIOMT) which synthesises melatonin in the pineal gland (Figure 1.64).

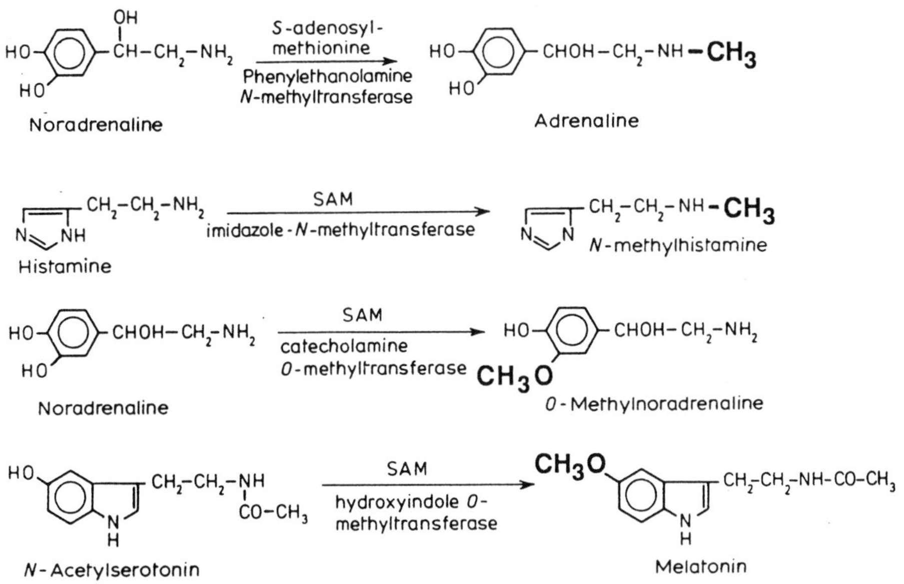

Figure 1.64 Examples of endogenous methyltransferases.

(d) *Other phase II reactions.* Acetylation and amino acid conjugation reactions are seen for endogenous compounds but are not widespread – the acetylation of serotonin in the biosynthesis of melatonin is one example, and the amino acid conjugation of bile acids is another (Figure 1.65).

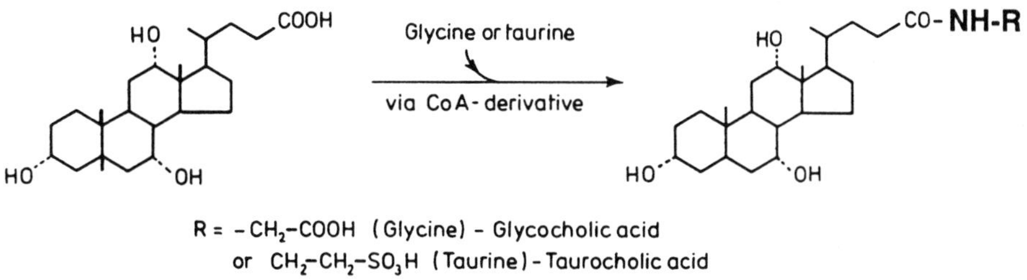

R = – CH$_2$–COOH (Glycine) – Glycocholic acid
   or CH$_2$–CH$_2$–SO$_3$H (Taurine) – Taurocholic acid

Figure 1.65 The amino acid conjugation of bile acids.

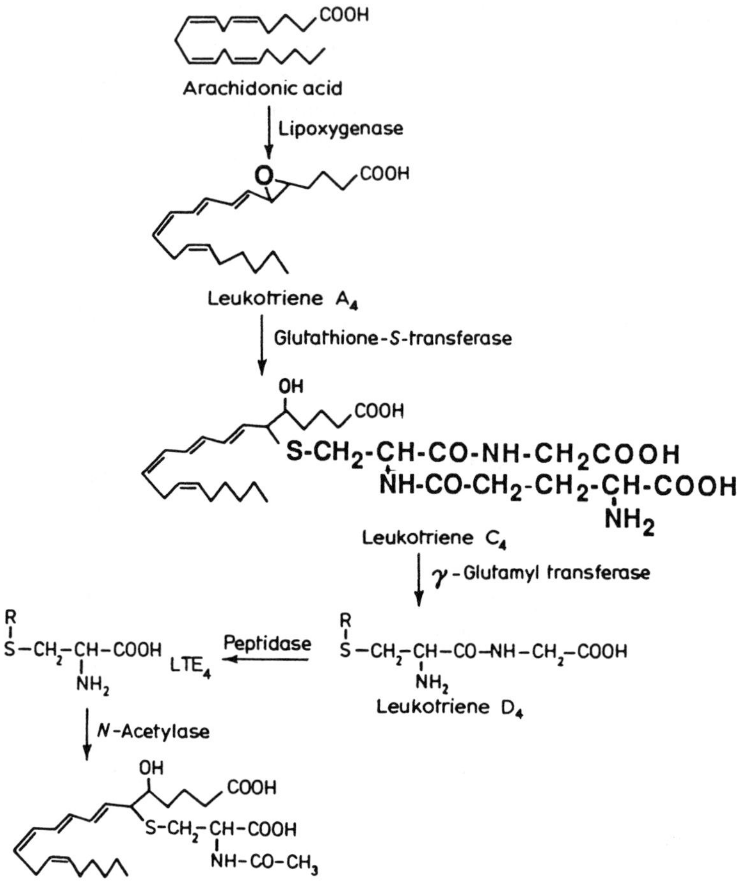

Figure 1.66 The biosynthesis of the leukotrienes.

Table 1.12 Phase II metabolism of endogenous compounds

Reaction	Substrates
Glucuronidation	Steroids Thyroxine Bilirubin Catecholamines
Sulfation	Steroids Carbohydrates
Methylation	Biogenic amines
Acetylation	Serotonin
Amino acid conjugation	Bile acids
Glutathione conjugation	Arachidonic acid metabolites (leukotrienes)

Glutathione conjugation, however, has been shown to be of major importance in the biosynthesis of the prostaglandin-like compounds, the leukotrienes. In fact, leukotriene synthesis involves phase I and II metabolism and is very similar to the metabolism of naphthalene (see Figure 1.47) involving epoxide formation, glutathione conjugation and breakdown of the conjugate to yield, finally, the cysteine conjugate and perhaps the mercapturic acid (Figure 1.66). A summary of phase II reactions involving endogenous compounds is given in Table 1.12.

1.6 General summary

It is apparent from this chapter that there are a large number of enzymes capable of metabolising drugs to many different products. Many of these enzymes have overlapping substrate specificities and will also metabolise endogenous compounds. There is, therefore, a great probability of competition between drugs and endogenous compounds for the same enzyme, between different enzymes for the same substrate and between two drugs for the same enzyme. These interactions are often the basis for the toxic or pharmacological actions of drugs. This is discussed in more detail in chapters 6 and 7.

It should also be emphasised that the reactions noted here are not a complete list of possible reactions but are those of general application. It would be impossible to give all reactions for all drugs, but a general appreciation of the most likely drug metabolic pathways has been given.

Further reading

Textbooks and symposia

Damani, L.A. (1989) *Sulphur-containing drugs and related compounds: Chemistry, biochemistry and toxicology. Vol. 1 and 2*, Ellis Horwood, Chichester.
Fishman, W.H. (1961) *Chemistry of drug metabolism*, Thomas, Springfield.
Hawkins, D.R. (1988–92) *Biotransformations: A survey of the biotransformations of drugs and chemicals in animals. Vols. 1-4*, Royal Society of Chemistry, London.
Jenner, P. and Tester B. (1980) *Concepts in drug metabolism*, Marcel Dekker, New York.
Lambie, J.W. (1983) *Drug metabolism and distribution*, Elsevier, Amsterdam.
Mulder, G.J. (ed) (1990) *Conjugation reactions in drug metabolism*, Taylor and Francis, London.
Parke, D.V. (1968) *The biochemistry of foreign compounds*, Pergamon, Oxford
Parke, D.V. and Smith, R.L. (1977) *Drug metabolism from microbe to man*, Taylor and Francis, London
Williams, R.T. (1959) *Detoxification mechanisms*, Chapman and Hall, London.

Reviews and original articles

Brenner, R.R. (1977) Metabolism of endogenous substrates by microsomes, *Drug Metab. Rev.*, **6** 155–212.
Burchell, B. and Coughtrie, M.W.H. (1989) UDP–Glucuronosyltransferases. *Pharmacol. Ther.*, **43** 261–89.
Capdevila, J.H. *et al.* (1992) Cytochrome P450 and the arachidonate cascade. *FASEB J.*, **6** 731–6.

Connelly, J.C. and Bridges, J.W. (1980) The distribution and role of cytochrome P450 in extrahepatic tissues. *Prog. in Drug Metab.*, **5** 1–109.

Conti, A. and Bickel, M (1977) History of drug metabolism: Discoveries of the major pathways in the 19th century. *Drug Metab. Rev.*, **6** 1–50.

DeLuca, H.F. (1980) Some new concepts emanating from the study of the metabolism and function of vitamin D. *Nutrition Rev.*, **38** 169–82.

Fitzpatrick, F.A. and Murphy, R.C. (1989) Cytochrome P450 metabolism of arachidonic acid. *Pharmacol. Rev.*, **40** 229–41.

George, J. and Farrell, G.C. (1991) Role of human hepatic cytochromes P450 in drug metabolism and toxicity. *Aust NZ J Med.*, **21** 356–62.

Gonzalez, F.J. and Nebert, D.W. (1990) Evolution of the P450 gene superfamily. *TIG* **6** 182–6.

Guengerich, F.P. (1988) *Mammalian cytochrome P450 Vol. 1 and 2*, CRC Press, Boca Raton, Florida.

Guengerich, F.P. (1989) Characterization of human microsomal P450 enzymes. *Ann Rev. Pharmacol. Toxicol.*, **29** 241–64.

Guengerich, F.P. (1990) Enzymatic oxidation of xenobiotic chemicals. *Biochem. Molec. Biol.*, **25** 97.

Guengerich, F.P. (1991) Reactions and significance of cytochrome P450 enzymes. *J. Biol. Chem.*, **266** 10019–22.

Guengerich, F.P. (1992) Human cytochrome P450 enzymes. *Life Sci.*, **50** 1471–8.

Ingelman-Sundberg, M. *et al.* (1990) Drug metabolising enzymes: Genetics, regulation and toxicology. *Proceedings of the VIIIth International Symposium on Microsomes and Drug Oxidations*, Stockholm.

Kappus, H. (1986) Overview of enzyme systems involved in bioreduction of drugs and other redox cycling. *Biochem. Pharmacol.*, **35** 1–6.

Koop, D.R. (1992) Oxidative and reductive metabolism by cytochrome P4502E1. *FASEB J.*, **6** 724–30.

Kroemer, H.K. and Klotz, U. (1992) Glucuronidation of drugs. *Clin. Pharmacokinet.*, **23** 292–310.

Kumar, R. (1984) Metabolism of 1,25-dihydroxy vitamin D_3 *Physiol. Rev.*, **64** 478–504.

Kupfer, D. (1980) Endogenous substrates of monooxygenases: fatty acids and prostaglandins. *Pharmac. Ther.*, **11** 469–96.

Mannervik, B and Danielson, U.H. (1988) Glutathione transferases – structure and catalytic activity. *CRC Crit. Rev. Biochem. Molec. Biol.*, **23** 283–320.

Meijer, J and DePierrre, J.W. (1988) Cytosolic epoxide hydrolase. *Chemico–Biol. Interact.*, **64** 207–49.

Paine, A.J. (1991) The cytochrome P450 gene superfamily. *Int. J. Exp. Path.*, **72** 349–63.

Parke, D.V. *et al.* (1991) The role of cytochrome P450 in the detoxication and activation of drugs and other chemicals. *Can. J. Physiol. Pharmacol.*, **69** 537–49.

Ryan, D.E. and Levin, W. (1990) Purification and characterisation of hepatic microsomal cytochrome P450. *Pharmacol. Ther.*, **45** 153–239.

Soucek, P. and Gut, I. (1992) Cytochromes P450 in rats. Structures, functions, properties and relevant human forms. *Xenobiotica* , **22** 83–103.

Takemori, S. and Kominami, S. (1984) The role of cytochrome P450 in adrenal steroidogenesis. *TIPS*, **9** 393–6.

Tephly, T.R. and Burchell, B. (1990) UDP–glucuronosyltransferases, a family of detoxifying enzymes. *TIPS*, **11** 276–9.

Testa, B. and Jenner, P. (1978) Novel drug metabolites produced by functionalization reactions: Chemistry and toxicology. *Drug Metab. Rev.*, **7** 325–70.

Waxman, D.J. (1988) Interactions of hepatic cytochrome P450 with steroid hormones. *Biochem. Pharmacol.*, **37** 71–84.

Wrighton, S.A. and Stevens, J.C. (1992) The human hepatic cytochromes P450 involved in drug metabolism. *Crit. Rev. Toxicol.*, **22** 1–21.

Ziegler, D.M. (1991) Unique properties of the enzymes of detoxification. *Drug Metab. Disp.*, **19** 847–52.

2 Enzymology and molecular mechanisms of drug metabolism reactions

2.1 Introduction

As described in chapter 1, drugs and xenobiotics are transformed by a variety of pathways in two distinct stages. The phase I (or functionalisation) reactions serve to introduce a suitable functional group into the drug molecule, thereby changing the drug in most cases to a more polar form and hence more readily excretable. In addition, the product of phase I drug metabolism may then act as the substrate for phase II metabolism, resulting in conjugation with endogenous substrates, increased water solubility and polarity, and drug elimination or excretion from the body. In a quantitative sense, the liver is the main organ responsible for phase I and phase II drug metabolism reactions, although this is by no means the only organ involved. Drug localisation, and hence probably metabolism, in a given tissue is dependent on many factors including the physico-chemical properties of the drug (pK_a, lipid solubility and molecular weight), chemical composition of the organ and the presence of uptake mechanisms which allow the drug to be 'trapped'. As drugs are often given several times per day in high doses for long periods, it is not surprising that the drug binding and metabolism sites become saturated in a given organ. This would then lead to drug diffusion to other sites in the body and may well explain extra-hepatic drug metabolism and some bizarre side effects observed after prolonged drug treatment. Other organs where drug metabolism reactions have been observed include skin, gastrointestinal tract, gastrointestinal flora, lung, blood, brain, kidney and placenta, amongst others.

Most of our fundamental knowledge regarding the molecular mechanisms of drug metabolism has been derived from studies on the liver. Although the molecular mechanisms of drug metabolism reactions can be studied at many levels of integration including the intact organism, liver perfusion, liver slices and hepatocyte cell cultures, most of our current knowledge has been derived from studies on isolated sub-cellular hepatocyte organelles and isolated enzymes. The morphological integrity of the hepatocyte can be disrupted by physical means and sub-cellular organelles may be isolated by consecutive differential centrifugation. With respect to drug metabolism reactions, two sub-cellular organelles are quantitatively the most important, namely the endoplasmic reticulum and the cytosol (or soluble cell sap fraction). The phase I oxidative enzymes are almost exclusively localised in the endoplasmic reticulum, along with the phase II enzyme, glucuronosyl transferase. By contrast, other phase II enzymes including the glutathione-S-transferases are predominantly found in the cytoplasm. In the intact cell, the endoplasmic reticulum consists of a continuous network of filamentous, membrane-bound channels and on physical disruption, results in the formation of 'microsomes' (literally small bodies). The microsomal fraction of liver cells is an operational term used to describe the 'pinched-off' and vesiculated fragments of the original endoplasmic reticulum, that retain most, if not all of their enzymatic activity. As shown in Tables 2.1 and 2.2, the hepatic endoplasmic reticulum serves many important functional roles including drug

Table 2.1 Morphological and biochemical characteristics of the hepatic endoplasmic reticulum (ER)

1. Membranes are 50–80 Ångströms in transverse plane.
2. ER occupies approximately 15% of total hepatocyte volume.
3. Volume of ER is 250% of nuclear and 65% of mitochondrial volumes.
4. Surface area of ER is $\times$ 37 of plasma membrane and $\times$ 9 of outer mitochondrial membrane.
5. ER of one hepatocyte has approximately 13×10^6 attached ribosomes.
6. ER contains 19% total protein, 48% total phospholipid and 58% of total RNA of rat hepatocyte.
7. ER membrane consists of 70% protein, 30% lipid, the majority of which is phospholipid, i.e. approximately 23 molecules of phospholipid per protein molecule.
8. Phospholipid of ER comprises of 55% phosphatidylcholine, 20–25% phosphatidylethanolamine, 5–10% phosphatidylserine, 5–10% phosphatidylinositol and 4–7% sphingomyelin.
9. The fatty acid content of above phospholipids mainly consist of palmitic, palmitoleic, stearic, oleic, linoleic and arachidonic acids.
10. ER also contains cholesterol (0.6 mg/g liver), triglycerides (0.5 mg/g liver) and small amounts of cholesterol esters, free fatty acids and vitamin K.
11. ER contains proteins that are 2% carbohydrate by weight containing the neutral sugars mannose and galactose.
12. ER can be induced by many drugs including phenobarbitone resulting in proliferation of protein and phospholipid.

Table 2.2 Enzymatic activities observed in hepatic endoplasmic reticulum

1. Synthesis of triglycerides, phosphatides, glycolipids and plasmalogens.
2. Metabolism of plasmalogens.
3. Fatty acid metabolism including oxidation, elongation and desaturation.
4. Cholesterol and steroid biosynthesis and metabolism.
5. Cytochrome P450-dependent drug oxidations, including hydroxylations, side chain oxidations, deamination, N- and S-oxidation and desulfuration.
6. L-Ascorbic acid synthesis.
7. Aryl- and steroid-sulfatases.
8. Epoxide hydrolase.
9. Cytochrome b_5.
10. NADH–cytochrome b_5 reductase.
11. NADPH–cytochrome c(P450) reductase.
12. Glucose-6-phosphatase.
13. UDP–glucuronosyltransferase.
14. L-Amino acid oxidase.
15. Azo reductase.
16. Cholesterol esterase.
17. 5'-Nucleotidase.
18. Lipid peroxidase.
19. 11ß- and 17ß-hydroxysteroid dehydrogenases.

metabolism reactions. Thus, drug metabolism reactions should not be considered in isolation, but rather as part of an integrated system.

Based on information gained from studies on both intact microsomal membranes, cytsolic fractions and purified enzyme components, it is the purpose of this chapter to clarify, on a molecular level, many of the enzyme-catalysed reactions of drug metabolism. This has been the subject of intense scientific research in recent years and the interested reader is referred to the section on further reading for more detailed information.

2.2 Cytochrome P450-dependent mixed-function oxidation reactions

The most intensively studied drug metabolism reaction is the cytochrome P450-catalysed mixed-function oxidation (M.F.O.) reaction. This reaction catalyses the hydroxylation of literally hundreds of structurally diverse drugs and chemicals, whose only common feature appears to be a reasonably high degree of lipophilicity. The M.F.O. reaction conforms to the following stoichiometry

$$NADPH + H^+ + O_2 + RH \xrightarrow{\text{Cytochrome P450}} NADP^+ + H_2O + ROH$$

where RH represents an oxidisable drug substrate and ROH the hydroxylated metabolite, the overall reaction being catalysed by the enzyme cytochrome P450. During the M.F.O. reaction, reducing equivalents derived from NADPH + H^+ are consumed and one atom of molecular oxygen is incorporated into the substrate, whereas the other oxygen atom is reduced to water. Studies using $^{18}O_2$ have unequivocally shown that the source of oxygen in the metabolite is derived from molecular oxygen and not from water. In addition to hydroxylation reactions, cytochrome P450 catalyses the N-, O- and S-dealkylation of many drugs (see chapter 1). These heteroatom dealkylation reactions can be considered as a specialised form of hydroxylation reaction in that the initial event is a carbon hydroxylation as described in chapter 1.

2.2.1 Components of the M.F.O. system

(a) *Cytochrome P450.* Cytochrome P450 is the terminal oxidase component of an electron transfer system present in the endoplasmic reticulum responsible for many drug oxidation reactions, and is classified as a haem-containing enzyme (a haemoprotein) with iron protoporphyrin IX as the prosthetic group (Figure 2.1). The enzyme consists of a family of closely related isoenzymes embedded in the membrane of the endoplasmic reticulum, and exists in multiple forms of monomeric molecular weight of approximately 45 000–55 000 Da (see chapter 3). The haem is non-covalently bound to the apoprotein and the name cytochrome P450 is derived from the fact that the cytochrome (or pigment) exhibits a spectral absorbance maximum at 450 nm when reduced and complexed with carbon monoxide. The haemoprotein serves as both the oxygen- and

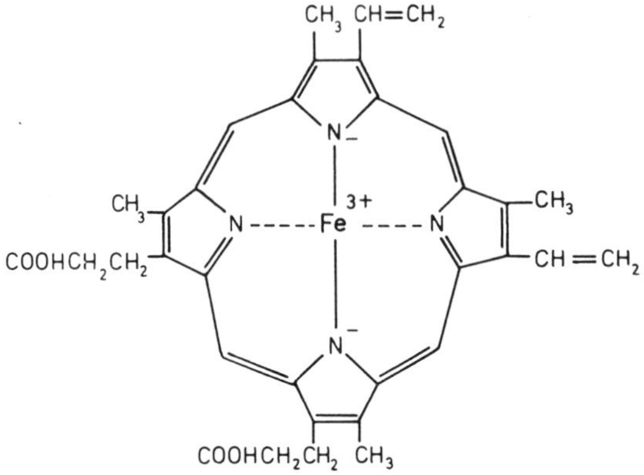

CH₃ CH=CH₂

[chemical structure of ferric protoporphyrin IX]

COOHCH₂CH₂⁻

COOHCH₂CH₂ CH₃

Figure 2.1 Structure of ferric protoporphyrin IX, the prosthetic group of cytochrome P450.

substrate binding locus for the M.F.O. reaction and in conjunction with the associated flavoprotein reductase, NADPH–cytochrome P450 reductase (see below), undergoes cyclic oxidation/reduction of the haem iron that is mandatory for its catalytic function.

Cumulative historical evidence and more recent studies on experimental manipulation of the cytochrome P450 genes are beginning to yield fascinating information on the structural and functional domains of the P450s. For example, for the cytochrome P4502B1 enzyme (Figure 2.2) particular regions of the proteins are thought to involve a membrane insertion segment, a multifunctional

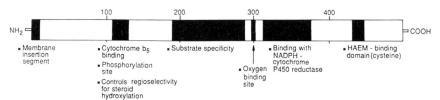

Figure 2.2 Putative functional domains of cytochrome P450. Many aspects of these functional domains remain to be clarified and this model is based on the CYP2B1 isoenzyme. Numbers represent the amino acid residues. Derived, in part, from Waxman, D.J. and Azaroff, L. (1992), *Biochemical Journal*, **281** 577–92.

site for the putative binding site for cytochrome b₅, a site of phosphorylation by cAMP-dependent protein kinases and several amino acid residues thought to be important for the regioselectivity of steroid hydroxylations, a hypervariable region thought to dictate substrate binding and hence substrate specificity, an oxygen-binding site (Threonine-301), an NADPH–cytochrome P450 reductase binding site and a highly conserved region near the carboxyl terminal responsible for haem binding via the invariant cysteine residue. Whereas many of those domains are still being confirmed for other cytochrome P450s, one thing that is absolutely clear is the presence of the invariant haem-binding segment (via a cysteine residue) of approximately 15 amino acid residues, a sequence that is conserved in all cytochrome P450s studied to date ranging from bacteria, through to lower mammals to man (Figure 2.3).

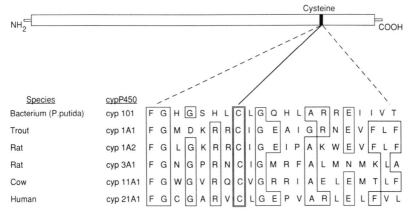

Species	cypP450																		
Bacterium (P.putida)	cyp 101	F	G	H	G	S	H	L	C	L	G	Q	H	L	A	R	R	E	I	I	V	T
Trout	cyp 1A1	F	G	M	D	K	R	R	C	I	G	E	A	I	G	R	N	E	V	F	L	F
Rat	cyp 1A2	F	G	L	G	K	R	R	C	I	G	E	I	P	A	K	W	E	V	F	L	F
Rat	cyp 3A1	F	G	N	G	P	R	N	C	I	G	M	R	F	A	L	M	N	M	K	L	A
Cow	cyp 11A1	F	G	W	G	V	R	Q	C	V	G	R	R	I	A	E	L	E	M	T	L	F
Human	cyp 21A1	F	G	C	G	A	R	V	C	L	G	E	P	V	A	R	L	E	L	F	V	L

Figure 2.3 The conserved haem-binding domain in cytochrome P450s. The cysteine residue that binds the haem prosthetic group as the 5th ligand is shown towards the carboxyl terminus of the polypeptide chain. The important cysteine residue is shown (C) and other amino acids are abbreviated by their one letter codes. The amino acid residues that are common between the various isoforms are boxed in.

(i) *Cytochrome P450 nomenclature and multiple forms.* Ever since its purification and isolation in a catalytically competent form in the late 1960s, many studies have emphasised that cytochrome P450 exists as multiple forms or isoenzymes, and several cytochrome P450s were isolated from various tissue sources. Unfortunately, this resulted in much confusion as to the identity of individual enzymes as no commonly agreed nomenclature system existed. In fact, particular cytochrome P450s would have several different names for the same enzyme if isolated in different laboratories – clearly an unsatisfactory situation. However, with the advent of gene cloning and sequencing, and the application of molecular biology techniques to cytochrome P450 structure analysis, the 1980s witnessed an explosion in the isolation and sequencing of cDNAs encoding multiple forms of the haemoprotein. This rapid accumulation of full-length cytochrome P450 amino acid sequences (predicted from open reading frames of the cognate cDNA nucleotide sequences) then allowed the development of a coherent nomenclature system which has now been universally accepted and uniquely identifies more than 200 different cytochrome P450s.

The basis of this unifying nomenclature system is divergent evolution and sequence similarity between the cytochrome P450s, resulting in the sub-classification of cytochrome P450s into gene families and gene sub-families. A cytochrome P450 sequence from one gene family is defined as usually having less than 40% resemblance to that from any other family (or put another way, within a given cytochrome P450 gene family, all the component genes in that family are greater than 40% identical in their sequence to each other). These gene families are further divided into gene sub-families where the nomenclature dictates that two cytochrome P450 proteins belong to the same gene sub-family when they are approximately 70% (or greater) similar in their sequence. Hence, cytochrome P4501A1 for example, usually describes only one particular gene encoding one particular isoenzyme (although some minor exceptions exist). This list of cytochrome P450 genes/enzymes is updated every two years and the number of identified genes continues to increase, for example, from 65 in 1987 to 221 in early 1993. For the development and detailed discussion of this nomenclature system, the reader is referred to the papers by Neberet *et al* and Nelson *et al* in the reading list.

This gene cloning/molecular biology approach to the structure, function and regulation of the cytochrome P450 gene superfamily has enabled considerable progress in the characterisation of human cytochrome P450 genes from human gene libraries, thus obviating the need for scarce human tissue for analysis. Over 30 human cytochrome P450s have now been isolated and unequivocally identified including the steroid hydroxylases (e.g. cytochrome P450s 11A1 and 21A2) and the major human drug metabolising cytochrome P450s including cytochrome P450s 2E1, 2C9, 2D6 and 3A4. The latter cytochrome appears to be the major hepatic cytochrome P450 in the majority of humans (up to 50% of the total), but it should be emphasised that the human hepatic drug-metabolising cytochrome P450 can show considerable inter-individual variation. This is clearly seen in variation in the cytochrome P4502D6 isoenzyme, and is responsible for the poor or extensive metaboliser phenotype towards debrisoquine and many other drugs (see chapter 7 for a fuller description of this phenomenon).

The ever increasing number of cytochrome P450 sequences has also stimulated computer-based molecular modelling of their tertiary structures. This modelling has been facilitated by the crystallisation and X-ray crystal structure determination of the soluble cytochrome P450 from the soil bacterium *Pseudomonas putida* (termed cytochrome P450101 in the new gene nomenclature and cytochrome $P450_{cam}$ in the old nomenclature). Thus, by using cytochrome P450101 as a 'template', other cytochrome P450s can be modelled based on sequence similarities. Because almost all the cytochrome P450s are membrane bound (and therefore inherently very difficult to crystallise), this matching to the cytochrome P450101 template is the only current method available to model the three-dimensional structures of these haemoproteins.

(b) *NADPH–cytochrome P450 reductase.* NADPH–cytochrome P450 reductase is a flavin-containing enzyme (a flavoprotein consisting of one mole of flavin adenine dinucleotide (FAD) and one mole of flavin mononucleotide (FMN) per mole of apoprotein (see Figure 2.4 for structures of these flavins). This makes NADPH–cytochrome P450 reductase unusual as most other flavoproteins have only FAD or FMN as their prosthetic group. The flavoprotein is sometimes termed NADPH–cytochrome c reductase because of the well-known ability of

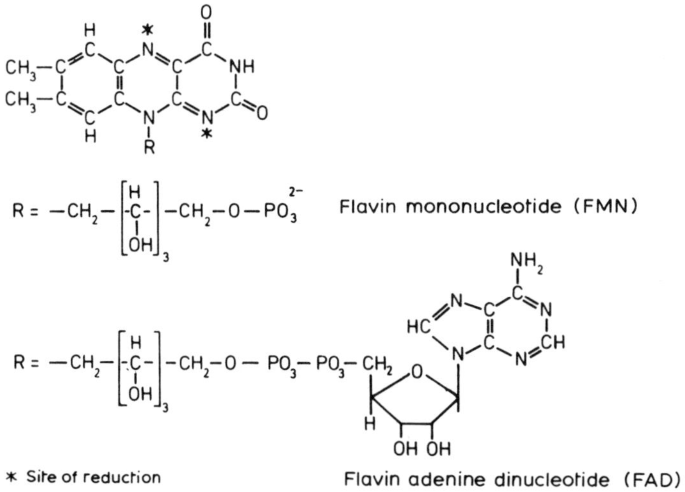

$R = -CH_2 - \left[\begin{array}{c} H \\ -C- \\ OH \end{array} \right]_3 -CH_2 - O - PO_3^{2-}$ Flavin mononucleotide (FMN)

$R = -CH_2 - \left[\begin{array}{c} H \\ -C- \\ OH \end{array} \right]_3 -CH_2 - O - PO_3 - PO_3 - CH_2$ Flavin adenine dinucleotide (FAD)

* Site of reduction

Figure 2.4 Structures of FAD and FMN, the prosthetic groups of NADPH–cytochrome P450 reductase.

the enzyme to reduce exogenous cytochrome c (an artificial electron acceptor in this instance) in the presence of NADPH + H$^+$. However, because cytochrome c is a mitochondrial haemoprotein and not present in the endoplasmic reticulum, the preferred terminology for this enzyme is NADPH– cytochrome P450 reductase in that cytochrome P450 is the endogenous acceptor of reducing equivalents from the flavoprotein. The enzyme has a monomeric molecular weight of approximately 78 000 Da and exists in close association with cytochrome P450 in the endoplasmic reticulum membrane. In addition to cytochrome P450, NADPH–cytochrome P450 reductase is an essential component of the M.F.O. system responsible for drug oxidations in that the flavoprotein transfers reducing equivalents from NADPH + H$^+$ to cytochrome P450 as

$$NADPH + H^+ \longrightarrow (FAD \xrightarrow[\text{P450 reductase}]{\text{NADPH–cytochrome}} FMN \longrightarrow \text{Cytochrome P450}$$

The need for an intermediary electron transfer flavoprotein is readily appreciated in light of the fact that NADPH + H$^+$ is a 2 electron donor and cytochrome P450 is a 2×1 electron acceptor. Accordingly, NADPH–cytochrome P450 reductase is thought to act as a 'transducer' of reducing equivalents by accepting electrons from NADPH and transferring them sequentially (one at a time) to cytochrome P450 (see above). The precise oxidation/reduction states of NADPH–cytochrome P450 reductase during cytochrome P450 dependent drug oxidations are not fully understood, as the redox biochemistry of the two flavins are complex (Figure 2.5 and Table 2.3), although there is strong evidence to support the role of FAD as the acceptor flavin from NADPH + H$^+$ and FMN as

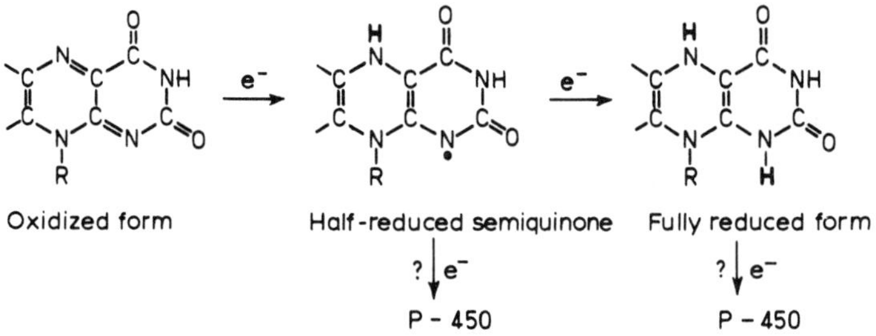

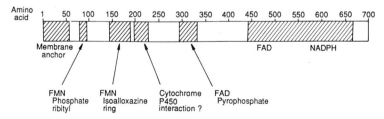

Figure 2.5 Flavin reduction.

Table 2.3 Redox biochemistry of the two flavin prosthetic groups present in NADPH–cytochrome P450 reductase[a]

$$F_1 + H^{\cdot} \rightleftharpoons F_1H^{\cdot}, E_m = -110\text{mV}$$

$$F_1H^{\cdot} = H^{\cdot} \rightleftharpoons F_1H_2, E_m = -270\text{mV}$$

$$E_m = -190\text{mV}$$

$$F_2 + H^{\cdot} \rightleftharpoons F_2H^{\cdot}, E_m = -290\text{mV}$$

$$F_2H^{\cdot} = H^{\cdot} \rightleftharpoons F_2H_2, E_m = -365\text{mV}$$

$$E_m = -320\text{mV}$$

[a] Abbreviations used are F_1, high potential flavin (probably FMN); F_2 low potential flavin (probably FAD); E_m, mid-point redox potential.

the donating flavin to cytochrome P450 in the electron transfer events (see steps 2 and 5 of the cytochrome P450 catalytic cycle, section 2.2.2).

Both the cDNA and genomic DNA encoding NADPH–cytochrome P450 reductase have been isolated from several sources. The rat gene has been extensively studied and consists of fifteen exons (i.e. the coding regions) spanning 20 kilobases of DNA. Comparison of the amino acid sequence of the reductase to several other flavoproteins of defined structure reveals that particular regions of the protein have specialised functions such as anchoring the reductase to the endoplasmic reticulum membrane and binding sites for FMN, FAD and NADPH, as shown in Figure 2.6.

Figure 2.6 Functional segments of the NADPH–cytochrome P450 reductase molecule.

(c) *Lipid.* Early studies on the resolution and reconstitution of M.F.O. activity in drug oxidations have shown the requirement of a heat-stable, lipid component. This component was originally identified as phosphatidylcholine and later studies showed the fatty acid composition of the phospholipid to be critical in determining functional reconstitution of M.F.O. activity. The precise mode of action of lipids is still unknown but it has been suggested that lipid may be required for substrate binding, facilitation of electron transfer or providing a 'template' for the interaction of cytochrome P450 and NADPH–cytochrome P450 reductase molecules.

2.2.2 Catalytic cycle of cytochrome P450

As mentioned above, cytochrome P450 is both the substrate- and oxygen-binding locus of the M.F.O. reaction. The central features of the cytochrome P450 catalytic cycle are the ability of the haem iron to undergo cyclic oxidation/reduction reactions in conjunction with substrate binding and oxygen activation, as outlined in Figure 2.7. The precise molecular details of this catalytic cycle have not all been fully elucidated and as the reaction cycle proceeds from step 1 to 6, less information is known.

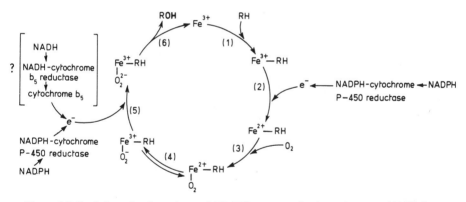

Figure 2.7 Catalytic cycle of cytochrome P450. RH represents the drug substrate and ROH the corresponding hydroxylated metabolite. Adapted from White and Coon, (1980) *Ann Rev. Biochem.*, **49** 315–56.

(a) *Step 1.* This is a relatively well characterised step and involves drug binding to the oxidised (Fe^{3+}, ferric) form of cytochrome P450. Early experiments in the late 1960s categorised drug binding to cytochrome P450 into three types, namely Type I, Type II and Modified Type II. At that time, these classifications were arbitrarily made on the basis of observed substrate induced changes in the absorbance spectrum of cytochrome P450 and subsequently many drugs and xenobiotics have been shown to bind to cytochrome P450, resulting in characteristic spectral perturbations of the haemoprotein (Table 2.4).

Table 2.4 Spectral interaction of drugs and other xenobiotics with cytochrome P450[a]

Type I	Type II	Reverse Type I
Aldrin	Aniline	Acetanilide
Aminopyrine	Amphetamine	Butanol
Benzphetamine	Cyanide	Diallyl barbituric acid
Caffeine	Dapsone	Ethanol
Chlorpromazine	Desdimethylimipramine	Methanol
Cocaine	Imidazole	Phenacetin
DDT	Metyrapone	Rotenone
Diphenylhydantoin	Nicotinamide	Theophylline
Ethylmorphine	Nicotine	Warfarin
Halothane	p-Phenetidine	
Hexobarbital	Pyridine	
Imipramine		
Phenobarbitone		
Propranolol		
Testosterone		

[a] Spectral changes of cytochrome P450 induced by xenobiotics have the following UV/visible characteristics in difference spectrum:

Type I, absorption peak at 385–390 nm and trough at approximately 420 nm.

Type II, absorption peak at 425–435 nm and trough at 390–405 nm.

Reverse type I (sometimes termed Modified Type II), absorption peak at 420 nm and trough at 388-390 nm.

Derived from Schenkman *et al.* (1981), *Pharmacol. Ther.*, **12** 43.

These spectral perturbations are the result of the ability of various drug substrates to perturb the spin equilibrium of cytochrome P450, which are best understood by considering haem ligation in cytochrome P450.

The bonding of the haem iron of cytochrome P450 to the four pyrrole nitrogen atoms of protoporphyrin IX and the two axial ligands lying normal to the porphyrin plane (Figure 2.8) may be described by ligand field theory. Thus, upon coordination of the ferric haem iron with these six ligands in an octahedral complex, the electrons occupying the d-orbitals of the ferric iron (which are energetically degenerate in the free ion) are, as a result of differences in their spatial arrangement, subjected to differential electron repulsion by the lone pair electrons of the ligands. Thus, the electrons occupying the d_{z^2} and $d_{x^2-y^2}$ orbitals (the lobes of which collectively exhibit octahedral symmetry and are oriented along the ligand bond axes), experience a greater electron repulsion than electrons occupying the d_{xy}, d_{yz} and d_{xz} orbitals (lying between the bond axes). This results in a splitting in the energy levels of the ferric ion d orbitals as shown in Figure 2.9.

The magnitude of the energy separation between the two higher energy orbitals (e_g) and the three lower energy orbitals (t_{2g}) is called the crystal field splitting (or stabilisation) energy, termed ΔE, and is a function of the strength of the ligand to ferric d orbital repulsion forces and thus the ligand field strength. The magnitude of ΔE has profound effects upon the distribution of the ferric d electrons. Thus if ΔE is greater than the energetic instability (C) resulting from electron–electron repulsion in a spin-paired d orbital, then a low spin d electron configuration of net spin $S = 1/2$ (one unpaired d electron) is predicted.

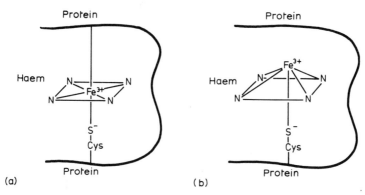

Figure 2.8 Haem iron coordination in cytochrome P450. (a) Hexa-coordinated, low-spin P450 with in-plane iron. (b) Penta-coordinated, high-spin P450 with out-of-plane iron. Note that the 5th ligand is a cysteine residue from the apoprotein and that cytochrome P450 exists as an equilibrium mixture of low-spin (6-coordinated) and high-spin (5-coordinated) forms. See text for detailed discussion of ligation and spin states.

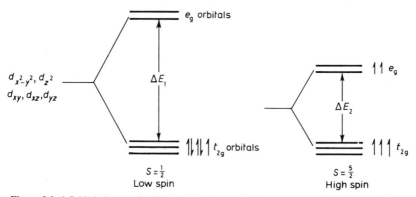

Figure 2.9 d-Orbital electron distribution in the low- and high-spin states of cytochrome P450.

Conversely, if C is greater than ΔE, a maximal paramagnetic configuration of $S = 5/2$ (5 unpaired d electrons) is predicted, as shown in Figure 2.9.

From this simplistic description, it is easily seen that a change in the spin state of the ferric haem iron is associated with a change in ΔE which could be envisaged as arising due to quantitative or qualitative alterations in the ligands coordinating to the haem iron. Since it is absolutely required that the four equatorial iron-to-pyrrole nitrogen bonds remain intact, the substrate induced spin state changes in cytochrome P450 may arise due to changes in axial ligand coordination.

Much effort has been spent by synthetic chemists in an attempt to understand the relationships between the spin state and geometric configuration of synthetic metal–porphyrin model complexes. It has generally been observed in such studies that most penta-coordinate haem models are high spin with an out-of-plane displacement of the haem iron, whereas hexa-coordinate complexes exhibit an in-plane, low spin iron (Figure 2.8). These observations therefore give support to the dogma of haemoprotein biochemistry that all high- and low-spin haemoproteins are penta- and hexa-coordinate respectively.

From such considerations, it is clear than an understanding of the immediate haem environment of cytochrome P450, and in particular the nature of the axial ligands, is crucial in understanding its mechanism of catalysis. The importance of the axial ligands as determinants of haemoprotein function is further substantiated when one considers that cytochrome P450 (a mixed-function oxidase), haemoglobin (an oxygen carrier), peroxidases and catalase all contain protoporphyrin IX as their prosthetic group, yet all of them perform vastly different biological functions.

Most cytochrome P450s exist in predominantly the low spin configuration with a ferric soret absorption at around 418 nm. When certain drug substrates (termed Type I substrates, including hexobarbitone and benzphetamine) bind to low spin cytochrome P450, they usually bind to the protein part of the molecule and change the conformation and hence the ligation of the haem prosthetic group with the protein. This results in a high spin configuration, and the change from a low spin to high spin configuration results in a characteristic spectral change (Type I spectral change), with an absorption maximum at around 390 nm and minimum around 420 nm in the difference spectrum (Figure 2.10). This difference spectrum arises due to the increase in absorbance at 390 nm (high spin form) and a decrease in absorbance at 420 nm, on binding of a Type I substrate.

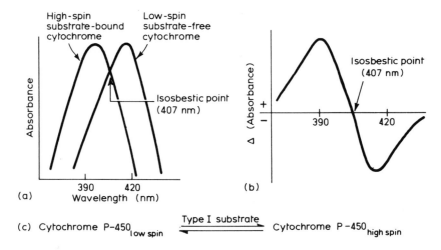

Figure 2.10 Spectral interaction of a Type I substrate with cytochrome P450. (a) Influence of substrate on the absolute spectrum of cytochrome P450. Note the increase in absorbance at 390 nm and decrease in absorbance at 420 nm upon substrate addition. (b) Substrate induced Type I difference spectrum. Note that the spectral change results from the absorbance changes in (a). (c) Influence of substrate on the spin equilibrium of cytochrome P450. Note that Type I substrates shift the spin equilibrium to the high-spin form.

Thus Type I substrates can be considered as those that modulate the spin equilibrium of cytochrome P450 towards the high spin form (Figure 2.10).

In contrast to Type I substrates, Type II substrates are mainly nitrogenous bases and are thought to ligate (via the lone pair electrons on the nitrogen atom) to the haem iron of cytochrome P450, resulting in a 6-coordinated, low spin haemoprotein.

An important *functional* consequence of these drug-induced spin state perturbations of cytochrome P450, is that the spin state shift is associated with changes in the mid-point redox potential of the haemoprotein. For example, a shift in the spin state of both bacterial and mammalian cytochrome P450s towards the high spin form is associated with a shift in the mid-point redox potential of the haemoprotein to a more positive value. This spin–redox coupling phenomenon is very likely to be of functional significance when one considers that the first electron reduction of ferric cytochrome P450 (step 2) by NADPH–cytochrome P450 reductase represents the committed step in cytochrome P450 dependent catalysis. A substrate induced shift in the haemoprotein mid-point redox potential to a more positive value results in a greater electromotive force for subsequent facile electron transfer between the flavoprotein and the cytochrome.

(b) *Step 2.* This involves the first electron reduction of substrate-bound ferric (Fe^{3+}) cytochrome P450 to the ferrous (Fe^{2+}) form of the haemoprotein. The reducing equivalent necessary for this reduction is originally derived from NADPH + H^+ and is transferred by the flavoprotein, NADPH–cytochrome P450 reductase. It is thought that the role of the flavins FMN and FAD in this electron transfer event are as shown in Figure 2.11.

In terms of the cytochrome P450 electron transfer proteins, there is a substantial difference between the mammalian microsomal system on the one

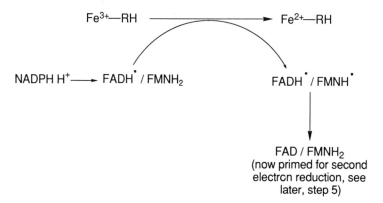

Figure 2.11 Role of flavins in the first electron reduction of cytochrome P450. Fe^{3+} and Fe^{2+} represents the oxidised (ferric) and reduced (ferrous) forms of cytochrome P450 haem iron respectively, bound to a substrate (RH).

hand and adrenal mitochondrial systems on the other. In the microsomal system, electron transfer occurs in the sequence NADPH + H$^+$/NADPH–cytochrome P450 reductase/cytochrome P450 as described above whereas there is an additional requirement for an iron–sulfur protein in the adrenal system, namely adrenodoxin.

In the adrenal mitochondrial system, electron transfer occurs in the sequence

NADPH + H$^+$ ⟶ NADPH–adrenodoxin reductase ⟶ adrenodoxin ⟶ cytochrome P450

It should be noted that unlike microsomal NADPH–cytochrome P450 reductase, adrenal mitochondrial NADPH–adrenodoxin reductase contains only FAD as the sole prosthetic group. In addition, the adrenal mitochondrial cytochrome P450 is different from its microsomal counterpart in that the former haemoprotein does not readily catalyse the oxidation of drugs. The endogenous roles for the cytochrome P450s have been discussed previously in chapter 1 and a more extensive consideration of the structure and regulation of the cytochrome P450 isoenzymes is presented in chapter 3.

As mentioned above, the high spin/low spin equilibrium of cytochrome P450 may well be important in this first electron reduction step. However, a full understanding of the spin–redox coupling in steps 1 and 2 of the catalytic cycle is not yet complete because of the inherent complexities associated with the redox biochemistry of the electron donor flavoprotein which contains both FAD and FMN as prosthetic groups, and is therefore a potential four electron carrier (see Table 2.3).

Although existing experimental data is strongly supportive of a spin–redox coupling event (with respect to haemoprotein reduction), extrapolations from thermodynamic data (spin state *equilibrium*) to the kinetic situation (one electron reduction *rate*) have to be treated with caution. This is primarily because the electromotive force for a redox reaction is a function of both the forward and backward rate constants for the electron transfer event.

(c) *Step 3.* This step involves the binding of molecular oxygen to the binary ferrous cytochrome P450–substrate adduct. This reaction is not well characterised in the mammalian system due to the unstable nature of the oxy–ferrous–substrate complex, but has been spectrally characterised in the adrenal system and the soluble bacterial system of *Pseudomonas putida* (P450$_{cam}$, so termed because the bacterium grows on camphor as a sole source of carbon and catalyses the 5-exo-hydroxylation of camphor).

(d) *Steps 4, 5 and 6.* These steps involve putative electron rearrangement, introduction of the second electron and subsequent oxygen insertion and product release. The precise oxidation states of iron and oxygen in these intermediates are not precisely known. Step 5 involves the input of a second electron, usually derived from NADPH–cytochrome P450 reductase (Figure 2.12), and possibly also derived from cytochrome b$_5$, although the precise role of cytochrome b$_5$ in cytochrome P450 catalysed drug oxidations remains the subject of much

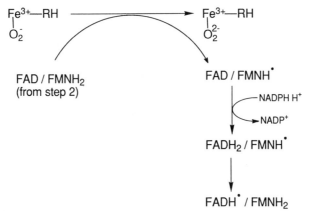

Figure 2.12 Role of the flavins in the second electron reduction of cytochrome P450.

controversy. Similarly, step 6 is not well understood and primarily concerns the actual chemical mechanism of oxygen insertion into the carbon substrate, resulting in product (metabolite) formation. However, the prevailing view of the chemistry of product formation involves two steps, namely abstraction of a hydrogen atom and oxygen rebound as

$$(FeO)^{3+} + RH \longrightarrow (FeOH)^{3+} \; R^{\bullet} \longrightarrow Fe^{3+} + ROH$$

A detailed discussion of the inorganic and organic chemistry involved in this reaction is outside the scope of this chapter and the interested reader is referred to the Further Reading section for more detailed information on this topic.

It should be pointed out that under certain conditions in the presence of particular drug substrates, the catalytic cycle of cytochrome P450 becomes 'uncoupled'. The uncoupling involves dissociation of the utilisation of reducing equivalents from product formation, resulting in the formation of reduced oxygen species instead of stoichiometric product formation as dictated by the M.F.O. equation described earlier. Accordingly, in producing hydrogen peroxide in an uncoupled system, cytochrome P450 functions as an NADPH–oxidase as

$$O_2 + NADPH + H^+ \xrightarrow{\quad P450 \quad} H_2O_2 + NADP^+$$

Although the precise source of hydrogen peroxide is not known, it is most likely that it arises from dismutation of one of the oxygenated cytochrome P450 intermediates produced during the catalytic cycle.

2.3 Microsomal flavin-containing monooxygenase

This enzyme was originally designated by the name microsomal mixed function amine oxidase in view of the fact that many tertiary amines were N-oxidised by this enzyme. It is also known as 'Ziegler's enzyme' in the older literature, so named after the scientist who discovered it. However, more recent work has shown that the enzyme additionally catalyses the S-oxidation of organic compounds (Figure 2.13). Accordingly, the enzyme is more appropriately termed the microsomal FAD-containing monooxygenase (F.M.O.). Using N,N-dimethylaniline as a representative substrate, the F.M.O. catalyses the following reaction

$$\text{NADPH} + \text{H}^+ + \text{O}_2 + \text{C}_6\text{H}_5 - \text{N(CH}_3)_2 \xrightarrow{\text{F.M.O.}} \text{NADP}^+ + \text{H}_2\text{O} + \text{C}_6\text{H}_5 - \text{N(CH}_3)_2$$

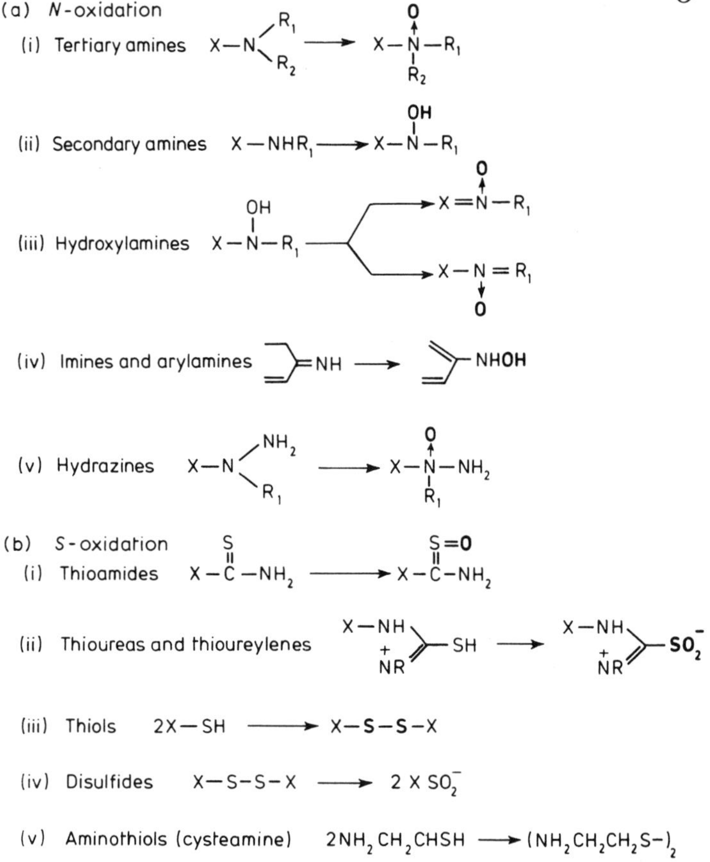

Figure 2.13 Substrates of the microsomal flavin-containing monooxygenase.

The F.M.O. enzyme is a polymeric protein exhibiting a monomeric molecular weight of 65 000 Da and containing one mole of FAD per protein monomer. The enzyme is found in many tissues, with highest concentrations being found in the microsomal fraction of the liver, and is present in substantial amounts in both man and hog, although lower amounts are present in smaller mammals such as the rat. The flavin monooxygenase uses either NADH or NADPH as a source of reducing equivalents in the above reaction, although the K_m for NADH is approximately ten times higher than that for NADPH; (i.e. NADPH half saturates the enzyme at one tenth the concentration of NADH and NADPH is therefore the preferred cofactor). As mentioned above, the F.M.O. catalyses the oxygenation of many nucleophilic organic nitrogen and sulfur compounds, including many drugs and xenobiotics such as the phenothiazines, ephedrine, N-methylamphetamine, norcocaine and the thioether- and carbamate-containing pesticides (Phorate and Thiofanox). This broad substrate specificity, coupled with the wide tissue distribution of the enzyme, suggests that the F.M.O. plays a major role in the oxidative metabolism of drugs and xenobiotics. The broad substrate specificity of the F.M.O. additionally suggests the presence of multiple forms (isoenzymes) and this has been substantiated by the cloning and sequencing of distinct genes from several species and tissues, including human liver.

Based on kinetic and spectral studies, the mechanism of flavin dependent monooxygenation is thought to occur as shown in Figure 2.14(a). The reaction mechanism involves flavin reduction (step 1), oxygen binding (step 2), internal electron transfer to oxygen forming the peroxy–flavin complex (step 3), substrate binding (step 4), oxygenated product release (step 5) and dissociation of

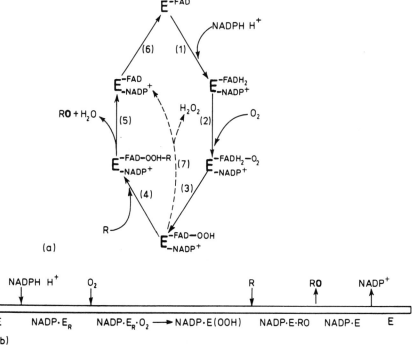

Figure 2.14 Oxidation of N- and S-containing xenobiotics by the microsomal flavin-containing monooxygenase. Abbreviations used are (a) E-FAD, oxidised enzyme; E-FADH$_2$ reduced enzyme; R, oxidisable substrate; RO, monooxygenated product. (b) E, oxidised enzyme; E$_R$, reduced enzyme.

NADP+ yielding the oxidised enzyme (step 6). In the absence of an oxidisable substrate, the peroxy–flavin intermediate slowly decomposes yielding H_2O_2 (step 7). The ordered reaction sequence is summarised in Figure 2.14(b). The peroxy–flavin intermediate is a strong electrophile and should therefore be capable of oxygenating any nucleophilic compound, such as N- and S-containing xenobiotics. As already seen in Figure 2.13 this is indeed the case, however, nucleophilic compounds containing an anionic group are effectively excluded from the active site of the enzyme and it has been suggested that this structural feature serves to exclude the futile oxidation of normal cellular components, since most endogenous nucleophiles contain one or more negatively charged groups.

It should be emphasised that this flavin monoxygenase is the only known *mammalian* flavoprotein hydroxylase, although many bacterial examples are known. In addition, the reaction mechanism described in Figure 2.14 dictates that substate binding occurs *after* pyridine nucleotide reduction, again an unusual feature of this enzyme.

2.4 Prostaglandin synthetase-dependent co-oxidation of drugs

Prostaglandin synthetase is an enzyme present in almost all mammalian cell types and catalyses the oxidation of arachidonic acid to prostaglandin H_2, the precursor to other important prostaglandins, thromboxanes and prostacyclin. The enzyme has two distinct catalytic functions, namely fatty acid cyclooxyge-nase activity forming prostaglandin G_2, and hydroperoxidase activity reducing prostaglandin G_2 to prostaglandin H_2. As shown in Figure 2.15(a), drugs and xenobiotics are co-oxidised during arachidonic acid metabolism by prosta-glandin synthetase, a biotransformation that is related to the hydroperoxidase component of prostaglandin synthetase. Several drugs are capable of undergoing this co-oxidation reaction including aminopyrine, benzphetamine, oxyphenbuta-zone and paracetamol as well as chemical carcinogens such as benzidine, benzo[a]pyrene, benzo[a]pyrene-7,8-dihydrodiol,7,12- dimethylbenzanthracene and N-(4-(5nitro-2-furyl)-2-thiazolyl) formamide.

The precise molecular mechanisms of the drug co-oxidation reactions are not clear at present, although some substrates such as the polycyclic aromatic hydro-carbons (benzo[a]pyrene and its diol metabolite) can incorporate oxygen into their carbon framework during the course of the reaction. In addition, several N-alkyl xenobiotics (including aminopyrine) are actively metabolised by an N-demethylation reaction.

Furthermore, other xenobiotics such as paracetamol appear to undergo a rad-ical-mediated mechanism resulting in the formation of glutathione conjugation of the drug (Figure 2.15(b)). This reaction probably involves a one electron oxidation resulting in hydrogen abstraction, yielding the phenoxy radical of paracetamol (step (i)). This radical may then have one of two fates. Firstly, the phenoxy radical may tautomerise forming the carbon-centred quinone radical which can then react with cellular glutathione, forming the glutathione conjugate of paracetamol (step (ii)). Alternatively, the phenoxy radical may be reduced with glutathione, reforming paracetamol (step (iii)). Support is given to this reaction mechanism by the rapid utilisation (oxidation) of glutathione during the reaction.

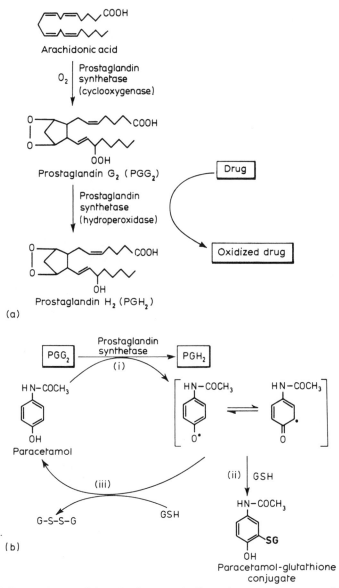

Figure 2.15 Co-oxidation of drugs by the prostaglandin synthetase enzyme system. (a) Role of prostaglandin synthetase in drug oxidations. (b) Postulated mechanism for the prostaglandin synthetase mediated metabolism of paracetamol. Adapted from Moldeus *et al.*, (1982) *Biochemical Pharmacology*, **31** 1363–8. GSH, glutathione.

It should be pointed out that paracetamol also undergoes substantial metabolism by the cytochrome P450-dependent M.F.O. system described earlier, although the relative contributions made by these two enzyme systems to the overall *in vivo* metabolism of paracetamol and related compounds is at present not known. Certainly, the prostaglandin synthetase-dependent co-oxidation of certain drugs is a significant metabolic pathway and could conceivably play a major role in drug biotransformation, particularly in those tissues that are rich in prostaglandin synthetase and low in M.F.O. activity, such as the kidney, urinary bladder, renal medulla, skin and lung.

2.5 Reductive drug metabolism

As with the oxidative drug metabolism reactions described above, the microsomal mixed function oxidase system makes a significant contribution to reductive drug metabolism pathways, and as shown in Table 2.5 many different chemical groups are susceptible to enzymatic reduction. Although our knowledge of reductive drug metabolism is not as developed as that of oxidation reactions, some reactions have been relatively well characterised. For example, tertiary amine oxides are extensively reduced by a cytochrome P450-dependent mechanism whereby amine formation is catalysed by the sequential two-electron reduction of the haemoprotein in a manner similar to mixed function amine oxidase activity as described above.

Table 2.5 Examples of reductive drug metabolism

Reduced chemical group	Reaction	Example
Nitro	$-NO_2 \longrightarrow -NH-OH$	Nitrofurantoin Chloramphenicol
Nitroso	$-N=O \longrightarrow -NH-OH$	Nitroso amantadine
Tertiary amine oxides	$-N \longrightarrow O \longrightarrow N-OH$	*N*-oxides of imipramine, tiaramide and indicine
Hydroxylamine	$-NH-OH \longrightarrow -NH_2$	*N*-hydroxyphentermine
Azo	$R^1-N=N-R^2 \longrightarrow R^1-NH_2+R^2-NH_2$	Prontosil, Amaranth
Quinone	quinone $\longrightarrow$ semiquinone	Adriamycin, Mitomycin C
Nitroso	denitrosation	CCNU (1-(2-chloroethyl)-nitrosourea)
Dehalogenation	$R-X \longrightarrow R^{\bullet} + X^-$ (X=halogen substituent)	Halothane Chloramphenicol

In addition, hydroxylamine reduction is catalysed by two separate enzyme systems. One involves cytochrome P450 and the other involves an NADH H⁺ dependent system as

$$NADH + H^+ \rightarrow NADH\text{-cytochrome } b_5$$
$$\text{reductase} \rightarrow \text{cytochrome } b_5 \rightarrow Fp$$

$$\begin{array}{c} R\text{--NH--OH} \\ \\ R\text{--NH}_2 \end{array}$$

In this latter system, NADH H⁺ serves as the preferred source of the necessary reducing equivalents that are then transferred by the cytochrome b_5 system to a terminal flavoprotein (Fp). This latter flavoprotein has been partially characterised from liver microsomes and actively catalyses the reduction of hydroxylamines, although the precise substrate specificity and hence overall contribution to drug metabolism still remains to be clarified. Similarly, although nitro reduction and azo reduction pathways have been recognised for many years, a full understanding of the enzymes involved is still developing. For example, the reduction of azo compounds such as amaranth and other food colourants/dyes is catalysed by several enzyme systems including cytosolic DT–diaphorase, NADPH–cytochrome P450 reductase and cytochrome P450, the latter two enzymes either acting in concert or separately catalysing azo reduction, depending on the substrate under consideration.

From the above discussion of the metabolism of amine-containing drugs it is clear that metabolic oxidation/reduction cycling of drugs may occur. This represents an interesting concept in drug biotransformation reactions as the balance between oxidative and reductive pathways can be important in determining both the overall pharmacological and toxicological profile of the drug. For example many drugs are active *per se* whereas others require metabolic activation to express their toxicity as is seen with many N-oxidised metabolites of drugs and xenobiotics.

Many anti-cancer drugs such as adriamycin and mitomycin C undergo reductive metabolism of the quinone moiety, a metabolic pathway that is thought to be a prerequisite for the anti-tumour properties of this class of compounds. As shown in Figure 2.16, the quinone undergoes a one-electron reduction reaction catalysed by the microsomal flavoprotein NADPH–cytochrome P450 reductase, resulting in the formation of the semi-quinone free radical species. This semi-quinone metabolite is unstable in the presence of oxygen and is rapidly reoxidised to form the parent quinone and the superoxide anion radical. This latter reduction product is central to the mode of action of these compounds and is involved in binding to nucleic acids, DNA strand scission and oxygen dependent cytotoxicity. In addition, the anti-cancer quinone drugs are also metabolised by other enzymes such as cytosolic DT–diaphorase, mitochondrial NADH–dehydrogenase and xanthine oxidase, although the relative contributions made by these enzymes still remains to be clarified. Furthermore, it has recently been shown that NADPH–cytochrome P450 reductase also is

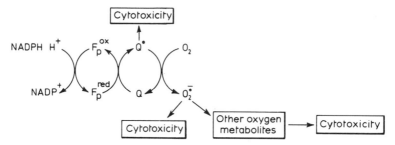

Figure 2.16 Role of NADPH–cytochrome P450 reductase in the activation of quinone anticancer drugs. Abbreviations used: $F_p ox$ and $F_p red$, oxidised and reduced forms of NADPH–cytochrome P450 reductase respectively; Q and Q', quinone and semiquinone forms respectively.

responsible for the reductive denitrosation of the nitrosourea anti-tumour drugs such as CCNU (lomustine). This reductive metabolism results in the formation of nitric oxide and the inactive, denitrosated parent urea and therefore represents a deactivation pathway.

The above two examples highlight the versatility of the enzyme NADPH–cytochrome P450 reductase. In addition to functioning as an intrinsic component of the mixed function oxidase system, this flavoprotein can independently catalyse the NADPH + H⁺ dependent one-electron reduction of quinones and nitrosoureas, thus utilising exogenous drugs as electron acceptors instead of the physiological acceptor, cytochrome P450.

Halothane is a widely used, volatile anaesthetic and this halogenated hydrocarbon is metabolised by both oxidative and reductive pathways in the liver. Whereas oxidative metabolism of halothane by the mixed function oxidase system is generally considered to be a detoxication pathway, reductive metabolism of this anaesthetic has been implicated in the well-documented toxicity of the drug. As shown in Figure 2.17(a), halothane is reductively metabolised by two successive dehalogenation reactions (debromination and defluorination), metabolic pathways that are stimulated by enzyme induction with phenobarbitone, thus implicating the cytochrome P450 dependent monooxygenase system in the biotransformation process. Further induction and inhibition studies pointed to a central role of cytochrome P450 in the reductive dehalogenation of halothane and the proposed participation of the haemoprotein is shown in Figure 2.17(b). This proposed mechanism has many features in common with the previously described mixed function oxidase reaction of cytochrome P450 in that the scheme proposes substrate binding and two $\times$ one-electron reduction steps (perhaps involving cytochrome b_5). However, the reaction mechanisms diverge in that during the *anaerobic* reduction of halothane, no oxygen is present and hence the reducing equivalents are not used to activate molecular oxygen, but rather are contributory to the formation of the radical and carbanion complexes of halothane, themselves the probable precursors of the dehalogenated metabolites. This reaction scheme may be superficially surprising in light of the high affinity

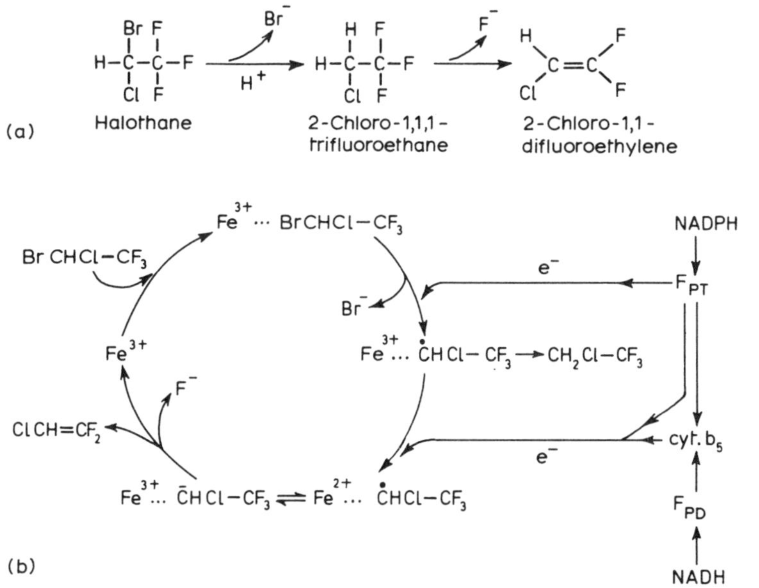

Figure 2.17 Reductive dehalogenation of halothane. (a) Halothane metabolism forming 2-chloro-1,1,1-trifluoroethane and 2-chloro-1,1-difluoroethylene. (b) Proposed reaction scheme of cytochrome P450 in the dehalogenation of halothane. Abbreviations used: Fe^{3+} and Fe^{2+}, the oxidised and reduced haem of cytochrome P450; F_{PT}, NADPH–cytochrome P450 reductase; cyt.b_5, cytochrome b_5; F_{PD}, NADH–cytochrome b_5 reductase. Derived from Ahr *et al.*, (1982) *Biochemical Pharmacology*, **31** 383–90.

of cytochrome P450 for oxygen and it may be predicted that oxygen would actively compete for the available reducing equivalents. However, certain cells have a very low oxygen tension, particularly in the centre of liver lobules and under these almost anaerobic conditions, it is plausible that cytochrome P450 would function in a reductive mode as described above. Accordingly, the prevailing tissue oxygen tension may very well be an important determinant of whether oxidative or reductive drug metabolism occurs.

2.6 Epoxide hydrolase

Among the many reactions catalysed by the microsomal mixed function oxidase system is the oxidation of a number of olefins and aromatic compounds forming epoxide (or oxirane) metabolites (i.e. oxygen is inserted across a carbon–carbon double bond). These epoxides are formed as metabolites of drugs such as carbamazepine, cyproheptadine and protriptyline and other xenobiotics including environmental pollutants of the polycyclic aromatic hydrocarbon class of compounds. The epoxides thus formed have several biological fates including direct excretion *in vivo*, non-enzymatic rearrangement forming phenols, irreversible binding to cellular nucleic acids and proteins, conjugation with endogenous glutathione, enzymatic hydration by epoxide hydrolase forming dihydrodiol metabolites, or undergo further oxidation to diol-epoxides. As shown in Figure 2.18(a), epoxidation can occur at various sites within the same molecule and resultant oxirane ring opening by epoxide hydrolase leads to the formation of both diol and diol-epoxide metabolites.

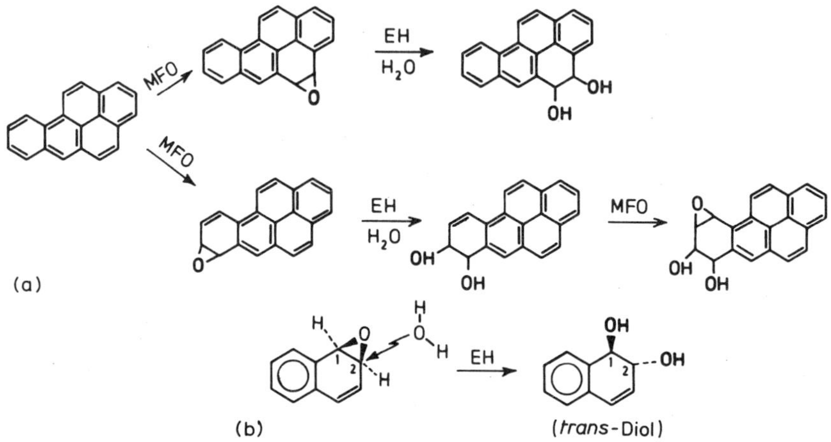

Figure 2.18 Epoxide formation and metabolism. (a) Scheme for the metabolism of the polycyclic aromatic hydrocarbon, benzo(*a*)pyrene resulting in the formation of epoxides, diols and diol-epoxides. (b) Stereospecific hydration of 1,2-naphthalene oxide by epoxide hydrolase. Abbreviations used: MFO, mixed function oxidase enzymes; EH, epoxide hydrolase.

Epoxides are reactive electrophilic species and epoxide hydrolase (sometimes termed epoxide hydratase) catalyses the nucleophilic attack of a water molecule on one of the two electron deficient carbon atoms of the oxirane ring. As shown in Figure 2.18(b), epoxide hydration of certain epoxide substrates can be highly stereoselective with respect to product formation, resulting in predominant formation of the *trans* diol isomer. However, the degree of stereospecific epoxide hydration is variable from one substrate to another and is governed by both steric and electronic characteristics of the substrate itself. In addition, it appears that the hydration reaction is also regioselective in that the less sterically hindered carbon in the 2 position (Figure 2.18(b)) incorporates water-derived oxygen far more readily than the one position.

Epoxide hydrolase is widely distributed throughout the animal kingdom, including Man. In the rat it occurs in almost every tissue examined, with highest activities being found in the liver and smaller, although significant, amounts being found in the testes, kidney, lung and adrenal gland. Hepatic epoxide hydrolase has been found to be non-uniformly distributed across the liver lobule. Similar amounts are present in mid-zonal and periportal hepatocytes with significantly more enzyme present in centrilobular hepatocytes in uninduced rat liver, a distribution that is in accord with the distribution of cytochrome P450. Thus, centrilobular hepatocytes appear to have the greatest capacity for both generating and hydrating epoxides. In the liver, epoxide hydrolase occurs predominantly in the endoplasmic reticulum fraction and recent studies have indicated the enzyme to be present in nuclear membranes and the cytosol of the hepatocyte and absent in peroxisomes, lysosomes and mitochondria.

The concentration of epoxide hydrolase is induced by most of the xenobiotic inducers of the mixed function oxidase system (chapter 3) and there is substantial evidence to suggest that the enzyme exists in multiple forms, with different substrate specificities. The highly purified enzymes derived from experimental animals exhibit a monomeric molecular weight of approximately 48 000–54 000 Da. The absorption spectra indicates that the enzyme is devoid of both haem and flavin chromophore prosthetic groups. It is of interest that human liver microsomes contain relatively high levels of epoxide hydrolase activity and the enzyme from this source has been purified and characterised. There is a substantial variation in the enzyme activity within the human population, suggesting that xenobiotic induction observed in animal studies may be relevant to the human situation. Furthermore, it has been proposed that human liver contains more than one form of epoxide hydrolase, some of which are immunochemically distinct from the rat liver enzyme.

In addition to metabolising epoxides of drugs and xenobiotics, it should be noted that epoxide hydrolase also catalyses the hydration of endogenous epoxides. These include 16α, 17α-epoxyandrosten-3-one (androstene oxide) and 16α, 17α-epoxyestratrienol (estroxide) at much higher rates than exogenous epoxides, suggesting a substantial role for this enzyme in endogenous metabolic reactions.

Much attention has focused on epoxide hydrolase, primarily because of the role played by the enzyme in the formation of chemical carcinogens from otherwise innocuous xenobiotics (see chapter 6 for a fuller discussion). In addition, epoxide hydrolase has been postulated to be a preneoplastic antigen, and therefore may prove useful as an early marker of liver cancer. The interested reader is referred to the bibliography at the end of this chapter for a fuller discussion of this latter phenomenon.

2.7 Glucuronide conjugation reactions

As indicated previously, phase I drug metabolism pathways represent a 'functionalisation' reaction in that the drug is chemically primed by oxidation to facilitate subsequent conjugation reactions with endogenous compounds, thus enhancing their excretion. One of the most important conjugation reactions (phase II) is that of glucuronide conjugation and many drugs are metabolised via this pathway. As shown in Table 2.6, many functional groups have the potential to be glucuronidated and it should be emphasised that the versatility of this

Table 2.6 Types of functional groups undergoing conjugation reactions with glucuronic acid

Functional group	Type	Example
Hydroxyl	Primary, secondary and tertiary, alcohols, phenols, hydroxylamines	Indomethacin, Paracetamol, 4-Hydroxy-coumarin, Aspirin, Chloromphen, Morphine
Carboxyl	Aromatic, arylalkyl	Nicotinic acid, Aminosalicylic acid, Clofibrate
Amino	Aromatic amines, sulfonamides, aliphatic tertiary amines	Meprobamate Dapsone Sulfafurazole
Sulphydryl	Thiols, dithioic acids	2-Mercapto-benzothiazole

pathway dictates that certain drugs can be directly conjugated with glucuronic acid (provided they have an existing functional group), thus bypassing the usual requirement for phase I metabolism. In a similar fashion to the mixed function oxidase enzymes, many endogenous compounds serve as substrates for the glucuronidation reaction and include bilirubin, many steroid hormones, thyroxine, triiodothyronine and catechols derived from catecholamine metabolism. This observation raises the intriguing question of whether glucuronide conjugation of drugs represents a late development by the organism and that the 'natural' role of this pathway is for physiological compounds.

The reaction mechanism for glucuronide formation and fate of the conjugates is shown in Figure 2.19. The early stages of this reaction are clearly involved in glycogen synthesis through the common intermediate of UDP–glucose and again highlights the intimate relationship between drug metabolism reactions and endogenous metabolic pathways. The readily available UDP–glucose may well explain the major role played by glucuronidation in drug metabolism. The key enzyme in glucuronidation reactions is UDP–glucuronosyl transferase (EC 2.4.1.17 sometimes abbreviated to glucuronyl transferase) and this enzyme catalyses the transfer of glucuronic acid to a suitable drug acceptor molecule, forming the glucuronide conjugate. It should be emphasised that the C-1 atom of glucuronic acid in UDP–glucuronic acid is in the α-configuration and during transfer to an acceptor drug substrate, inversion occurs resulting in formation of the β-configuration. The resulting drug conjugate is then excreted either in the urine or faeces (Figure 2.19) and it appears that the molecular weight of the drug is a critical determinant in dictating the route of excretion. For example, in the rat, glucuronide conjugates of molecular weight greater than 400 Da are excreted predominantly in the bile (i.e. drugs with molecular weight greater than approximately 200 Da), whereas lower molecular weight conjugates primarily undergo urinary excretion. Thus high molecular weight drugs such as morphine, chloramphenicol and glutethimide and glucuronide conjugates of

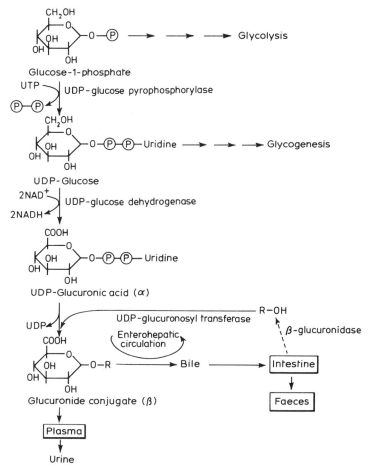

Figure 2.19 Enzymes involved in glucuronide formation and biological fate of conjugates. From Bowman and Rand, *Textbook of Pharmacology, Second Edition,* Blackwell (1980).

both endogenous and exogenous steroids are excreted in the bile and hence into the intestine. However, the intestine contains significant amounts of the enzyme β-glucuronidase, an enzyme that catalyses the hydrolysis of the glucuronide conjugate, resulting in the formation of free drug which may then be reabsorbed, transported to the liver and then undergo re-conjugation and re-excretion. This behaviour is termed *enterohepatic recirculation* and may make a significant contribution to prolonging the half-life of the drug in the body, with the obvious result of potentiating the pharmacological action of the drug, providing that sufficiently high blood levels of drug are achieved.

The enzyme UDP–glucuronosyltransferase is found in almost all mammalian species with the notable exceptions of the cat and a mutant strain of rat called the

Gunn rat. Cats are particularly susceptible to the pharmacological actions of morphine, an observation that is readily rationalised by the fact that the major route of morphine metabolism is by glucuronidation. The Gunn rat is an interesting example of enzyme deficiency in that this strain is completely incapable of forming glucuronide conjugates of bilirubin whereas glucuronosyl transferase activity towards most other substrates is apparently normal. The reason for this low transferase activity is now becoming clearer as it has recently been reported that the Gunn rat has a –1 frameshift mutation as determined by isolation and sequence comparison of the genes in the Wistar rat (normal activity) and the Gunn rat (deficient). As shown in Figure 2.20, the crucial region is at nucleotide 1239 or 1240 where a G residue is missing, thus generating a new TGA stop codon. Thus a truncated version of the transferase is generated by this new stop codon and is missing 115 amino acids compared to the Wistar rat gene. This new carboxyl terminal has no hydrophobic character, is not inserted into the microsomal membrane and the truncated enzyme is degraded/secreted in the Golgi apparatus.

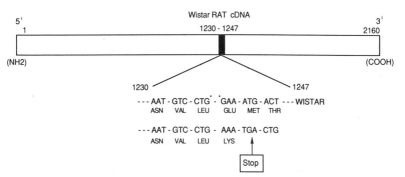

Figure 2.20 Frameshift mutation in the Gunn rat UDP–glucuronosyltransferase gene.

This early observation coupled to the fact that glucuronosyl transferase activity is induced by many drugs and xenobiotics (resulting in altered substrate specificities) has led to the theory that this enzyme exists in multiple forms. Although investigation of UDP–glucuronosyltransferase isoenzymes has not been as extensively described as for cytochrome P450, there is much evidence to suggest that multiple forms do indeed exist. The most investigated species has been the rat and recently a *tentative* classification has been proposed based on substrate specificities (Table 2.7).

UDP–glucuronosyltransferase enzymes are present in many tissues, mostly in the liver but also in kidney, small intestine, lung, skin, adrenals and spleen. The enzyme is mainly localised in the membrane of hepatic endoplasmic reticulum fractions and is therefore ideally positioned to glucuronidate the products of the mixed function oxidase reactions. The enzyme has no prosthetic group and the monomeric molecular weight of highly purified enzyme preparations varies from approximately 50 000 to 60 000 Da. The catalytic activity of the

Table 2.7 Substrate specificities of hepatic microsomal
UDP–glucuronosyltransferase in the rat

Form of enzyme	Substrate glucuronidated
A	2-Aminobenzoate
	2-Aminophenol
	3-Hydroxybenzo(a)pyrene
	N-Hydroxy-2-naphthylamine
	1-Naphthol
	4-Nitrophenol
	Testosterone
B	Bilirubin
	Morphine
C	Oestrone
	4-Nitrophenol
D	Chloramphenicol
	4-Hydroxy biphenyl
	Morphine

Derived from Burchell, B. (1981) in *Reviews in Biochemical Toxicology 3*, E.Hodgson, J.R. Bend and R.M. Philpot), Elsevier, pp.1–32.

glucuronosyltransferases is substantially influenced by the presence of lipids, and although the specific mode of action of lipids has not been elucidated, this may well be an important observation with respect to the existence of proposed multiple forms of the enzyme. An interesting feature of UDP–glucuronosyltransferase activity is that the microsomal, membrane-bound enzyme exhibits 'latency', i.e. full enzyme activity is only expressed in the presence of membrane perturbants such as detergents. The physiological and pharmacological significance (if any) of this enzyme latency has not been fully elucidated yet.

2.8 Glutathione-*S*-transferase

The glutathione-*S*-transferase family of enzymes are soluble proteins predominantly found in the cytosol of hepatocytes and catalyse the conjugation of a variety of compounds with the endogenous tripeptide glutathione (glutamyl-cysteinylglycine, abbreviated to GSH) as follows

$$R-CH_2-X \xrightarrow[\text{Glutathione--}S\text{-transferase}]{\text{GSH}} R-CH_2-SG$$

where $R-CH_2-X$ represents literally hundreds of electrophilic substrates, and $R-CH_2-SG$ represents the glutathione adduct. In addition to their ability to catalyse the above conjugation reaction, certain glutathione-*S*-transferases have the ability to bind a variety of endogenous and exogenous substrates without metabolism. Examples of these two distinct roles of glutathione-S-transferase are given in Table 2.8. It should be emphasised that glutathione conjugation is possible with either unchanged drugs or their electrophilic metabolites, the only apparent chemical prerequisite being the presence of a suitably electrophilic centre enabling reactivity with the nucleophilic glutathione. In this respect, glutathione conjugation significantly differs from both glucuronide and sulfate conjugation, in that in the latter two reactions, both the glucuronide and sulfate moieties must first be 'activated' in the form of UDP–glucuronic acid and 3'-phosphoadenosine-5'-phosphosulfate respectively, prior to conjugation. Such chemical reactivity of glutathione and electrophiles can, in some cases, allow the conjugation reaction to proceed non-enzymatically. As with the high molecular weight glucuronide conjugates, glutathione metabolites are infrequently removed from the body by urinary excretion and preferential elimination occurs in the bile.

Table 2.8 Role of glutathione-S-transferases in the conjugation and binding of endogenous and exogenous compounds

Binding function	Conjugation function
Bilirubin	Vitamin K_3
Oestradiol	Oestradiol-17ß
Cortisol	Paracetamol
Testosterone	Sulfobromophthalein
Tetracycline	Parathion
Penicillin	Urethane
Ethacrynic acid	1-Chloro-2,4-dinitrobenzene

Many glutathione conjugates are not excreted *per se* but rather undergo further enzymatic modification of the peptide moiety, resulting in the urinary or biliary excretion of cysteinyl-sulfur substituted N-acetylcysteines, more commonly referred to as mercapturic acids. As shown in Figure 2.21 for an arene oxide metabolite, mercapturic acid formation is initiated by glutathione conjugation, followed by removal of the glutamate moiety by glutathionase and subsequent removal of glycine by a peptidase enzyme, the latter two enzymes being present in both liver, gastrointestinal tract and kidney. In the final step, the amino group of cysteine is acetylated by a hepatic N-acetylase resulting in formation of the mercapturic acid derivative. This latter acetylation reaction is reversible and deacetylases can reform the amino metabolite.

The cysteine conjugate of xenobiotics can undergo an alternative metabolic pathway by serving as a substrate for the cysteine conjugate β-lyase enzyme (see chapter 1) which catalyses the following β-elimination reaction

$$R-S-CH_2-CH \begin{array}{c} COOH \\ \\ NH_2 \end{array} \xrightarrow{\beta\text{-lyase}} RSH + CH_3-CO-COOH + NH_3$$

where R is a xenobiotic.

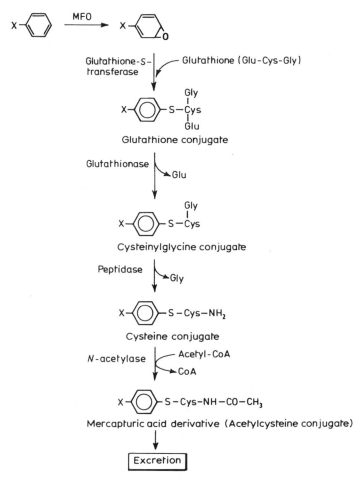

Figure 2.21 Role of the glutathione in mercapturic acid biosynthesis. Abbreviations used: MFO for oxidase enzymes; Glu, glutamate; Cys, cysteine; Gly, glycine; CoA, Coenzyme A.

The cysteine conjugate β-lyase enzymes occur in several tissues including the gastro-intestinal tract, liver and kidney and the renal and hepatic forms have been the most extensively studied. All β-lyase enzymes studied to date contain pyridoxal phosphate, and as such, the enzyme *additionally* functions as a transaminase and therefore exhibits a sophisticated level of regulation. The monomeric molecular weights of the β-lyases are around 48 000 Da and the liver form is also known as kynureninase and the kidney form as glutamine transaminase K. It appears that multiple forms of cysteine conjugate β-lyase exist and certainly the liver and kidney forms are distinct proteins.

From the above discussion it is clear that glutathione conjugation serves as a protective mechanism whereby potentially toxic, electrophilic metabolites are 'mopped-up' either as glutathione conjugates or mercapturic acids. However it is becoming increasingly recognised that glutathione conjugation is not exclusively a detoxification reaction and that certain xenobiotics are toxicologically activated by this conjugation route, either as such or as a result of further processing of the glutathione conjugate, a concept that is further developed in chapter 6. As will be discussed in chapter 6, cellular levels of glutathione are an important determinant of xenobiotic toxicity.

The glutathione-S-transferase enzymes exist in multiple forms as heterodimers or homodimers of two sub-units, of approximate monomeric molecular weights in the range 20 000-25 000 Da. The nomenclature system has been confusing for this group of enzymes as several different systems have been used. Recently, a unifying nomenclature for the human transferases has been suggested, primarily based on the four major classes of soluble enzymes (Alpha, Mu, Pi and Theta) and reflecting their sub-unit compositions. Thus GSTA1-1 is a glutathione-S-transferase (GST) of the Alpha class, consisting of a homodimer of two '1'- type sub-units.

The transferases are inducible by various xenobiotics, including phenobarbital and polycyclic aromatic hydrocarbons, and in the case of heterodimers, each sub-unit may be differently and independently regulated by transcriptional gene activation mechanisms.

2.9 Sulfate conjugation

Many drugs are oxidised to a variety of phenols, alcohols or hydroxylamines which can then serve as excellent substrates for subsequent sulfate conjugation, forming the readily excretable sulfate esters. However, inorganic sulfate is relatively inert and must first be 'activated' by ATP as in the following mechanism

$$ATP + SO_4^{2-} \xrightarrow{\text{ATP–sulfurylase}} \text{adenosine-5'-phosphosulfate + pyrophosphate}$$
$$\text{(APS)}$$

$$APS + ATP \xrightarrow{\text{APS–phosphokinase}} \text{3'-phosphadenosine-5'-phosphosulfate + ADP}$$
$$\text{(PAPS)}$$

$$PAPS + R\text{–}OH \xrightarrow{\text{Sulfotransferase}} R\text{–}O\text{–}SO_3H + \text{3'-phosphoadenosine-5'}$$
$$\text{-phosphosulfate}$$

For phenolic metabolites, the key enzyme in this sequence is sulfotransferase (phenol–sulfotransferase, EC 2.8.2.1). The sulfotransferase enzymes are soluble enzymes found in many tissues including liver, kidney, gut and platelets and catalyse the sulfation of drugs such as paracetamol, isoprenaline and salicylamide and many steroids. It appears that the sulfotransferases exist in multiple enzyme forms with the steroid sulfating enzymes being distinct from the sulfotransferases responsible for drug conjugation reactions. It should be emphasised that sulfation conjugation reactions are not as widespread or as of quantitative importance as glucuronide conjugation reactions, due in part to the limited bioavailability of inorganic sulfate and hence PAPS. This is particularly true when a drug is actively metabolised to phenolic products or when high body burdens of phenolic drugs are reached (for example, in overdosage), resulting in effective saturation of this metabolic pathway.

2.10 Amino acid conjugation

Many classes of drugs including anti-inflammatory profens, hypolipidaemics, diuretic and analgesic agents have a carboxylic acid as part of their structure and as such are susceptible to conjugation with endogenous amino acids prior to excretion. In a similar manner to both glucuronide and sulfate conjugation, amino acid conjugation of free carboxylic acid groups in drugs requires metabolic activation, according to the following scheme

$$R–COOH + ATP \longrightarrow R–CO–AMP + H_2O$$

$$R–CO–AMP + CoASH \longrightarrow R–CO–SCoA + AMP$$

$$R\text{-}CO\text{-}SCoA + NH_2–R'–COOH \longrightarrow R–CONH–R'–COOH + CoASH$$

where R–COOH represents the drug, CoASH is coenzyme A and NH_2–R'–COOH is an endogenous amino acid. In this scheme, the inert carboxyl group is activated to its acyl coenzyme-A derivative prior to amide formation with the amino function of the donating amino acid. As shown in Table 2.9, this

Table 2.9 Amino acids utilised in the conjugation of carboxylic acids

Amino acid	Species	Acid
Glycine	Mammals, non-primate mammals	Aromatic, heterocyclic and acrylic acids, arylacetic acids
Glutamine	Primates, rat, rabbit, ferret	Arylacetic acids, 2-naphthylacetic acid
Taurine	Mammals, pigeon	Arylacetic acids
Ornithine	Birds	Aromatic and arylacetic acids
Glutamic acid	Fruit bats	Benzoic acid
Aspartic acid	Rat	o,p'-DDA
Alanine	Mouse, hamster	p,p'-DDA
Histidine	African bats	Benzoic acid

Derived from Caldwell, J. (1980). In *Concepts in Drug Metabolism, Part A*, P. Jenner, and B. Testa, Marcel Dekker, New York, p. 221.

conjugation reaction occurs in many species, utilising a variety of amino acids and appears to be a complementary pathway to the glucuronidation of carboxyl groups.

This conjugation reaction occurs extensively in hepatic mitochondria and has been used to advantage in chemical tests of liver function. For example benzoic acid is conjugated with glycine, resulting in excretion of the benzyl glycine conjugate, sometimes referred to as hippuric acid. Under conditions of normal liver function, a specified amount of hippuric acid is excreted within a few hours after either oral administration or slow intravenous injection. In parenchymal liver disorders such as hepatitis or cirrhosis, the urinary output of hippuric acid is low (assuming normal renal function) and therefore constitutes a useful indicator of hepatic viability.

2.11 Control and interactions of drug metabolism pathways

From the previous chapter and the above discussion, it is clear that ingested drugs can be metabolised by a variety of chemical pathways, catalysed by different enzyme systems (Figure 2.22). As with most biotransformation pathways, drug metabolism reactions do not usually occur at random and specific biological control mechanisms are operative at several stages in the overall process. In addition, a particular drug metabolism pathway does not usually operate in isolation and the activity of one pathway can influence the activity in another. Furthermore, many drug biotransformation pathways are intimately related to endogenous metabolic pathways sharing both the same source of co-factors, co-substrates, prosthetic groups and even enzyme systems, thereby imposing an additional level of control on drug metabolism. The above concepts will be developed in this section, and where possible, specific examples will be given.

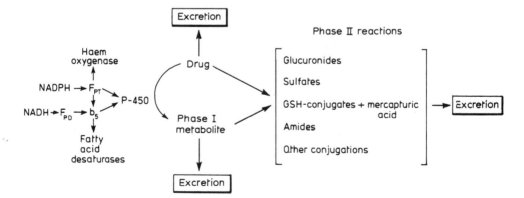

Figure 2.22 Drug metabolism pathways. Abbreviations used. F_{PT}, NADPH–cytochrome P450 reductase; F_{PD} NADH–cytochrome b_5 reductase; P450, cytochrome P450; b_5, cytochrome b_5.

2.11.1 Substrate and oxygen availability

The majority of drugs are lipophilic in nature and therefore metabolism represents an efficient means of clearing the drug from the body. If metabolism is a prominent feature of clearance, then the 'bioavailability' of the drug assumes an important role in that the more readily accessible the drug is to the drug metabolising enzymes, then the greater will be its metabolism. Accordingly, the physico-chemical properties of the drug such as degree of ionisation or lipophilicity are important in dictating the absorption of the drug and access to the membrane-bound or soluble drug-metabolising enzymes. As most of the phase I oxidation enzymes are located in the lipid rich, and therefore lipophilic membrane of the hepatic endoplasmic reticulum, it then follows that a substantial degree of drug lipophilicity is required to ensure adequate substrate availability. Many studies have shown that this is indeed the case and significant correlations have been repeatedly found between the lipid–water partition coefficient of drugs and and their extent of binding to and metabolism by the phase I enzymes in general, and cytochrome P450 in particular. Therefore, the physico-chemical nature of the drug itself is an important determinant of drug availability and hence potential to be metabolised.

As discussed previously, molecular oxygen is an essential requirement for cytochrome P450-dependent monooxygenation of drugs. In most body tissues, oxygen is freely available and in sufficiently high concentrations to ensure adequate drug oxidation. However, tissue concentrations of oxygen may well be very low under certain pathophysiological conditions and in the relatively hypoxic centre of the liver mass, thus placing a possible constraint, and therefore control on drug oxidations. The availability of oxygen is an important determinant of the route or pathway of drug metabolism. For example, halothane is metabolised by both oxidative and reductive anaerobic pathways, yielding metabolites that are quite different from each other, and more importantly, these metabolites have been postulated to have different toxicities. Although our understanding of the role of tissue levels of oxygen in drug metabolism is still in its infancy, it remains an area of fundamental importance.

2.11.2 NADPH supply

NADPH is an obligatory requirement for cytochrome P450-dependent drug oxidations, therefore the availability of this reduced pyridine nucleotide is an important control mechanism in drug oxidations. As shown in Figure 2.23, hepatic NADPH is derived from two sources, the major pathway being the pentose phosphate pathway (sometimes referred to as the hexose monophosphate shunt), further augmented by reducing equivalents derived from the mitochondrial translocation of NADPH. In addition to supplying the necessary reducing equivalents for drug oxidations, NADPH is required in endogenous biosynthetic pathways including fatty acid biosynthesis. For example, during the biosynthesis

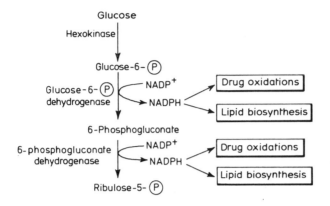

(a)

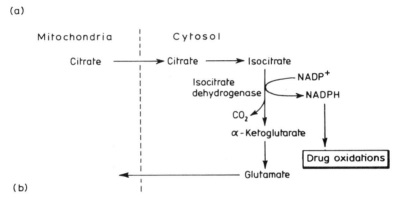

(b)

Figure 2.23 Biosynthesis of NADPH utilised in drug oxidations. (a) Pentosephosphate pathway. (b) NADP⁺-linked, isocitrate dehydrogenase.

of palmitic acid starting from acetyl-CoA, 14 moles of NADPH are consumed per mole of palmitic acid formed, thus placing a substantial demand on the availability of cellular NADPH during active lipid biosynthesis. In addition, the availability of NADPH for drug oxidations is critically influenced by the cellular NADP⁺/NADPH ratio, which in turn, is linked to the activity of the NADP⁺ linked dehydrogenases such as isocitrate dehydrogenase and glucose-6-phosphate dehydrogenase. Accordingly, the availability of NADPH in drug oxidations is substantially influenced by prevailing metabolic conditions forming a coupled, interactive system and therefore constitutes a control point in drug oxidations.

2.11.3 Synthesis and degradation of cytochrome P450

In any enzyme catalysed reaction, the absolute amount of active enzyme contributes to the overall reaction, thus the concentration or amount of the drug metabolising enzymes are clearly important. As the amount of enzyme present is a dynamic balance between enzyme synthesis and enzyme degradation, factors that alter the steady state level of the enzymes then make a significant contribution to the regulation of drug metabolism. Of all the enzymes responsible for drug metabolism, cytochrome P450 has been the most intensively studied and the biogenesis and catabolism of this haemoprotein will now be considered with particular emphasis placed on the role of haemoprotein turnover as a control mechanism in drug oxidations. It must be emphasised that the following concepts are also applicable to the regulation of the other drug metabolising enzymes, and that cytochrome P450 is only being used here as a well-documented example.

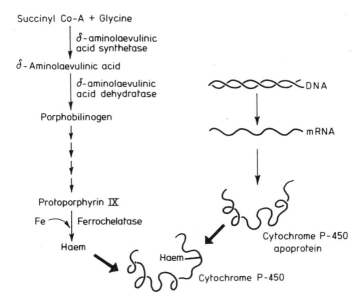

Figure 2.24 Biosynthesis of cytochrome P450.

(a) *Synthesis of cytochrome P450.* The holoenzyme of cytochrome P450 consists of both haem and protein moieties, and therefore are subjected to different control mechanisms in their biosynthesis, both of which contribute to the final, steady-state level of the enzyme. As shown in Figure 2.24, the biosynthesis of intact cytochrome P450 is a complex, coordinated process and involves different sub-cellular compartments of the hepatocyte during assembly of the intact holoenzyme. A major point of control is the utilisation of the haem prosthetic group. Not only is haem inserted into cytochrome P450, but it is also inserted into mitochondrial cytochromes and other hepatic haemoproteins such as catalase and cytochrome b_5. Accordingly, the total hepatic demand for haem is dictated not only by cytochrome P450 but by other cellular haemoproteins, again illustrating the interrelationship between drug oxidations and normal cellular processes. In addition, many drugs and chemicals have the ability to influence haem biosynthesis by either inducing the enzyme delta-aminolaevulinic acid synthetase, the rate limiting step in haem biosynthesis, or by causing a depletion of existing free haem. This latter point is noteworthy because delta-aminolaevulinic acid synthetase is subjected to negative feedback inhibition by haem, therefore certain drugs that initiate haem depletion, can cause a 'rebound' effect in haem synthesis resulting in acute attacks of porphyria in genetically predisposed individuals.

Synthesis of the apoprotein moiety of cytochrome P450 is also subjected to control by the ability of drugs (such as the barbiturates) to induce protein synthesis. Although drug induction of cytochrome P450 is considered in more detail in chapter 3, it is relevant to point out that not only is cytochrome P450 induced by drugs, but different isoenzymes (or multiple forms) are induced by different drugs. These cytochrome P450 isoenzymes exhibit substantial differences in their respective abilities to catalyse the oxidation of structurally diverse drugs, and it is then quite clear that the isoenzyme complement of individual haemoproteins is an important determinant of the ability of the liver to metabolise a specific drug. In view of the common occurrence of polypharmacy where patients are exposed to more than one drug (one of which may be an enzyme inducer), this 'drug-induced control mechanism' has significant ramifications in both clinical pharmacology and toxicology (see chapters 6 and 7).

(b) *Degradation of cytochrome P450.* The major pathway of haem degradation involves an enzyme termed haem oxygenase, resulting in the eventual formation of bile pigments such as bilirubin. The complete microsomal haem oxygenase system requires both the haem oxygenase protein and the flavoprotein, NADPH–cytochrome P450 reductase. The participation of this latter flavoprotein is interesting in that NADPH–cytochrome P450 reductase is also a necessary component of the cytochrome P450-dependent drug oxidation system, as discussed previously. Therefore during the normal course of drug oxidations, the flow of reducing equivalents through the reductase is not exclusively channeled to cytochrome P450 and during periods of active hepatic haem oxidation, there is competition exerted on the oxidation reaction by haem oxygenase activity, thus exerting another level of control on drug oxidation. In addition, many drugs and chemicals, especially those with an olefinic moiety, have the ability to covalently bind and inactivate the haem group in cytochrome P450. This would then constitute another control mechanism whereby cytochrome P450 activity (and hence certain drug oxidation reactions) is substantially inhibited by prior or concomitant exposure to this class of drugs.

2.11.4 Control of drug metabolism by endogenous co-substrates

As shown in Table 2.10, many of the enzymes of drug metabolism also catalyse the metabolism of a plethora of endogenous substrates. Some of these enzymes are relatively specific for endogenous substrates, such as a variant of

Table 2.10 Endogenous co-substrates of the drug metabolising enzymes

Cytochrome P450	Glucuronosyl transferase	Glutathione transferase
Fatty acids	Bilirubin	Bilirubin
Leukotrienes	Serotonin	Cortisol
Prostaglandins	Testosterone	Testosterone
Steroids		Glutathione
Cholesterol		Leukotrienes
Vitamin D_3		
Thyroxine		

cytochrome P450 (termed cytochrome $P450_{scc}$ or CYP11A in the new terminology) responsible for the side chain cleavage of cholesterol in the adrenals, whereas others such as hepatic cytochrome P450 are less specialised and catalyse steroid, fatty acid and prostaglandin hydroxylation in addition to drug oxidations. For this latter type of drug metabolising enzyme, there is therefore a competition for available enzyme between the drug and the endogenous substrate. Many factors are important in determining which substrate will be preferentially metabolised including the tissue levels, the effective local concentration at the active site and the relative affinities of the competing substrates for the enzyme in question. As many endogenous substrates are in a constant state of flux due to synthesis, utilisation and degradation reactions, it is obvious that a precise analysis of the role of the endogenous co-substrates as competitors for the enzyme systems *in vivo* is difficult. Nevertheless, it is absolutely clear that competition does occur *in vitro* and therefore represents another mechanism whereby drug metabolism is subjected to a degree of control.

2.11.5 Participation of cytochrome b_5

As indicated earlier, the precise role of cytochrome b_5 in drug oxidation reactions is far from clear, as no uniform effect has been observed. For example, cytochrome b_5 has been reported to either stimulate, inhibit, have no effect or even be an obligatory component of cytochrome P450-dependent oxidations, dependent on both the nature of the drug undergoing metabolism and the isoenzyme of cytochrome P450 under consideration. In those reactions dependent on cytochrome b_5 electron flow probably occurs as

NADH $\longrightarrow$ NADH–cytochrome b_5 reductase $\longrightarrow$

cytochrome $b_5 \longrightarrow$ cytochrome P450

It should also be noted that cytochrome b_5 is also reduced by NADPH–cytochrome P450 reductase, thereby placing another 'drain' on the reducing equivalents of this flavoprotein. The main endogenous biological function of hepatic microsomal cytochrome b_5 is to participate in the desaturation of long-chain, fatty acid acyl-CoA derivatives, by providing reducing equivalents for the terminal desaturase enzymes. The desaturation of fatty acids in the endoplasmic reticulum is an active process and includes the delta 5-, delta 6- and delta 9-desaturases, and therefore constitutes a potent drain on cytochrome b_5-mediated reducing equivalents, and consequently, significantly influences those drug oxidation reactions mediated by cytochrome b_5. In addition, unlike cytochrome P450, cytochrome b_5 is relatively insensitive to induction by exogenous drugs and chemicals. In uninduced, liver microsomes, the molar ratio of cytochrome P450:cytochrome b_5 is approximately 2:1 and during induction this can increase to around 6:1. Therefore the molecular association between these two haemo-proteins is almost certainly influenced by induction and may then significantly alter both quantitative and qualitative aspects of drug metabolism.

2.11.6 Glucuronidation

As indicated in Figure 2.19, the conjugation of drugs and their metabolites with glucuronic acid is intimately related to carbohydrate metabolism, via UDP–glucuronic acid (UDPGA), the donor of the glucuronide moiety. The synthesis of UDPGA is not the sole metabolic pathway for glucose-1-phosphate and UDP–glucose and these two intermediates are important in both glycolysis and glycogenesis pathways. From the viewpoint that glucuronidation is both an extensive and a not readily saturable reaction, it would appear that under normal metabolic conditions, the supply of UDPGA is not rate-limiting in conjugation reactions. However, under conditions of excessive utilisation of carbohydrate or glycogenesis, the flux of UDPGA through glucuronidation-based mechanisms is impaired, again illustrating the interaction of drug metabolism with normal metabolic processes. In addition, like cytochrome P450, the UDP–glucuronosyl-transferases are subjected to induction by clinically used drugs and are important in the metabolism of endogenous compounds. Therefore the concepts discussed for cytochrome P450 are equally applicable to the UDP–glucuronosyltrans-ferases leading to altered substrate specifity after induction and subjected to competition by endogenous substrates.

2.11.7 Cellular competition for glutathione

In addition to acting as a co-substrate for the glutathione-S-transferase-calatysed conjugation of electrophilic drugs and chemicals, glutathione has other cellular functions. Two molecules of glutathione are oxidised by the enzyme glutathione peroxidase (in the presence of an oxidised substrate such as lipid peroxides) forming the disulfide of glutathione. The glutathione disulfide may then in turn, be reduced back to glutathione by the enzyme glutathione reductase, thus setting up a cycle of glutathione utilisation coupled to the detoxication of cellular peroxides. However, under conditions of oxidative stress when peroxide con-centrations are high, the formation of glutathione disulfide exceeds the capacity of the reductase, and high glutathione disulfide levels build up, are removed from the hepatocyte and excreted in the bile. The net result of this process is to deplete the hepatocyte of glutathione and thereby reduce the availability of this co-substrate for the glutathione-S-transferase-catalysed conjugation of drugs.

Another major cellular utilisation of glutathione is in the biosynthesis of the leukotrienes, including leukotrienes LTD_4 and LTE_4. These leukotrienes are derived originally from arachidonic acid and condensation of leukotriene A_4 (an epoxide of arachidonic acid) with glutathione (catalysed by glutathione-S-transferase) results in formation of LTC_4 and subsequently, LTD_4 and LTE_4. Accordingly, it is clear that when there is a high cellular demand for glutathione in leukotriene biosynthesis, the available levels of glutathione for xenobiotic conjugation are decreased and may become limiting under certain patho-physiological situations.

In conclusion, it must be emphasised that both phase I and phase II drug metabolism pathways cannot be considered in isolation, but rather as part of a coupled, interactive system, interfacing directly with many endogenous metabolic pathways. As our knowledge of the pathways and enzymology of drug metabolism advances, then so too must our knowledge of their control and interaction with other enzyme systems.

Further reading

Textbooks and symposia

Archakov, A.I. and Bachmanova, G.I. (1989). *Cytochrome P450 and Active Oxygen*, Taylor and Francis, London.

Benford, D.J. *et al.* (1987). *Drug Metabolism: from Molecules to Man*, Taylor and Francis, London.

Damani, L.A. (1989). *Sulphur-containing Drugs and Related Organic Compounds, Volumes 1,2 and 3*, Ellis Horwood, Chichester.

Gorrod, J.W. *et al.* (1988), *Metabolism of Xenobiotics*, Taylor and Francis, London.

Guengerich, F.P. (1987). *Mammalian Cytochromes P450, Volumes 1 and 2*, CRC Press, Boca Raton.

Hutson, D.H. *et al.* (1989). *Intermediary Xenobiotic Metabolism in Animals: Methodology, Mechanisms and Significance*.

Kalow, W. (1992), *Pharmacogenetics of Drug Metabolism*, Pergamon Press, New York.

Kato, R. *et al.* (1989). *Xenobiotic Metabolism and Disposition*, Taylor and Francis, London.

Reviews and original articles

Coughtrie, M.W.H. (1992). Role of molecular biology in the structural and functional characterisation of the UDP-glucuronosyl transferases. In: *Progress in Drug Metabolism, Volume 13* (ed., G.G. Gibson), Taylor and Francis, London, p35–72.

Dolphin, C.T. *et al.* (1992). Cloning, primary sequence and chromosomal location of human FM02, a new member of the flavin-containing mono-oxygenase family. *Biochem. J.*, **287** 261–7.

Eling, T.E. and Curtis, J.F. (1992) Xenobiotic metabolism by prostaglandin H synthetase. *Pharmac. Ther.*, **53** 261–73.

Falany, C.N. *et al.* (1990). Purification and characterisation of human liver phenol-sulfating phenol sulfotransferases. *Arch. Biochem. Biophys.*, **278** 312–8

Gibson, G.G. and Tamburini, P.P. (1984). Cytochrome P450 spin state: inorganic biochemistry and functional significance. *Xenobiotica*, **14** 27–47.

Gonzalez, F.J. (1990). Molecular genetics of the P450 superfamily. *Pharmac. Ther.*, **45** 1–38.

Gonzalez, F.J. and Nebert, D.W. (1990). Evolution of the P450 gene superfamily. Animal–plant 'warfare', molecular drive and human genetic differences in drug oxidation. *Trends in Genetics*, **6** 182–6.

Grant, D.M. *et al.* (1992). Polymorphisms of N-acetyltransferase genes. *Xenobiotica*, **22** 1073–81.

Guengerich, F.P. (1990). Enzymatic oxidation of xenobiotic chemicals. *Critical Reviews in Biochemistry and Molecular Biology*, **25** 1990–2153.

Guengerich, F.P. (1991). Reactions and significance of cytochrome P450 enzymes. *J. Biol. Chem.*, **266** 10019–22.

Henderson, C.J. and Wolf, C.R. (1992). Molecular analysis of cytochrome P450s in the CYP2 gene family. In: *Progress in Drug Metabolism, Volume 13* (ed., G.G. Gibson), Taylor and Francis, London, p73–139.

Hodgon, E. and Levi, P.E. (1992). The role of the flavin-containing monooxygenase (E.C. 1.14.13.8) in the metabolism and mode of action of agricultural chemicals. *Xenobiotica*, **22** 1175–83.

Iyanagi, T. (1987). On the mechanisms of one- and two- electron transfer by flavin enzymes. *Chemica Scripta*, **27A** 31–6.

Iyanagi, T. (1991). Molecular basis of multiple UDP-glucuronosyltransferase isoenzyme deficiencies in the hyperbilirubinemic rat (Gunn rat). *J. Biol. Chem.*, **266** 24048–52.

Iyanagi, T. *et al.* (1989). The 3-methylcholanthrene-inducible UDP–glucuronosyltransferase deficiency in the hyperbilirubinemic rat (Gunn rat) is caused by a –1 frameshift mutation. *J. Biol. Chem.*, **264** 21302–7.

Jakoby, W.B. and Ziegler, D.M. (1990). The enzymes of detoxication. *J. Biol. Chem.*, **265** 20715–8.

Johnson, E.F. (1992). Mapping determinants of the substrate selectivities of P450 enzymes by site-directed mutagenesis. *TIPS*, **13** 122–6.

Levine, W.G. (1992). Azoreduction of drugs and other xenobiotics. In: *Progress in Drug Metabolism, Volume 13* (ed., G.G. Gibson), Taylor and Francis, London, p179–216.

Lewis, D.F.V. and Moereels, H. (1992). The sequence homologies of cytochromes P450 and active-site geometries. *J. Comp-Aided Mol. Design*, **6** 235–52.

Mannervik, B. *et al.* (1992). Nomenclature for human glutathione transferases. *Biochem. J.*, **282** 305–8.

Nebert, D.W. *et al.* The P450 Gene Superfamily: Recommended nemenclature and updates. *DNA Cell Biol.* (1987), **6** 1–11; (1989), **8** 1–13; (1991), **10** 1–14; (1993), **12** 1–51.

Porter, T.D. *et al.* (1990). NADPH–cytochrome P450 oxidoreductase gene organisation correlates with structural domains of the protein. *Biochem.*, **29** 9814–8.

Porter, T.D. and Coon, M.J. (1991). Cytochrome P450 multiplicity of isoforms, substrates and catalytic and regulatory mechanisms. *J. Biol. Chem.*, **266** 13469–74.

Shaw, P.N. and Blagborough, I.S. (1989). Cysteine conjugate β-lyase, II: isolation, properties and structure–activity relationships. In: *Sulphur-containing Drugs and Related Organic Compounds, Volume 2, Part B* (ed., L.A. Damani), Ellis-Horwood, Chichester, p136–55.

Smith, D.A. and Jones, B.C. (1992). Commentary: Speculations on the substrate structure activity relationship (SSAR) of cytochrome P450 enzymes. *Biochem. Pharmacol.*, **44** 2089–98.

Strolin-Benedetti, J. *et al.* (1988). Contributions of monoamine oxidase to the metabolism of xenobiotics. In: *Progress in Drug Metabolism, Volume 11* (ed., G.G. Gibson), Taylor and Francis, London, p149–74.

Tateishi, M. and Tomisawa, H. (1989). Cysteine conjugate β-lyase, I: Toxic thiol production. In: *Sulphur-containing Drugs and Related Organic Compounds, Volume 2, Part B* (ed., L.A. Damani), Ellis-Horwood, Chichester, p121–33.

Ziegler, D.M. (1990). Flavin-containing monoxygenases: enzymes adapted for multi-substrate specificty. *TIPS*, **11** 321–4.

3 Induction and inhibition of drug metabolism

3.1 Introduction

The study of drug metabolism in experimental animals in general and man in particular is ideally studied under strictly controlled conditions, such that we only observe the influence of the normal physiological and biochemical processes that contribute to the metabolism of the drug in question. However, this ideal situation is rarely achieved and the metabolism of drugs is substantially influenced by the deliberate or passive intake of many chemical substances that man is increasingly being exposed to either in his environment, for medical reasons or as a result of his lifestyle. These chemical substances are derived from a variety of sources and include pharmaceutical products, cosmetics, food additives and industrial chemicals. As summarised in Table 3.1, the magnitude of the various chemicals in use today, and hence the potential exposure to man, is staggering.

While it is clear that the ingestion of drugs, and to a certain extent food additives, is a predetermined, conscious act, many of the chemicals in Table 3.1 enter the body by more subtle means as exemplified by the pollution of food chains by insecticides and the accidental (sometimes, intentional) exposure to industrial chemicals and solvents from the environment. The magnitude of this latter problem is clearly seen in a recent study in the United States, where the Environmental Protection Agency reported that 288 different classes of chemical compounds were identified in domestic drinking water supplies. The food supply also represents an abundant source of chemical additives such as anti-oxidants, colourants, flavour enhancers and stabilisers that the human population is continually exposed to on a daily basis. For example, a recent UK government survey analysed approximately 5000 food products which contained 7000 chemical additives. Put another way, the average dietary intake of food additives in the UK is approximately 8 g/person/day or 2.9 kg/person/year.

Table 3.1 Estimated chemicals in use today

Classification	Number
Active ingredients of pesticides	1 500
Pharmaceutical products (drugs)	6 000
Food additives with nutritional value	2 500
Food additives to promote product life	3 000
Additional chemicals in use (including industrial chemicals)	50 000

From the above considerations, it is clear that man is either intentionally or accidently exposed to many chemical substances that have the potential to alter drug metabolism. Accordingly, it is the purpose of this chapter to outline the induction and inhibition of drug metabolism by these chemicals, and to rationalise wherever possible, their mode(s) of action on a molecular basis. Other factors affecting drug metabolism (including species, genetic, sex, age and dietary factors) are considered in the following two chapters and the pharmacological, toxicological and clinical implications of altered drug metabolism are considered in subsequent chapters.

3.2 Induction of drug metabolism

3.2.1 Induction of drug metabolism in man

Many currently used drugs of diverse pharmacology and chemical structure are well known to induce either their own metabolism or the biotransformation of other drugs in man (Table 3.2). The list of drugs shown in Table 3.2 is by no

Table 3.2 Therapeutic drugs that induce their own metabolism or the biotransformation of other drugs in man

Classification	Examples
Analeptics	Nikethamide
Analgesic, antipyretic and anti-inflammatory drugs	Antipyrine Phenylbutazone
Antibiotics	Rifampicin
Anticonvulsants	Carbamazepine, Phenytoin
Antifungal drugs	Griseofulvin
Antilipidaemics	Halofenate
Antimalarials	Quinine
Diuretics	Spironolactone
Psychotropic drugs	Chlorimipramine
Sedatives and hypnotics	Amylobarbitone, Barbitone, Chloral hydrate, Cyclobarbitone, Dichloralphenazone, Glutethimide, Hexobarbitone, Mandrax (a mixture of methaqualone and diphenyhydramine) Meprobamate, Phenobarbitone
Steroids	Testosterone
Vitamins	Vitamin C

Adapted from Bowman and Rand, *Textbook of Pharmacology, Second Edition*, Blackwell, London (1980).

means complete and only reflects those drugs for which there is a reasonably strong body of evidence for their ability to induce drug metabolism in man, and almost certainly this list is much longer in reality.

As indicated in chapter 1, the liver is the major organ responsible for drug metabolism in most species, and as far as man is concerned, a major problem is how to assess the extent of induction of hepatic drug metabolism. Several methods have been proposed to study induction in man and these include increased drug clearance, decreased drug plasma half life, increased plasma γ-glutamyl transferase, increased urinary excretion of D-glucaric acid, increased urinary 6β-hydroxycortisol and plasma bilirubin levels. Although none of these methods can unequivocally substantiate the induction of drug metabolism in man, taken collectively, they provide a reasonable indication of induction. Although the mechanism(s) involved in the induction of drug metabolism in man are not clearly defined, the induction of specific liver enzymes (particularly the mixed function oxidase enzymes of the endoplasmic reticulum, chapter 1) play a substantial role and have profound implications in clinical pharmacology, as discussed in chapters 5 and 7.

Clearly then, there are many problems associated with both the assessment and understanding of the basic mechanisms involved in the induction of drug metabolism in man, not the least of which are the ethical considerations. As a consequence of these limitations, much attention has focused on the use of experimental animals in drug induction studies. Although animal studies have proved extremely useful in characterising the phenomena of drug metabolism and its induction, it must always be borne in mind that animal experiments only given an indication of the situation in man.

3.2.2 Induction of drug metabolism in experimental animals

The duration and intensity of pharmacological action of many drugs is primarily dictated by their rate of metabolism, and as a corollary, chemical inducers that modify drug metabolism would be expected to alter the pharmacological effects of drugs. A good example of this phenomenon is the influence of phenobarbitone and benzo[a]pyrene on the metabolism and duration of action of the muscle relaxant, zoxazolamine. As shown in Figure 3.1, zoxazolamine undergoes metabolic hydroxylation at the 6-position by liver homogenates and as shown in Table 3.3, pretreatment of experimental animals with either phenobarbitone or the polycyclic aromatic hydrocarbon, benzo[a]pyrene, results in a substantial increase in zoxazolamine metabolism and consequently, a significant decrease in the paralysis time by the drug.

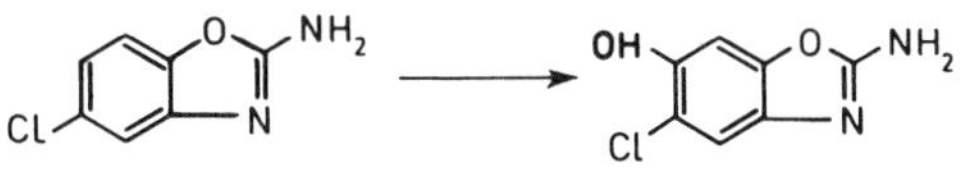

Figure 3.1 Metabolism of zoxazolamine by rat liver homogenates.

Table 3.3 Influence of phenobarbitone or benzo[a]pyrene pretreatment on the metabolism and pharmacological action of zoxazolamine in the rat

Parameter	Control (saline treated)	Phenobarbitone treated[a]	Benzo[a]pyrene treated[b]
Paralysis time (min)	137	62	20
Whole body decay ($t_{1/2}$, min)	102	38	12
Zoxazolamine metabolism (nmol/mg protein/h)	3	14	15

[a] Animals were treated with phenobarbitone (30 mg/kg. i.p.) twice daily for 4 days and killed 24h after the last injection.
[b] Animals were treated with a single i.p. injection of benzo[a]pyrene (20mg/kg) 24h prior to sacrifice.
Adapted from Trevor, A. (1972), in *Fundamentals of Drug Metabolism and Drug Disposition* (B.N. La Du *et al.*), Williams and Wilkins, Baltimore.

Clearly, the range of drugs and chemicals that have the ability to induce similar hepatic drug metabolism has been more thoroughly investigated in laboratory animals than in man, and as documented in Table 3.4, many structurally diverse drugs and chemicals have been shown to induce liver drug metabolism in various species.

There is apparently no structure–activity relationship in the ability of these various inducers to stimulate drug metabolism, and the only common physico-chemical property is that the majority of these compounds are relatively lipophilic in nature. Whereas no general conclusions can be made, it will be shown later that there is a well-defined structure–activity relationship for some of these classes of compounds (see section 3.2.7).

3.2.3 Role of cytochrome P450 in the induction of drug metabolism

In an attempt to localise the site of induction of drug metabolism, significant advances have been made in considering the role of the liver. As outlined in chapter 1, the liver serves as the main organ responsible for drug metabolism and it was not entirely unexpected that significant hepatic alterations in the drug metabolising enzyme systems were noted in response to inducing agents. Of particular importance is the hepatic cytochrome P450 enzyme system. Early studies in the mid 1960s clearly showed that both cytochrome P450 and its associated flavoprotein reductase, NADPH–cytochrome P450 reductase were substantially induced in response to phenobarbitone pretreatment and that this was paralleled by induction of drug metabolism. This observed inductive effect of phenobarbitone was not, however, confined to the enzymes of drug metabolism and other enzymes of the hepatic endoplasmic reticulum were induced (Figure 3.2), indicative of a general proliferation of this subcellular organelle.

Nevertheless it soon became clear that induction of drug metabolism was generally accompanied by increases in liver microsomal cytochrome P450

Table 3.4 Inducers of hepatic drug metabolism in experimental animals

Classification	Example	Use or occurrence
Drugs	Phenobarbitone and most barbiturates	Sedative/hypnotic
	Phenytoin	Anti-convulsant
	Pregnenolone-16α-carbonitrile	Catatoxic steroid
	Rifampicin	Antibiotic
	Triacetyloleandomycin	Antibiotic
	Clofibrate	Hypolipidaemic
Alcohols	Ethanol	Beverage, skin disinfectant
Flavones	5,6-Benzoflavone	Synthetics, citrus fruits
Food additives and anutrients	Butylated hydroxyanisole (BHA), Butylated hydroxytoluene (BHT) Ethoxyquin	Food antioxidants
	Isosafrole	Oils of sassafras, nutmeg and cinnamon
Halogenated hydrocarbons	2,3,7,8-Tetrachlorodibenzo-*p*-dioxin (TCDD)	Contaminant of herbicides and defoliants (2,4,5-T)
	3,3',4,4'-Tetrachlorobiphenyl	Insulator in capacitors/trans-formers
	3,3',4,4',5,5'-Hexabromobiphenyl	Flame retardant
Insecticides	DDT (dichlorodiphenyl trichloroethane)	Agricultural pesticide
	Chlordecone (Kepone)	Organochlorine pesticide
	Piperonyl butoxide	Insecticide synergist
Polycyclic aromatic hydrocarbons	Including 3-methylcholanthrene, phenanthrene, chrysene, 1-2,benzanthracene and benzo[*a*]pyrene	Environmental pollutants found in industrial and domestic combustion products, cigarette smoke and oil contaminants
Solvents	Toluene and xylenes	Solvents, cleaning agents and degreasers

content, and in addition, different inducers did not uniformly increase the metabolism of all drugs to the same extent, i.e. certain inducers did indeed substantially increase drug metabolism, other inducers had little or no effect and paradoxically, certain 'inducers' actually decreased the metabolism of some drugs investigated. An example of this diversity of drug metabolism responses to various inducers is shown in Table 3.5.

The inducers shown in Table 3.5 are all well known to induce liver micro-somal cytochrome P450 and their influence on the rate of drug metabolism depends on the substrate being examined. In addition to exhibiting a certain degree of substrate specificity, inducers are well documented to exhibit both stereo- and regioselectivity towards the metabolism of several drugs. This is exemplified by the influence of inducers on the metabolism of the *R*- and *S*-isomers of warfarin, both isomers of warfarin being hydroxylated at various positions in the molecule by the cytochrome P450-dependent mixed function oxidase system of the liver endoplasmic reticulum (Table 3.6).

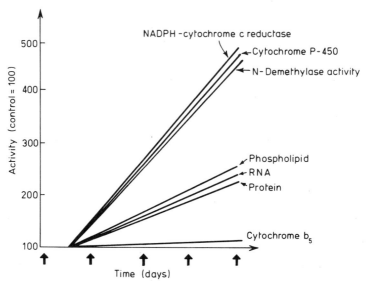

Figure 3.2 Induction of hepatic endoplasmic reticulum enzymes by phenobarbitone. Bold arrows indicate the daily injection of phenobarbitone. Adapted from Ernster and Orrenius (1965) *Fed. Proc.*, **24** 1190.

Table 3.5 Influence of various inducers on the metabolism of various model drug substrates

Drug	Control	Inducer [a,b]			
		PB	PCN	MC	ARO
Ethylmorphine	13.7 ± 0.8	16.8 ± 4.3	24.9 ± 3.5	6.4 ± 0.5	9.5 ± 1.2
Aminopyrine	9.9 ± 0.8	13.9 ± 1.7	9.7 ± 1.3	7.6 ± 1.8	13.7 ± 1.2
Benzphetamine	12.5 ± 1.2	45.7 ± 14.0	6.6 ± 0.7	5.7 ± 1.1	15.8 ± 2.7
Caffeine	0.5 ± 0.1	0.7 ± 0.1	–	0.5 ± 0.1	0.6 ± 0.1
Benzo[a]pyrene	0.1	0.1	0.1	0.3	–

[a] Abbreviations of inducers used: PB, phenobarbitone; PCN, pregnenolone-16α-carbonitrile; MC, 3-methylcholanthrene; ARO, Arochlor 1254.

[b] All drug metabolising activities are expressed as nmol product formed/min/nmol cytochrome P450 (V_{max} values).

Adapted from Powis, G., Talcott, R.E. and Schenkman, J.B. (1977). In: *Microsomes and Drug Oxidations*, (V. Ullrich, *et al.*) Pergamon Press, pp. 127–35.

Table 3.6 Influence of cytochrome P450 induction on the *in vitro* metabolism of *R*- and *S*- warfarin

Inducer	Hydroxylated warfarin metabolites[a]			
	R-isomer		*S*-isomer	
	7-OH	8-OH	7-OH	8-OH
Uninduced	0.22	0.04	0.04	0.01
Phenobarbitone	0.36	0.07	0.09	0.02
3-Methylcholanthrene	0.08	0.50	0.04	0.04

[a] Metabolism is expressed as nmol warfarin metabolite formed/nmol cytochrome P450/min

3.2.4 Induction of multiple forms (isoenzymes) of cytochrome P450

In view of the extremely broad substrate specificity of liver microsomal cytochrome P450 towards the metabolism of drugs, and the diversity of responses to inducers as outlined above, it was initially proposed that these observations could be rationalised by assuming the existence of more than one form (or isoenzyme) of cytochrome P450. Thus different inducers would have the potential to elevate the levels of a specific sub-population of cytochrome P450, each with a characteristic substrate specificity towards the metabolism of drugs. This concept of cytochrome P450 multiplicity has now been firmly established in recent years and has had a profound influence on drug metabolism studies. Validation of this latter hypothesis has been achieved largely by the development of techniques enabling the cytochrome P450 isoenzymes to be solubilised and purified from liver endoplasmic reticulum fragments such that structural and functional comparisons of highly purified cytochrome P450 preparations can be assessed and compared.

The exact number of cytochrome P450 isoenzymes is not known with certainty, but approximately 220 are known at present. There are strain differences and tissue differences in expression of these isoenzymes, in addition to the presence of more than one form in a given tissue of a given species. The reason for this uncertainty in the exact number of cytochrome P450 variants is that the characterisation of the multiple forms is a relatively recent occurrence, with the first successful (partial) purification being achieved in 1968. Another problem associated with the exact number of cytochrome P450 variants is the different criteria used by different laboratories in assessing cytochrome P450 heterogeneity and a lack of standard techniques in assessing their structural and functional properties. However, it must be emphasised that with the newly accepted gene nomenclature described in chapter 2, this confusion on the identity of multiple forms has largely been resolved and each new cytochrome P450 identified and assigned a particular name, must have its complete amino acid sequence known (either from classical N-terminal sequencing studies or predicted from the cognate cDNA or gene).

The unequivocal assignment of unique 3-dimensional structure to cytochrome P450 isoenzymes is not possible at present because of the difficulty in crystallising membrane-bound proteins for X-ray crystallography studies. Currently accepted criteria for cytochrome P450 heterogeneity are shown in Table 3.7.

The most intensively studied cytochrome P450s are those derived from the endoplasmic reticulum of rat and rabbit liver. Advantage has been taken of the fact that phenobarbitone and 3-methylcholanthrene (and other polycyclic aromatic hydrocarbons) induce different cytochrome P450 proteins in both of these species and the structural and functional properties of these isoenzymes have been studied in detail. In general, most of the criteria outlined in Table 3.7 have been satisfied for these induced haemoproteins, and therefore on this basis,

Table 3.7 Distinctive criteria for the assignment of cytochrome P450 heterogeneity in highly purified preparations.

1. Spectral properties of the ferric, ferrous and carbon monoxy–ferrous states.
2. Spectral interactions with drug substrates.
3. Substrate specificities in reconstituted enzyme systems.
4. Immunological properties including lack of cross-reactivity of antibodies to heterologous cytochrome P450 antigens.
5. Monomeric molecular weights.
6. Amino acid composition.
7. Peptide fragmentation patterns by chemical or enzymatic means.
8. Partial or complete amino acid sequences.

Table 3.8 Substrate specificities of two forms of rat liver cytochrome P450 induced by either phenobarbitone or 3-methylcholanthrene

Substrate	Form of cytochrome P450	
	Phenobarbitone induced Form (2B1)	3-Methylcholanthrene induced Form (1A1)
Benzphetamine	52.0[a]	2.5
Benzo[a]pyrene	0.2	3.9
Ethoxycoumarin	4.1	56.0
Testosterone		
6ß-hydroxylation	0.2	0.3
7α-hydroxylation	0.7	1.0
16α-hydroxylation	1.5	0.2

The activities of the two induced cytochrome P450 variants shown in the above table determined in the presence of highly purified forms of each isoenzyme and therefore reflect catalytic activities of each enzyme variant.

[a] Activities are expressed as nmol metabolite formed per min per nmol cytochrome P450.

it is widely believed that phenobarbitone and 3-methylcholanthrene are representative of two distinct classes of inducers of drug metabolism. Apart from the biochemical diversity between these induced variants of cytochrome P450, there is substantial pharmacological evidence for the existence of multiple forms in that enzyme variants exhibit substantially different substrate specificities with respect to drug metabolism (oxidation) reactions. This metabolic diversity towards drug oxidations is readily seen in Table 3.8, which shows the substrate specificities of specific phenobarbitone- and 3-methylcholanthrene-induced rat liver cytochromes P450 (CYP2B1 and CYP1A1).

Table 3.8 clearly shows that the nature of the induced cytochrome P450 isoenzyme is important in determining the extent of drug oxidation. For example, benzphetamine serves as an excellent substrate for the phenobarbitone-induced variant whereas the 3-methylcholanthrene form only poorly metabolises this substrate. In contrast, ethoxycoumarin is rapidly metabolised by the polycyclic aromatic hydrocarbon-induced isoenzyme whereas the barbiturate-induced variant does not oxidise ethoxycoumarin as efficiently. It should be further emphasised that the liver of a particular species (including man) usually contains more than one cytochrome P450 variant and therefore the overall ability of the liver to metabolise drugs (i.e. those drugs whose metabolism is cytochrome P450-dependent) is dictated by both the type and amount of the cytochrome P450 sub-populations.

Information is now beginning to accumulate indicating that human liver contains similar cytochrome P450 isoenzymes as are observed in experimental animals. The purification and characterisation of several human liver cytochrome(s) P450 has already been reported and it has been shown that the hepatic haemoproteins from human and rat share certain features of structural, functional and immunological similarity.

3.2.5 Significance of multiple forms of cytochrome P450

The existence of multiple forms of cytochrome P450 is not solely a biochemical curiosity, but has profound ramifications in both pharmacology and toxicology. Some of the more important consequences of cytochrome P450 heterogeneity include

(1) The existence of cytochrome P450 isoenzymes may, in part, rationalise the substantial differences in drug metabolism that are observed as a function of sex, species, age, nutritional status and inter-subject variability as discussed in chapters 4 and 5.

(2) Multiple forms of cytochrome P450 may provide an explanation of why only certain tissues are susceptible to chemically dependent toxicity. For example, many chemicals that are known to cause cancer in experimental animals are biologically inert *per se* and require metabolic oxidation by the cytochrome P450 enzyme system before they can ultimately express their carcinogenicity. An excellent example of the role of cytochrome P450 in the activation of innocuous chemicals to potent carcinogens is shown in Figure 3.3. In this example, inert benzo[a]pyrene (a ubiquitous environmental contaminant) is first metabolised by cytochrome P450 forming the 7,8-epoxide derivative which subsequently serves as the substrate for another microsomal enzyme, epoxide hydrolase, to form the 7,8-diol derivative of benzo[a]pyrene. This latter diol is further metabolised by cytochrome P450 to the potent, ultimate carcinogen, benzo[a]pyrene 7,8-diol-9,10-epoxide, which can then bind to nucleic acids and initiate the complex series of events leading to cancer. Therefore it is clear that any tissue that contains the appropriate cytochrome P450 isoenzymes to catalyse the two oxidation reactions in Figure 3.3 (and of course epoxide hydrolase) may be susceptible to carcinogenesis by this chemical. In reality, the biological situation is much more complex than outlined above and other factors including, for example, the role of detoxifying, conjugating (phase II) enzymes and the role of

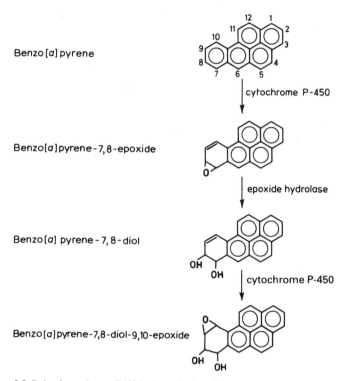

Benzo[a]pyrene

cytochrome P-450

Benzo[a]pyrene-7,8-epoxide

epoxide hydrolase

Benzo[a]pyrene-7,8-diol

cytochrome P-450

Benzo[a]pyrene-7,8-diol-9,10-epoxide

Figure 3.3 Role of cytochrome P450 in the activation of the precarcinogen benzo[a]pyrene.

DNA repair mechanisms are important in determining tissue susceptibility to chemical carcinogens. However, it is clear from the above considerations that cytochrome P450 has a substantial role to play in chemical carcinogenesis.

(3) The induction of cytochrome P450 isoenzymes by commonly used drugs such as phenobarbital has important ramifications in clinical pharmacology. For example it is not an uncommon clinical practice to use combination drug therapy where a patient is being treated with more than one drug at a time, and many drug–drug interactions have been observed, particularly with enzyme (cytochrome P450) inducers such as phenobarbitone. A well-documented drug–drug interation has been observed in patients who are being treated with both phenobarbitone (a sedative) and warfarin derivatives (anticoagulents). Because phenobarbitone induces the cytochrome P450 enzymes in the liver that are responsible for the metabolism of warfarin, the effective pharmacological levels of warfarin are thereby reduced and the dose of warfarin has to be substantially increased to maintain effective, therapeutic levels. The problem arises when the phenobarbitone treatment is withdrawn and the metabolism of warfarin is accordingly reduced, resulting in increased, toxic plasma levels of

warfarin because of the low therapeutic index of this drug (i.e. effectively a warfarin overdosage in this latter situation).

(4) As discussed in chapter 1, cytochrome P450 is not only responsible for the metabolism of drugs and xenobiotics but actively plays a role in the oxidation of many endogenous compounds such as steroids, prostaglandins, fatty acids and vitamin D_3. Although our understanding of the cytochrome P450 isoenzymes involved in endogenous compound metabolism is not as well developed as compared to those cytochrome P450s responsible for drug metabolism, it is clear that a substantial alteration of the former group of cytochrome P450 isoenzymes by drug and environmental inducers may well influence many aspects of intermediary metabolism where cytochrome P450 is involved.

Therefore it is clear that the induction of the drug-metabolising enzymes is particularly important in the areas of clinical pharmacology and toxicology and the reader is referred to chapters 6 and 7 for a more detailed discussion of these phenomena.

3.2.6 Induction of extrahepatic drug metabolism

Although the liver is the main organ responsible for drug metabolism in most species, significant activities are present in extrahepatic tissues including lung, kidney, skin, intestinal mucosa, and many other tissues. Whereas the liver appears to be a particularly sensitive target organ for the induction of the drug metabolising enzymes in general and cytochrome P450 in particular, the inductive response in extrahepatic tissues is more variable. Extrahepatic enzyme induction depends not only on the nature of the inducing agent and the extra-hepatic tissue but also on the particular drug substrate under investigation. For example, Table 3.9 shows that cigarette smoke (containing polycyclic aromatic hydrocarbon-inducing agents) substantially increases the hydroxylation of benzo[a]pyrene in lung and placenta and is a less effective inducing agent in the intestine. Similarly, induction of phenacetin metabolism in the lung was only 5% of that observed with benzo[a]pyrene metabolism in the same tissue.

Although many extrahepatic cytochrome P450s are induced by drugs and chemicals, it is absolutely clear that many extra-hepatic isoenzymes of cytochrome P450 are regulated by endogenous compounds and hormones (Table 3.10). Practically all of these cytochrome P450s are involved with the

Table 3.9 Induction of phenacetin and benzo[a]pyrene metabolism by cigarette smoke in extrahepatic tissues of the rat

Enzyme activity	Induction (% of control value)			
	Liver	Intestine	Lung	Placenta
Phenacetin de-ethylation	20	100	60	–
Benzo[a]pyrene hydroxylation	120	120	1200	500

Table 3.10 Constitutive cytochrome P450s regulated by endogenous compounds[1]

Tissue	P450 species induced	Endogenous inducer/regulator[2]
Adrenal	CYP11A1, CYP11B1, CYP17, CYP21A1	ACTH
Ovary	CYP11A1	FSH
Ovary	CYP17	LH
Ovary	CYP19	FSH
Testis	CYP11A1	LH
Leydig Cell	CYP17	LH
Kidney	250HVITD$_3$1α	PTH

[1] Derived from Okey, A.B. (1990) *Pharmacol. Therapeut.*, **45** 241–98.

[2] Abbreviations used are ACTH, adrenocorticotrophic hormone; FSH, follicle stimulating hormone; LH, lutenising hormone; PTH, parathyroid hormone; 250HVITD$_3$1α, 25-hydroxy-vitamin D$_3$-1α-hydroxylase.

biotransformation of physiologically important compounds and the regulatory mechanisms seem to involve ACTH-dependent, increased levels of cAMP in many instances, and a cAMP-dependent transcriptional activation of the cognate genes. At present, it is not clear if cAMP directly activates P450 gene transcription or if cAMP-regulatable proteins are necessary for induction. These SHIP (steroid hydroxylase inducing proteins) mediators have remained elusive to isolate and characterise but remain a conceptually attractive hypothesis involving *trans*-activation of an enhancer element in the regulatory (5'-flanking) region of the corresponding cytochrome P450 genes. In general terms, the cytochrome P450s discussed above are usually not induced by xenobiotics and this is a very useful separation as these endogenous cytochrome P450s are essential to survival and reproduction of the organism.

3.2.7 Mechanisms of cytochrome P450 induction

Although the precise molecular mechanisms of cytochrome P450 induction are not fully understood at present, much effort has been expended in trying to rationalise the inductive response of the drug-metabolising enzymes in hepatic tissue. Figure 3.4 shows the functional components of the hepatic mixed function oxidase system responsible for cytochrome P450-dependent drug metabolism. Accordingly, induction of drug metabolism may arise as a consequence of increased synthesis, decreased degradation, activation of pre-existing components or a combination of these three processes. More specifically, Table 3.11 summarises some of the biochemical effects noted on response to enzyme inducers. From this table, it is clear that enzyme inducers have a variety of effects on the functional components of the mixed function oxidase system, particularly on the terminal haemoprotein, cytochrome P450, as summarised in Table 3.11.

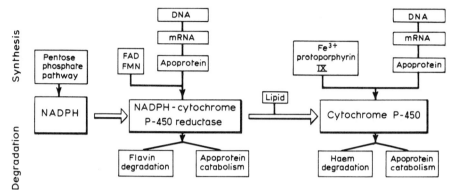

Figure 3.4 Synthesis and degradation of the functional components of the hepatic mixed function oxidase system.

Table 3.11 Differences in induction mechanisms for cytochrome P450s[1]

P450 isoenzyme	Representative inducer	Main induction mechanism
1A1	Dioxin	Transcriptional activation by ligand activated Ah receptor
1A2	3-Methylcholanthrene	mRNA stabilisation
2B1/2B2	Phenobarbital	Transcriptional gene activation
2E1	Ethanol, acetone isoniazid	Protein stabilisation (in part)
3A1	Dexamethasone	Transcriptional gene activation
4A6	Clofibrate	Transcriptional activation, mediated by peroxisome proliferator activated receptor

[1] Modified from Waxman, D.J. and Azaroff, L. (1992) *Biochem. J.*, **288** 577–92.

Table 3.12 Drugs and chemicals that act as phenobarbitone-type inducers of cytochrome P450s

Phenobarbitone and several barbiturates
Phenytoin
DDT
Pentamethylbenzene
Polychlorinated biphenyls (PCBs) with *ortho* chlorines
2-Acetylaminofluorene

Derived from Okey, A.B. (1990) *Pharmacol. Therapeut.*, **45** 241–98.

Phenobarbitone induction of cytochrome P450s. Treatment of experimental animals with phenobarbitone (and related agents, Table 3.12) results in a substantial increase in the hepatic levels of translatable polysolmal mRNA for some cytochrome P450s, particularly CYP2B1 and CYP2B2. Specific complementary

DNA probes (cDNA) to cytochrome P450 mRNA have been synthesised and using cDNA–mRNA hybridisation techniques, it has been shown conclusively that a few hours after phenobarbitone pretreatment, a substantial increase in the level of mRNA coding for cytochrome P4502B1 is observed. This mRNA induction is accompanied by increases in intranuclear RNAs that represent precursors to cytochrome P450 and mRNA.

An interesting example of phenobarbitone-dependent gene regulation is in the differential regulation of cytochrome P4502B1 and P4502B2. These two closely related isoenzymes share an overall 97% amino acid sequence similarity with only 14 residues different out of a total of 491. One of these variable regions is in exon 7 in residues 344 to 349, as

CYP 2B2 – Ser – His – Arg – **Leu** – Pro – **Thr** –
CYP 2B1 – Ser – His – Arg – **Pro** – Pro – **Ser** –

Knowing these small differences in amino acid sequence, specific oligonucleotide probes can be chemically synthesised for the above two isoenzymes, thus yielding an analytical method to determine the influence of phenobarbitone on these closely related isoenzymes. This type of molecular analysis has yielded the information that even although the sequences of CYP2B1 and 2B2 are almost identical, their regulation by phenobarbitone is very different (CYP2B1 is induced, CYP2B2 is not) with the functional importance that CYP2B1 and 2B2 exhibit different rates of substrate biotransformation (CYP2B1 is usually more active than CYP2B2) and hence contribute to differential activation/deactivation of xenobiotics.

Although cytochrome P4502B1 is the major phenobarbitone-inducible cytochrome P450, several other cytochrome P450 sub-families are also induced (Table 3.13). Accordingly, it would appear that the major inductive effect of phenobarbitone in the liver is to increase specific mRNA levels by augmenting transcription, rather than stabilising pre-existing levels of protein precursors or increased translational efficiency. At present, no specific cytoplasmic or nuclear receptors for phenobarbitone have been identified.

Table 3.13 Phenobarbitone-inducible cytochrome P450s in the rat[1]

P450 isoenzyme	Approximate fold-induction[2]	Comments
2A1	2–4	Also induced by CYP1A1 inducers
2B1	50–100	Major phenobarbitone-induced form
2B2	20	Only slightly induced
2C6	2–4	–
2C7	20	Developmentally regulated
3A1	10	Also inducible by dexamethasone and macrolide antibiotics
3A2	10	Male-specific expression in adult rats

[1] Derived from Waxman, D.J. and Azaroff, L. (1992) *Biochem. J.*, **281** 577-92.
[2] Induction assessed as either increase in apoprotein or relevant mRNA.

Table 3.14 Polycyclic aromatic hydrocarbon-like inducers of cytochrome P450

Polycyclic aromatic hydrocarbons
 3-methylcholanthrene
 benzo(a)pyrene
 benz(a)anthracene
 dibenz(a,h)anthracene
Phenothiazines
β-Naphthoflavone and other flavones
Plant indoles
 indole-3-acetonitrile
 indole-3-carbinol
Ellipticine
Charcoal-broiled beef
Cigarette smoke
Crude petroleum
Polychlorinated biphenyls
Polybrominated biphenyls
Halogenated dibenzo-p-dioxins
Halogenated dibenzofurans

Derived from Okey, A.B. (1990) *Pharmacol. Therapeut.*, **45** 241–98.

Polycyclic aromatic hydrocarbon induction of cytochrome P450s. In contrast to phenobarbitone induction of hepatic drug metabolising enzymes, induction by environmental polycyclic aromatic hydrocarbons such as 3-methylcholanthrene, β-naphthoflavone, benzo[a]pyrene, 2,3,7,8-tetrachlorodibenzo-p-dioxin (TCDD, dioxin) (see also Table 3.14) is thought to be associated with a specific cytosolic receptor, termed the Ah receptor. As shown in Figure 3.5, polycyclic aromatic hydrocarbon inducers combine with this specific protein receptor in a similar fashion to hormone receptors. The inducer–receptor complex is then translocated to the nucleus of the hepatocyte whereupon induction-specific mRNA is transcribed from DNA. The interaction of this Ah receptor–inducer complex with the regulatory elements of cytochrome P450 responsive genes (primarily CYP1A1) is now beginning to be understood at the molecular level and is a complex interactive system of positive control elements (drug responsive elements, DREs or sometimes called xenobiotic responsive elements, XREs) which function as transcriptional enhancers and negative control elements, all situated at approximately −1 kilobase upstream of the transcriptional start site in the 5' flanking region of the gene. Large amounts of newly translated, specific cytochrome P450 are then incorporated into the membrane of the hepatic endoplasmic reticulum, resulting in the observed induction of metabolism of certain drugs and xenobiotics. It should be noted that although the extent of induction of the drug-metabolising enzymes by polycyclic aromatic hydrocarbons is not as pronounced as observed for phenobarbitone, the gross levels of cytochrome P450 do not represent the induction of specific forms of cytochrome P450. For example, one of the specific isoenzyme variants of cytochrome P450 inducible by these environmental pollutants (CYP1A1) is

Hepatocyte

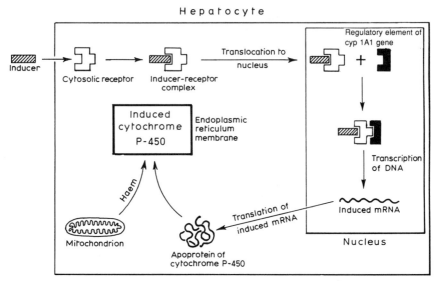

Figure 3.5 Receptor-mediated induction of cytochrome P450 by polycyclic aromatic hydrocarbons. Adapted from Okey, A.B. (1990) *Pharmacol. Therapeut.*, **45** 241–98.

present in very low amounts in non-induced liver (approximately 2–5%) and increases approximately 8 to 16-fold on induction. This observation is similar to that seen with phenobarbitone induction, except that the absolute level of cytochrome P450 upon phenobarbitone induction is much larger, due in part, to the exaggerated proliferative response to this barbiturate.

Extensive studies have been carried out on the ability of various polycyclic aromatic hydrocarbons to interact with the above cytosolic receptor and hence induce specific cytochrome P450 variants. For example, Table 3.15 shows the rank order potency of various compounds to inhibit the binding of 3-methylcholanthrene to the cytosolic receptor. From this table it is seen that 2,3,7,8-tetrachlorodibenzo-*p*-dioxin is a potent inhibitor of 3-methylcholanthrene binding to the cytosolic receptor and in general, the data in Table 3.15 correlates well with the relative potency of these compounds to induce cytochrome P450 in the 1A sub-family. In addition, it should be noted that certain strains of mice are non-responsive to these inducers and are characterised by an absence of the cytosolic receptor.

The Ah receptor protein has been purified to homogeneity from the liver of B6 mice. Apparently the native receptor is a labile 95 KDa protein, which can be easily proteolysed to yield a 70 KDa fragment. The cDNA for this receptor has been isolated and completely sequenced and analysis of the deduced amino acid sequence reveals a region with similarity to the basic region/helix–loop–helix motif found in many transcription factors that undergo dimerisation before they are functionally active. Thus the Ah receptor is very likely a ligand (i.e. inducer) activated transcription factor.

Table 3.15 Potency of various compounds as competitors of binding of 3-methylcholanthrene to the mouse hepatic cytosolic receptor

Competitor	Competitor concentration giving 50% inhibition of 3-methylcholanthrene binding (M)[a]
2,3,7,8-Tetrachlorodibenzo-*p*-dioxin	0.3×10^{-9}
Dibenz[*a,h*]anthracene	0.1×10^{-8}
Dibenz[*a,c*]anthracene	0.3×10^{-8}
ß-Naphthoflavone	0.1×10^{-7}
Benzo[*a*]pyrene	0.1×10^{-7}
Benz[*a*]anthracene	0.5×10^{-7}
6-Aminochrysene	0.8×10^{-7}
Pregnenolone-16α-carbonitrile	0.1×10^{-6}
Anthracene	0.8×10^{-6}

[a] 3-Methylcholanthrene concentration was 10 nM.
Adapted from Okey, A.B. and Vella, L.M. (1982). *Eur. J. Biochem.*, **127** 39–47.

Ethanol inducible cytochrome P4502E1. Feeding ethanol to experimental animals results in the induction of the biotransformation of drugs and the oxidation of ethanol itself, suggesting that ethanol induces a specific isoform of cytochrome P450. This turned out to be the case and ethanol (and other compounds such as imidazole, isoniazid, acetone and pyrazole) induces the cytochrome P4502E1 isoenzyme. Interestingly, the induction of the CYP2E1 isoenzyme arises through multiple mechanisms, depending on the induction stimulus (Figure 3.6), although the predominant xenobiotic-dependent induction appears to be via stabilisation and inhibition of degradation of the CYP2E1 apoprotein.

Clofibrate induction of cytochrome P450s. Clofibrate is a clinically used hypolipidaemic drug and appears to have specificity for induction of cytochrome P450s in the CYP4 gene family, inducing isoenzymes that do not readily metabolise drugs but prefer lipids (particularly fatty acids) as substrates. Recent work has identified, cloned and sequenced a member of the steroid hormone superfamily of receptors, termed the peroxisome proliferator activated receptor (PPAR), so-called because clofibrate belongs to a large class of compounds known as the peroxisome proliferators. This PPAR consists of two domains, a ligand-binding region that binds clofibrate and a DNA-binding region that binds to the regulatory elements of the responsive genes in the CYP4 family (the interaction with CYP4A6 has been relatively well characterised) as demonstrated in Figure 3.7. It is interesting to note that fatty acids can act as natural ligands for this PPAR and at present, it is not clear if the CYP4 family induction arises solely from drug–PPAR interaction or clofibrate-dependent perturbation of lipid homoeostasis and subsequent lipid activation of the receptor or a combination of these two mechanisms (Figure 3.7).

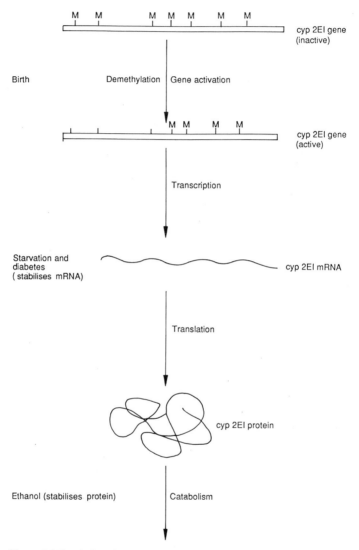

Figure 3.6 Regulation of the cytochrome P4502E1 gene. M represents methylated cystosine residues.

The above discussion was centred on different types of cytochrome P450 inducers as if every inducer only induces one particular sub-family of enzymes. Whereas this is true for some inducers it most certainly is not true for all of the inducers known to date and it must be borne in mind that certain xenobiotics will induce several sub-families within the same family and even in totally different families.

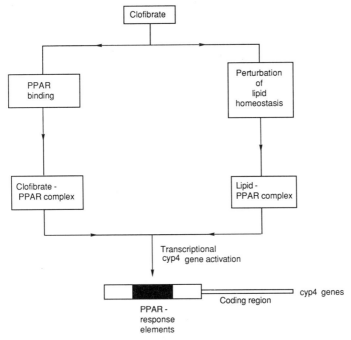

Figure 3.7 Regulation of cytochrome P4504 family genes by the peroxisome proliferator activated receptor (PPAR).

3.2.8 Induction of non-cytochrome P450 drug-metabolising enzymes

Although cytochrome P450 is an important enzymatic determinant of drug metabolism, it is by no means the only drug-metabolising enzyme whose levels are induced in response to a chemical or drug challenge. Indeed, most of the enzymes involved in drug metabolism are induced to various extents by a structurally diverse group of chemicals and drugs and some examples of this are shown in Table 3.16.

In general, the above inducers are relatively non-specific in that they cause a general proliferation of the hepatic endoplasmic reticulum membrane or of the enzymes of drug metabolism. However, it should be pointed out that some of the enzymes shown in Table 3.16 exist in multiple forms (e.g. the glucuronosyl transferases) or as homo/hetereodimers of two sub-units (e.g. the glutathione-*S*-transferases). Accordingly, the induction of UDP–glucuronosyl transferase is highly dependent on the nature of the inducer under consideration. Induction of this latter enzyme with phenobarbitone results in the induction of a form of the transferase that preferentially utilises chloroamphenicol as substrate whereas induction with 3-methylcholanthrene results in a transferase that has a specificity for 3-hydroxy benzo[*a*]pyrene as substrate. In a similar manner, there is evidence to suggest that the different sub-units of glutathione-*S*-transferase are

Table 3.16 Induction of drug-metabolising enzymes

Enzyme	Inducer
Epoxide hydrolase	2-Acetylaminofluorene, aldrin, Arochlor 1254, dieldrin, ethoxyquin, isosafrole, 3-methylcholanthrene, phenobarbitone, *trans*-stilbene oxide.
Glucuronosyl transferase	Dieldrin, isosafrole, 3-methylcholanthrene, phenobarbitone, polychlorinated biphenyls, 2,3,7,8-tetrachlorodibenzo-*p*-dioxin
NADPH–cytochrome P450 reductase	2-Acetylaminofluorene, dieldrin, isosafrole, phenobarbitone, polychlorinated biphenyls, *trans*-stilbene oxide.
Glutathione-*S*-transferase	2-Acetylaminofluorene, 3-methylcholanthrene, phenobarbitone, 2,3,7,8-tetrachlorodibenzo-*p*-dioxin, *trans*-stilbene oxide.
Cytochrome b_5	2-Acetylaminofluorene, butylated hydroxytoluene, griseofulvin

differentially induced by phenobarbitone. Therefore, the induction of non-cytochrome P450 enzymes responsible for drug metabolism (particularly the UDP–glucuronosyl transferases and the glutathione-*S*-transferases) impose another level of control on the overall metabolic fate of a drug.

3.3 Inhibition of drug metabolism

A major concern of clinical pharmacologists is the area of drug–drug interactions in which two or more drugs are co-administered resulting in either therapeutic incompatibility or toxic reactions. Although the 'blunderbuss' approach to polypharmacy has significantly diminished in recent years, many patients are still treated simultaneously with a combination of different drugs. For example a recent study of 138 randomly selected i.v. solutions has shown that 24% of these solutions contained two drugs and 14% contained five or more drugs. Just as one drug can induce the metabolism of a second drug as discussed in the previous section, the inhibition of drug metabolism by other drugs or xenobiotics is a well-recognised phenomenon. Accordingly, it is the purpose of this section to focus on well-defined examples of the inhibition of drug metabolism, particularly at the level of liver cytochrome P450. This inhibition of drug metabolism by drugs or xenobiotics can take place in several ways including the destruction of pre-existing enzymes, inhibition of enzyme synthesis or by complexing and thus inactivating the drug-metabolising enzyme. The reader is also referred to chapters 4 and 5 where additional consideration is given to inhibition of drug metabolism and to chapters 6 and 7 where the pharmacological, toxicological and clinical implications of this phenomenon are discussed in detail.

3.3.1 Inhibition of drug metabolism by destruction of hepatic cytochrome P450

Many therapeutic drugs and environmental xenobiotics have the ability to destroy cytochrome P450 in the liver by a variety of mechanisms. For example it has been known for several years that xenobiotics containing an olefinic (C=C) or acetylenic (C≡C) function are porphyrinogenic, resulting in the formation of 'green pigments' in the liver. Some representative examples are given in Table 3.17. The chemical nature of these green pigments has recently been identified in most instances as alkylated or substrate–haem adducts derived from cytochrome P450. Interestingly, the majority of these olefinic and acetylinic compounds are relatively inert *per se* and require metabolic activation by cytochrome P450 itself (prior to adduct formation), and are therefore classified as 'suicide substrates', of the haemoprotein. It should be pointed out that the above suicide substrates are relatively selective towards cytochrome P450 in that cytochrome b_5 concentrations (the other haemoprotein of the hepatic endoplasmic reticulum membrane) are usually not affected by these porphyrinogenic xenobiotics.

Table 3.17 Inhibitors of the drug-metabolising enzymes: drugs and xenobiotics that destroy hepatic cytochrome P450

Olefinic derivatives	Acetylenic derivatives
Allobarbital	Acetylene
Allylisopropylacetamide	Ethchlorvynol
Aprobarbital	Ethynyloestradiol
Ethylene	Norethindrone
Fluoroxene	
Secobarbital	
Vinyl chloride	

A major consequence of haem modification by the above compounds is a significant and sustained drop in the levels of functional cytochrome P450, which in turn, results in a reduction in the capacity of the liver to metabolise drugs (Table 3.18). In addition, it would appear likely that the isoenzymes of hepatic cytochrome P450 exhibit differential susceptibilities to destruction by olefinic xenobiotics as exemplified by the pronounced susceptibility of the phenobarbiotone-induced variant (Table 3.18). The primary target of olefinic drug-induced loss of functional activity is at the haem locus and is substantiated by the observation that the administration of exogenous haem substantially restored both the hepatic cytochrome P450 content and drug-metabolising activity after allylisopropylacetamide treatment, a compound well known to destroy cytochrome P450.

The above suicidal activation of olefinic and acetylenic drugs to active metabolites resulting in cytochrome P450 haem destruction has profound pharmacological implications. For example, pretreatment of experimental animals with allylisopropylacetamide results in a significant increase in both hexobarbitone-induced sleeping time and zoxazolamine-induced paralysis time (Table 3.19), both these drugs undergoing cytochrome P450-dependent metabolism.

Table 3.18 Influence of allylisopropylacetamide (AIA) on hepatic drug metabolism, cytochrome b_5 and cytochrome P450[a]

Parameter	Source of liver microsomes		
	Control	Phenobarbital induced	3-Methylcholanthrene induced
		(% of activity in non-AIA treated animals)	
Cytochrome P450[b]	84	33	74
Cytochrome b_5[b]	ND[c]	113	ND[c]
Ethylmorphine N-demethylase [d]	62	8	35
p-Chloro-N-methyl-aniline N-demethylase [d]	75	51	75
Hexobarbital 3'-hydroxylase [d]	80	22	62

[a] Male rats were treated with either phenobarbital, 3-methylcholanthrene or without pretreatment (control). After an overnight fast, animals were then injected with allylisopropylacetamide (200 mg kg^{-1}), killed 1 h later and hepatic microsomes prepared by ultracentrifugation.

[b] nmol haemoprotein/mg protein.

[c] ND = not determined.

[d] Metabolism is expressed as nmol product formed/mg protein/15 min.

Derived from Farrell and Correia (1980), *J.Biol.Chem.*, **255** 10128–33.

Table 3.19 Influence of allylisopropylacetamide (AIA) on the pharmacological activity of hexobarbitone and zoxazolamine

	Control	AIA pretreated
Hexobarbitone sleeping time (min)	37.8+2.0	235.6+27.8
Zoxazolamine paralysis time (min)	257.6+10.5	477.8+31.5

Rats were given either hexobarbitone (150 mg/kg, i.p.) or zoxazolamine (100 mg/kg, i.p.) 11 h after allylisopropylacetamide (300 mg/kg, s.c.).

Adapted from Unseld and DeMatteis (1978). *Int. J.Biochem.*, **9** 865–9.

These results also support the concept that allylisopropylacetamide preferentially destroys the phenobarbitone-inducible cytochrome P450 isoenzyme in that hexobarbitone (a preferred substrate of this isoenzyme) sleeping time was increased six-fold, whereas zoxazolamine (not readily metabolised by this cytochrome P450 variant) paralysis time was only increased two-fold.

Accordingly, inhibition of drug metabolism by olefinic and acetylenic drugs and xenobiotics depends not only on the chemical nature of the drug itself but also on the prevailing complement of cytochrome P450 isoenzymes and their substrate specificities. It should be pointed out that although the above examples have highlighted the ability of allylisopropylacetamide to destroy cytochrome P450 and consequently inhibit drug metabolism, many drugs (listed in Table 3.17) have similar properties. In view of the common occurrence of olefinic and acetylenic groups in pharmaceutical products in use today, it is clear that many drug–drug interactions may be rationalised at the level of cytochrome P450 destruction.

Table 3.20 Acute effects of cobalt-haem on hepatic drug metabolism and haem biosynthesis

Activity	Saline control	Cobalt–haem treated
Ethylmorphine demethylase (pmol HCHO/mg/h)	0.56 ± 0.06	0.06 ± 0.02
Aniline hydroxylase (nmol 4-aminophenol/mg/h)	89.4 ± 6.9	32.8 ± 3.0
Microsomal haem (nmol/mg)	1.85 ± 0.04	0.89 ± 0.05
Cytochrome P450 (nmol/mg)	0.80 ± 0.04	0.19 ± 0.03
Cytochrome b_5 (nmol/mg)	0.35 ± 0.01	0.23 ± 0.01
Haem oxygenase (nmol bilirubin/mg/h)	2.65 ± 0.11	15.62 ± 0.09
δ-Aminolevulinate synthetase (nmol product/mg/h)	0.20 ± 0.05	0.02 ± 0.01

A single dose of cobalt–haem (125 pmol/kg, s.c.) was given to rats and the above data determined 72 h later.

Adapted from Drummond and Kappas (1982). *Proc. Nat. Acad. Sci. (USA).*, **79** 2384–8.

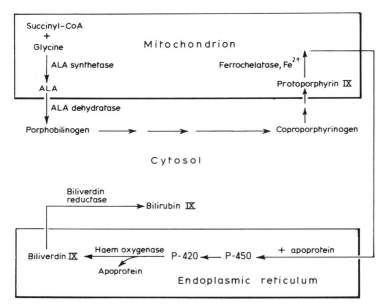

Figure 3.8 Biosynthesis of hepatic cytochrome P450–haem. ALA; α-aminolevulinic acid. Adapted from Testa and Jenner (1981) *Drug Metab. Rev.*, **12** 1–117.

3.3.2 Metal ions and hepatic cytochrome P450

Related to the above inhibitory effects of olefinic and acetylenic compounds on drug metabolism, is the ability of metal ions to substantially inhibit functional oxidase activity. The influence of metal ions on drug metabolism activities is considered in chapter 5 and it is informative to concentrate on the role of cobalt in drug biotransformation reactions. As shown in Table 3.20, cobalt (in the form of cobalt–haem) has a pronounced influence on both drug metabolism and the biosynthesis/degradation of hepatic haem. In particular, subsequent to cobalt pretreatment, drug metabolism was substantially decreased as was the hepatic microsomal content of cytochrome P450 and total haem. These results can be rationalised by the observation that cobalt has a pronounced inhibitory effect on the rate-limiting step of haem biosynthesis (delta-amino-levulinate synthetase) and additionally causes a substantial increase in haem catabolism, as reflected in the six-fold increase in haem oxygenase activity. The importance of these latter two enzymes in the synthesis and degradation of cytochrome P450–haem is shown in Figure 3.8.

Therefore in contrast to the olefinic and acetylenic drugs described above that act primarily by modifying existing cytochrome P450–haem, metal ions such as cobalt exert their inhibitory influences on drug metabolism by modulating both the *synthesis* and *degradation* of the haem prosthetic group of cytochrome P450.

3.3.3 Inhibition of drug metabolism by compounds forming inactive complexes with hepatic cytochrome P450

In addition to modulating the synthesis/degradation of hepatic cytochrome P450, certain classes of drugs and xenobiotics can inhibit drug metabolism by totally different means, e.g. by forming spectrally detectable, inactive complexes with the haemoprotein. These compounds are substrates of cytochrome P450 and require metabolism to exert their full inhibitory effects, in a similar manner to the olefinic and acetylenic drugs described earlier. However, unlike the latter group of drugs, inhibitors forming complexes are metabolised by cytochrome P450 forming a metabolic intermediate (or product) that binds tightly to the haemoprotein, thus preventing its further participation in drug metabolism and forming the basis of the observed inhibition. Examples of this class of inhibitors are shown in Table 3.21.

A direct comparison of the inhibition of drug metabolism by many of the drugs shown in Table 3.21 is complicated by the observation that the parent drugs themselves exhibit some degree of competitive or non-competitive inhibition, however it is clear that pre-incubation of the inhibitor with liver homogenates (i.e metabolism) results in a substantial increase in the inhibitory action of these drugs. Furthermore, the above observations are reflected *in vivo* where it has been observed that pretreatment of experimental animals with these inhibitors results in a substantial increase in both hexobarbital narcosis and zoxazolamine paralysis times.

Mechanistic studies on the inhibition by the above xenobiotics have mainly been attempted with amphetamine and methylenedioxybenzene compounds. Although the precise nature of the inhibitory, reactive metabolites responsible

Table 3.21 Drugs and xenobiotics inhibiting drug metabolism by complexing with cytochrome P450

Nitrogenous compounds	Non-nitrogenous compounds
Amphetamine	Isosafrole
Benactyzine	Piperonal
Cimetidine	Piperonyl butoxide
Dapsone	Safrole
Desimipramine	Sesamol
2-Diethylaminoethyl-2,2-diphenylvalerate (SKF 525 A)	
2,5-Dimethoxy-4-methylamphetamine (STP)	
Diphenhydramine	
Fenfluramine	
Isoniazid	
Methadone	
Methamphetamine	
Nortriptyline	
Oleandomycin	
Phenmetrazine	
Propoxyphene	
Sulfanilamide	
Triacetyloleandomycin	

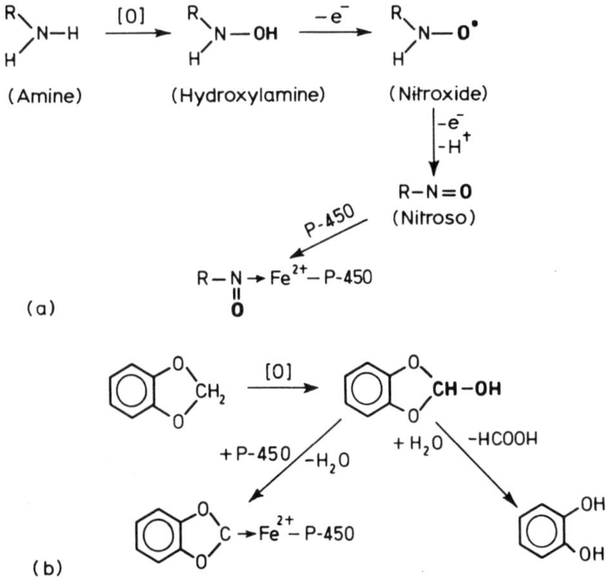

Figure 3.9 Proposed scheme for the formation of inhibitory cytochrome P450 complexes. (a) Amphetamines, (b) methylenedioxybenzene compounds. Adapted from Testa and Jenner (1981) *Drug Metab. Rev.*, **12** 1–117.

for the observed inhibition has not been absolutely delineated, there is strong evidence to support the theory that amphetamines act through the nitro (or nitroxide) metabolite and the methylenedioxybenzene derivatives are activated to a reactive carbene, and subsequent ligation to cytochrome P450 (Figure 3.9).

The complexes thus formed exhibit distinctive spectral characteristics and normally absorb maximally to 448 at 456 nm with the reduced (ferrous) form of cytochrome P450.

An interesting example of the above inhibition of drug metabolism is seen with the antibiotic, triacetyloleandomycin. Triacetyloleandomycin (similar in structure to erythromycin) is widely used in man to treat patients who are sensitive to penicillin and several reports have appeared where the administration of this antibiotic produces severe drug–drug reactions. For example, concomitant administration of triacetyloleandomycin with oral contraceptives may produce liver cholestasis, ischemic incidents with ergotamine, neurologic signs of carbamazepine intoxication and theophylline intoxication, suggesting that triacetyloleandomycin may somehow decrease the metabolism of these drugs in humans. Triacetyloleandomycin is interesting in that it induces its own demethylation and subsequent oxidation to a metabolite that forms a stable complex which absorbs at 456 nm with ferrous cytochrome P450 in the liver. On prolonged usage, this compound then inhibits drug oxidation and modulates the pharmacological activity of hexobarbitone (Table 3.22).

Table 3.22 Influence of triacetyloleandomycin on hexobarbitone metabolism and sleeping time

Drug pretreatment	Hexobarbitone hydroxylase activity (nmol/min/mg)	Hexobarbitone sleeping time (min)
None	1.8 ± 0.7	22 ± 8
1 h after TAO [a], 1 mmol/kg	1.7 ± 0.7	27 ± 9
24 h after TAO, 1 mmol/kg	1.2 ± 0.7	40 ± 18
TAO, 1 mmol/kg daily, for 4 days	0.3 ± 0.1	168 ± 58

[a] TAO; triacetyloleandomycin.

From Pessayre et al. (1981), Biochem. Pharmacol., **30** 559–64.

Accordingly, it has been postulated that the drug–drug reactions referred to above, can be rationalised by complexation and subsequent inhibition of cytochrome P450. Interestingly, a related antibiotic, oleandomycin (three free hydroxyl groups, not N-acetylated), shows similar properties to triacetyl-oleandomycin in that oleandomycin can also induce its own cytochrome P450-dependent metabolism. However, compared to triacetyloleandomycin, oleandomycin is both a weaker inducer of microsomal enzymes and also a much poorer substrate for the induced cytochrome P450, resulting in diminished inactive cytochrome P450 complex formation. This reduced activity of oleandomycin is consistent with the observation that no severe drug–drug interactions have been reported in man, and indicates that oleandomycin may be a safer substitute for triacetyloleandomycin in patients who receive other drugs metabolised by cytochrome P450.

Table 3.23 Miscellaneous drugs and xenobiotics that inhibit drug metabolism

Drug/xenobiotic	Use or occurrence	Nature of inhibitory action
Amantadine	Anti-viral drug	Specific mode of action unknown, may alter synthesis or degradation of cytochrome P450.
7,8-Benzoflavone	Plant consituent	Complex action, relatively specific competitive inhibitor of cytochrome P4501A sub-family.
Carbon disulfide	Vulcanisation of rubber, intermediate in rayon manufacture, occupational exposure significant	Denaturation and loss of hepatic cytochrome P450, sulfur binding to microsomal proteins possibly induces lipid peroxidation.
Carbon tetrachloride	Solvent	Loss of liver microsomal enzymes, lipid peroxidation, activated by cytochrome P450-dependent metabolism (carbon–halogen bond cleavage).
Cimetidine	Anti-ulcer drug	Binds to cytochrome P450 (competitive inhibitor?)
Chloramphenicol	Broad spectrum antibiotic	Competitive inhibitor of cytochrome P450, also non-competitive inhibition due to covalent binding to apoenzyme of cytochrome P450 (suicide substrate).
Cyclophosphamide	Anti-cancer and immunosuppressant drug	Denaturation of cytochrome P450 by alkylation of sulphydryl groups in active site.
Disulfiram	Therapy of alcoholics	Blocks ethanol oxidation at stage of acetaldehyde by inhibiting aldehyde oxidase.
Ellipticine	Anti-cancer drug	Potent competitive inhibitor of cytochrome P4501A sub-family.
Indomethacin	Anti-inflammatory drug	Depletes cytochrome P450 by unknown mechanism.
MAO inhibitors	Anti-depressant drugs	Inhibits monoamine oxidase (MAO) and enzymes of drug metabolism.
Metyrapone	Diagnosis of pituitary function	Binds tightly to and inhibits cytochrome P450.
Parathion	Insecticide	Haem loss and binding of atomic sulfur to cytochrome P450.
Tilorone	Anti-viral agent (interferon inducer)	Alters cytochrome P450 turnover, probably by increasing its degradation, or inhibition of synthesis.

3.3.4 Inhibition of drug metabolism: miscellaneous drugs and xenobiotics

The inhibition of drug metabolism is by no means confined to the above groups of compounds, and as shown in Table 3.23, many drugs and xenobiotics of diverse chemical structure can act through a variety of mechanisms to decrease the biotransformation of drugs. Again, the liver appears to be the most important and susceptible target organ for inhibition of drug metabolism and the data shown in Table 3.23 are only representative of the many reported instances of decreased drug metabolism.

It must always be remembered that the drug metabolising enzymes are also regulated by 'internal factors' involving endogenous or constitutive mechanisms. For example, interferons and interleukin cytokines produced by viral infections can lead to a down-regulation of cytochrome P450 mRNA, probably at the transcriptional level. In addition, the activity of the cytochrome P450 isoenzymes is substantially reduced by cAMP-dependent protein kinases and phosphorlyation of serine resides. This short-term regulation of the cytochrome P450s is thought to arise from phosphorlyation-dependent destruction of the cytochrome P450s, some isoenzymes being more susceptible to destruction than others. This general concept of 'internal factors' regulating drug metabolism is dealt with in much more detail in the next chapter.

3.4 Conclusions

The study of drug metabolism is both a complex and challenging one. This chapter has highlighted some of the *chemical* factors that are responsible for either the induction or inhibition of drug metabolism and it is clear that these factors make a significant and complex contribution to modulating drug biotransformation. Awareness of the extent of induction and inhibition of drug metabolism is complicated by the observation that the body burden of potentially regulatory chemicals is unknown to any degree of accuracy, primarily because of the significant role played by environmental chemicals. Because of the variable exposure of man to pharmaceutical products and environmental chemicals, it is not absolutely certain that we can define 'basal levels' of drug metabolism in any given population or ethnic group. However with the refinement of epidemiological and animal studies in drug metabolism, we can confidently look forward to the the future when at least we will have fully catalogued and largely understood the influence of pharmaceuticals and chemicals on drug metabolism. Whether or not this information will be acted upon however, is a different matter.

Further reading

Textbooks and symposia

Ruckpaul, K. and Rein, H. (1990) *Principles, mechanisms and biological consequences of induction. Frontiers in Biotransformation, Volume 2*, Taylor and Francis, London.

Reviews and original articles

Bababny, G. *et al.* (1988) Macrolide antibiotics as inducers and inhibitors of cytochrome P450 in experimental animals and man. In *Progress in Drug Metabolism, Volume 11* (G.G. Gibson), Taylor and Francis, London, pp. 61–98.

Bock, K.W. *et al.* (1990) Induction of drug-metabolising enzymes by xenobiotics. *Xenobiotica*, **20** 1101–11.

Boobis, A.R. *et al.* (1990) Species variation in the response of the cytochrome P450-dependent monooxygenase system to inducers and inhibitors. *Xenobiotica*, **20** 1139–61.

Bradfield, C.A. *et al.* (1991) Purification and *N*-terminal amino acid sequence of the Ah receptor from the C57BL/6J mouse. *Mol. Pharmacol.*, **39** 13–19.

Burbach, K.M. *et al.* (1992) Cloning of the Ah receptor cDNA reveals a distinctive ligand-activated transcription factor. *Proc. Nat. Acad. Sci. (USA)*, **89** 8185–9.

Chen, Y.L. *et al.* (1992) Effects of interleukin-6 on cytochrome P450-dependent mixed function oxidases in the rat. *Biochem. Pharmacol.*, **44** 137–48.

Craig, P.I. *et al* (1989) Rat but not human interferons suppress hepatic oxidative drug metabolism in rats. *Gastroenterology*, **97**, 999–1004.

Gibson, G.G. (1992) Co-induction of cytochrome P4504A1 and peroxisome proliferation: a causal or casual relationship? *Xenobiotica*, **22** 1101-9.

Green, S. (1992) Commentary: receptor-mediated mechanisms of peroxisome proliferators. *Biochem. Pharmacol.*, **43** 393–401.

Hankinson *et al.* (1991) Genetic and molecular analysis of the Ah receptor and CYP1A1 gene expression. *Biochimie*, **73** 61–6.

Issemann, I. and Green, S. (1990) Activation of a member of the steroid hormone receptor super-family by peroxisome proliferators. *Nature*, **347** 645–50.

Jansson, I. *et al* (1990) Relationship between phosphorylation and cytochrome P450 destruction. *Arch. Biochem. Biophys.*, **283** 285–92.

Landers, J.P. and Bunce, N.J. (1991) Review: the Ah receptor and the mechanism of dioxin toxicity. *Biochem. J.*, **276** 273–87.

Moochhala, S.M. *et al.* (1989) Induction and depression of cytochrome P450-dependent mixed function oxidase by a clonal consensus α-interferon (IFN-αCON$_1$) in the hamster. *Biochem. Pharmacol.*, **38** 439–47.

Murray, M. (1992) P450 enzymes: inhibition mechanisms, genetic regulation and effects of liver disease. *Clin. Pharmacokin.*, **23** 132–46.

Murray, M. and Reidy, G.F. (1990) Selectivity in the inhibition of mammalian cytochromes P450 by chemical agents. *Pharmacol. Rev.*, **42** 85–101.

Nebert, D.W. (1989) The Ah locus: genetic differences in toxicity, cancer, mutation and birth defects. *Crit. Rev. Toxicol.*, **20** 137–152.

Nelson, D.R. *et al* (1993). The P450 superfamily: update on new sequences, gene mapping, accession numbers, early trivial names of enzymes and nomenclature. *DNA Cell Biol*, **12** 1–51.

Oesch-Bartlomowicz, B. and Oesch, F. (1990) Phosphorlyation of cytochrome P450 isoenzymes in intact hepatocytes and its importance for their function in metabolic processes. *Arch. Toxicol.*, **64** 257–61.

Okey, A.B. (1990) Enzyme induction in the cytochrome P450 system. *Pharmacol. Therapeut.*, **45** 241–98.

Ortiz de Montallano, P.R. (1988) Suicide substrates for drug metabolising enzymes: mechanisms and biological consequences. In *Progress in Drug Metabolism, Volume 11* (G.G. Gibson), Taylor and Francis, London, pp. 99–148.

Park, B.K. and Kitteringham, N.R. (1990) Assessment of enzyme induction and enzyme inhibition in humans: toxicological implications. *Xenobiotica*, **20** 1171–85.

Poland, A. *et al.* (1991) Characterisation of polyclonal antibodies to the Ah receptor prepared by immunisation with a synthetic peptide hapten. *Mol. Pharmacol.*, **39** 20–6.

Postlind, H. *et al.* (1993) Response of human cyp1-luciferase plasmids to 2, 3, 7, 8 - tetrachlorobidenzo-*p*-dioxin and polycyclic aromatic hydrocarbons. *Toxicol, App. Pharmacol.*, **118** 255–62.

Saatcioglue, F. *et al.* (1990) Multiple DNA-binding factors interact with overlapping specificities at the aryl hydrocarbon response element of the cytochrome P4501A1 gene. *Mol. Cell. Biol.*, **10** 6408–16.

Testa, B. (1990) Mechanisms of inhibition of xenobiotic-metabolising enzymes. *Xenobiotica*, **20**, 1129–37.

Watson, A.J. and Hankinson, O. (1992) Dioxin- and Ah receptor-dependent protein binding to xenobiotic responsive elements and G-rich DNA studied by *in vivo* foot printing. *J. Biol. Chem.*, **266** 6874–8.

Waxman, D.J. and Azaroff, L. (1992) Review: phenobarbital induction of cytochrome P450 gene expression. *Biochem. J.*, **281** 577–92.

4 Factors affecting drug metabolism: internal factors

4.1 Introduction

Drugs can be metabolised by many different pathways (see chapter 1) and many factors can determine which pathway is used by which drug and to what extent a particular drug is biotransformed by a particular pathway. These factors range from the species of organism studied to the environment in which that organism lives. In order to discuss this topic, the factors affecting drug metabolism will be split into internal (i.e. physiological and pathological) factors (discussed in this chapter) and external factors (i.e. diet and environment) (discussed in chapter 5). These are, of course, purely arbitrary divisions and much interaction exists between the various factors (cf. hormonal, sex and age influences) – such interactions will be pointed out where they are important. The factors discussed here are also not an exhaustive list and other factors that play a role in controlling drug biotransformation will be found in the Further Reading section at the end of chapter 5. The factors to be discussed here are:

internal
- species
- genetic (strain)
- age
- sex
- hormones
- disease

external
- diet
- environment

Each of these factors will be examined in turn giving examples of the differences seen. Internal factors are discussed in this chapter, while external factors are discussed in chapter 5.

4.2 Species differences

There are many examples of species differences in drug metabolism. They can be found for both phase I and phase II metabolism and can be either quantitative

Table 4.1 The species variation in hexobarbitone metabolism, half-life and sleeping time

	Sleeping time (min)	Hexobarbitone half-life (min)	Hexobarbitone metabolism (units)
Mice	$12 \pm 8^\dagger$	19 ± 7	16.6
Rats	90 ± 15	140 ± 54	3.7
Dog	315 ± 105	260 ± 20	1
Man		~360	

†mean ± (standard deviation)
(Data from Quinn, G. P. *et al.* (1958) *Biochem. Pharmacol.*, **1** 152–9. Reprinted with permission of Pergamon Press.)

Table 4.2 Species differences in caffeine metabolism

Parameter	Man	Monkey	Rat	Rabbit
Total metabolism	322	235	160	137
Theobromine	28	13	15	19
Paraxanthine	193	11	20	42
Theophylline	16	190	20	30

Results expressed as pmoles of product per min.mg protein.
Data taken from Berthou *et al.* (1992) *Xenobiotica*, **22** 671–80

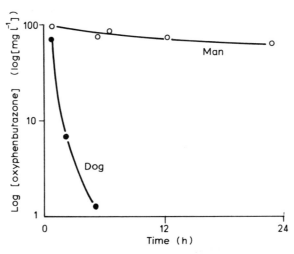

Figure 4.1 Plasma levels of oxyphenobutazone in man and dog. (From Burns, J.J. (1962) In *Metabolic factors controlling duration of drug action* (B.B. Brodie and E.G. Erdos), Pergamon, Oxford, p. 278. Used with permission of Pergamon Press.)

(same metabolic route but differing rates) or qualitative (differing metabolic routes). A few examples of each of these cases are given below.

The data in Table 4.1, for example, show that the oxidative metabolism of hexobarbitone varies widely between species and is inversely related to the half-life and duration of action of the drug. It should be noted that there is not always a direct relationship between metabolism, half-life and action of a drug. These problems are further discussed in chapter 7. In this case however, this would seem to indicate that man metabolises hexobarbitone at a slower rate than the dog and that the rate of elimination of the drug from the body is dependent on metabolism of the drug. Other species differences in phase I metabolism can be seen for caffeine (Table 4.2) where the formation of paraxanthine is highest in man and lowest in monkey, whereas theophylline production is highest in monkey and lowest in man, and with flunarizine metabolism which is higher in rat than in dog or human. As can be seen from Figure 4.1 oxyphenbutazone is rapidly cleared in the dog ($T_{1/2}$ 30 min) whilst, in man, the rate of metabolism is rather slow ($T_{1/2}$ 3 days). This is an extreme example but clearly indicates the possible range of species differences.

In terms of phase II metabolism, it is seen that sulfadimethoxine is converted to the glucuronide in man but no glucuronide formation is evident in rat, guinea-pig or rabbit. Phenol is metabolised by conjugation to glucuronic acid and/or sulfate and the relative proportion of each metabolite depends on the species studied (Table 4.3).

Table 4.3 The species variation in the relative proportions of phenol conjugation to glucuronide and sulfate

	Phenol conjugation[†]	
	Glucuronide	Sulfate
Cat	0	87
Man	23	71
Rat	25	68
Rabbit	46	45
Pig	100	0

[†] Expressed as excretion of a particular conjugate as a percentage of total excretion of drug.

(Data from various sources; see further reading section in chapter 5.)

All the above are simple examples of one or two enzymes acting on one compound. The situation can, however, become quite complex when a larger number of reactions are involved in the metabolism of one compound. Such a compound is amphetamine, the overall metabolism of which is shown in Figure 4.2.

The rat mainly hydroxylates amphetamine leading to conjugated products on the phenol group whereas the rabbit and guinea-pig (and man) mainly deaminate amphetamine. The guinea-pig further oxidises the ketone to benzoic acid and excretes conjugates of benzoic acid. The rabbit has been shown to reduce the ketone and excrete the subsequent conjugates of the alcohol.

It is clear from the information given above that different species can differ in their routes of metabolism as well as in the rates at which the metabolism occurs. Many other species have now been tested for drug-metabolising ability such as farm species (sheep, goats, cattle), fish, birds and even microorganisms and plants. In general, drug metabolism in non-mammalian species is lower than in mammals. Species differences in drug metabolism are important to industries involved in testing new chemicals, such as drugs, in order to achieve a suitable model of human toxicity. For such purposes an animal model is required that as nearly as possible mimics the metabolism of the compound seen in man. This animal model may be different for the different compounds under study.

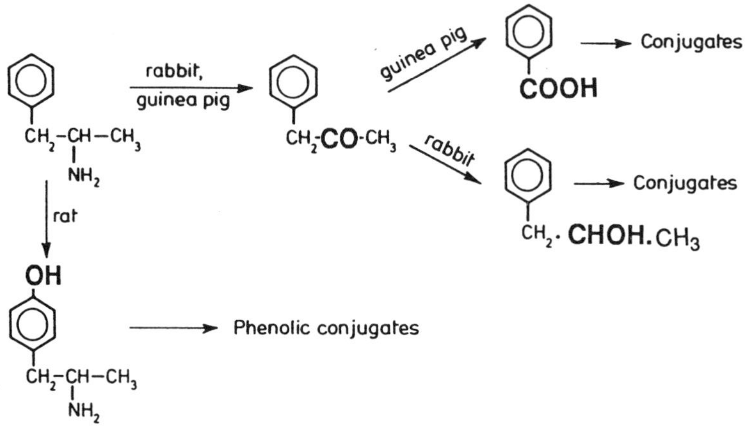

Figure 4.2 The metabolism of amphetamine in rabbit, guinea-pig and rat.

4.3 Genetic (strain/racial) differences

It has been noted above that significant differences in drug metabolism are found between species – it is equally true, however, that such differences exist within species. This is most easily seen in the inbred populations of rats and mice used in many studies but is also being found for other species, including man. The inbred strains of rodents, however, remain a model for genetic differences in other species. Such strain differences are referred to as genetic polymorphism.

The classical example of strain differences in drug metabolism is that of hexobarbitone metabolism in the mouse (see Table 4.4). It is seen that there is up to a 2.5-fold difference in sleeping time between one strain of mouse and another and that the values for the animals in the inbred groups are close to each other whereas the outbred group shows a wide variation in sleeping time. This is clear evidence for a genetic control of drug metabolism. The marked strain differences in the mouse have also been extended to include differences in the induction of drug metabolism (see chapter 3). Using two strains of mouse it was shown that one (strain C57) responds to treatment with 3-methylcholanthrene (3-MC, a polycyclic hydrocarbon inducer of aryl hydrocarbon hydroxylase) whilst the other (strain DBA) does not. Cross-breeding of the strains (see Table

Table 4.4 Hexobarbitone sleeping time in various strains of mouse

Strain	Sleeping time (min)
A/NL	48 ± 4[†]
BALB/cAnN	41 ± 2
C57L/HeN	33 ± 3
C3HFB/HeN	22 ± 3
SWR/HeN	18 ± 4
Swiss (outbred)	43 ± 15

[†]mean ± (standard deviation)

All animals were age-matched males and were given a standard dose of hexobarbitone.

(Data from various sources; see further reading section in chapter 5.)

Table 4.5 Effect of cross-breeding on the inducibility of polycyclic hydrocarbons of aryl hydrocarbon hydroxylase in mice

Strain	% Inducible
C57 (Ah^dAh^d)[†]	100
DBA (Ah^bAh^b)[†]	0
F1 (C57 × DBA) (Ah^bAh^d)[†]	100
F1 × C57	100
F1 × DBA	50
F1 × F1	75

[†]Ah is the gene for inducibility for polycyclic hydrocarbons Ah^d - inducible, Ah^b - not inducible

(Data from various sources; see further reading section in chapter 5.)

4.5) has shown that the inheritance of inducibility is an autosomal dominant (Ah_d) and accounted for by the presence of the Ah receptor. Inducibility by phenobarbital has also been shown to be under genetic control in the mouse. The biochemical mechanism of this induction is discussed in chapter 3.

In the rat, strain differences are reported to be less common and have, until recently, centred mainly around the genetically deficient Gunn rat which is unable to form many of the glucuronides produced by other strains of rat. Interbreeding of Gunn and normal rat strains leads to glucuronidation capacities intermediate between the two, indicating that neither trait is dominant. Genetic polymorphism in phase I metabolism has also been seen, notably with the rats showing other genetic deficiencies – the hyperbilirubinaemic EHBR rats have lower N-demethylase but higher aromatic hydroxylase activities whereas the obese Zucker rats show a lower aryl hydrocarbon hydroxylase activity compared to lean controls. These 'genetic differences' in drug metabolism, however, may be secondary to the primary genetic lesion.

Such genetic control of drug metabolism can only be studied in genetically pure (i.e. inbred) animals and such experiments cannot ethically be performed in man. Some observations on possible genetic control of drug metabolism in out-bred populations can, however, be done using breeding experiments (in animals) and family epidemiological data (in humans).

In man the possibility of showing a pure genetic influence on drug metabolism is hampered by interfering influences from environmental sources as it is impossible to keep humans in controlled conditions of environment, diet, etc. during their life-span. It has, however, been possible to show probable genetic effects on drug metabolism which have subsequently been proved using molecular biological techniques.

It has been recognised for a long time that large variations in drug metabolism occur in man and that discrete genetic sub-populations are apparently present in the human population. One such sub-population is the group of 'isoniazid slow acetylators'. The acetylation of isoniazid in the human population exhibits a bimodal distribution with about half the Caucasian population 'fast acetylators' and half 'slow acetylators'. Family studies show that 'slow acetylation' is an autosomal recessive trait. The unusually high incidence of this recessive trait in the population indicates that 'slow acetylation' must confer some sort of advantage or be closely linked to a gene giving such an advantage.

With respect to phase I metabolism by cytochrome P450, it has long been thought that some sort of genetic control was in operation based on the 'twin' studies of Vessell and others. It was found that identical twins resembled each other very closely in terms of drug metabolism whereas fraternal twins (twins developed from two different eggs) showed variations similar to the general population. Also the rates of metabolism of desmethylimipramine, nortriptyline, phenylbutazone and dicoumarol show good mutual correlation, indicating a common mechanism of control of their metabolism. Recently a definite genetic polymorphism in cytochrome P450-dependent drug oxidation has been seen using the marker substrate, debrisoquine. The 4-hydroxylation of this compound shows a bimodal distribution in the population (Figure 4.3). Again twin, family and population studies have indicated that the 'poor metaboliser' (PM) trait is recessive. In this case, however, no advantage appears to be linked to the PM trait as these are in low frequency in the population. The metabolism of a number of other drugs has now been linked to debrisoquine 4-hydroxylation so that poor metabolisers of debrisoquine also show low metabolism of sparteine, phenytoin, phenformin and phenacetin. If these correlations hold true then it can be seen that a simple test (debrisoquine 4-hydroxylation) could be used to pinpoint patients at risk due to low metabolism of the drug to be administered. Other individual differences in oxidative drug metabolism do not correlate to debrisoquine metabolism and may represent other genes controlling cytochrome P450 such as that for the metabolism of dextromethorphan, cytochrome P450dbl, and that for mephenytoin 4-hydroxylation. These polymorphisms are becoming regarded as of great clinical significance – a topic which is discussed in greater detail in chapter 7.

Another aspect of genetic control of drug metabolism is the appearance of racial differences. Differences between the metabolism of propranolol in Negro

and Caucasian populations exist as do differences in the glucuronidation of paracetamol between Caucasians and Chinese. Genetic differences within a population
can affect the rate at which drugs are metabolised and there is convincing evidence
to support a direct genetic control of some oxidative and conjugative reactions.

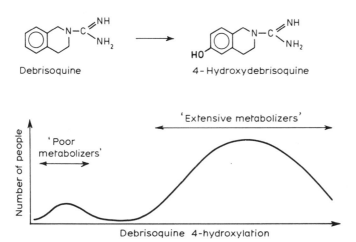

Figure 4.3 The distribution of the rate of metabolism of debrisoquine in the Caucasian population.

4.3.1 Mechanism of control of species and genetic differences

With the advent of powerful molecular biological techniques, it is becoming
apparent that most species and genetic differences in drug metabolism arise
because of the presence of genes coding for different enzymes. The inability of
the cat to glucuronidate phenol is due to the absence of a phenol glucuronosyltransferase whereas the bilirubin glucuronosyltransferase is still present
allowing the cat to clear the endogenous compound, bilirubin. The Gunn rat is
deficient in a number of glucuronosyltransferase activities and also has defective
glucuronosyltransferase enzymes. The species and strain differences in glucuronidation are thus due to the presence of different isoenzymes. Different
enzymes are also responsible for the 'fast' and 'slow' acetylators. The abnor-
mality has been traced to a defective gene both in the rat and in man.

Species differences in phase I oxidative metabolism are also thought to be
based on the different complement of cytochrome P450 in the different species.
Over 200 different isoenzymes of cytochrome P450 are now recognised, some
having widespread distribution (e.g. isoenzymes 1A1 and 2E1) whereas others
appear to be found only in one species (e.g. the human specific 2B7). The complement of cytochrome P450 isoenzymes determines, therefore, the range of
oxidative processes seen for individual drugs. For a further discussion of isoenzyme forms of drug-metabolising enzymes and their nomenclature see chapter 2.

A great deal of research has been performed on the polymorphism of cytochrome P450, particularly related to debrisoquine hydroxylation and it has been found that one isoenzyme of cytochrome P450 (2D6) is responsible for this enzyme activity in man. In the 'poor metaboliser' phenotype this isoenzyme was absent from the liver and three mutant alleles of CYP2D6 have been identified in 'poor metabolisers'.

In one instance at least, however, differences in the enzyme are not responsible for a species difference – and this is the inability of dog liver to acetylate sulfonamides (Figure 4.4). It has been suggested that a reversing enzyme, a deacetylase, converts the acetyl derivative back to the original compound or that a natural inhibitor exists in the dog.

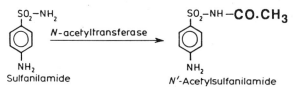

Figure 4.4 The acetylation of sulfanilamide.

A great deal of progress has been made in recent years in the understanding of the genetic control of drug metabolism but much work still needs to be done particularly at the molecular level to fully elucidate the mechanisms involved in this control.

4.4 Age

It has long been recognised that the young, and particularly the newborn, and the old of many animals are more susceptible to drug action. Studies on the development of drug-metabolising capacity have indicated that this increased sensitivity of neonates may be related to their very low or, at times, unmeasurable drug-metabolising capacity which subsequently develops in a species, strain, substrate and sex-dependent manner until adult levels of enzyme activity are achieved. The decrease in drug-metabolising capacity in old age also appears to be dependent on these factors.

4.4.1 Development of phase I metabolism

The activity of phase I drug metabolism may develop in many different ways between birth and adulthood and, indeed, may start developing at different times during gestation. The pattern of development varies according to the species and sex of the animal and on the substrate being investigated (and, thus, the particular isoenzyme being studied). A general idea of the patterns of development is shown in Figure 4.5.

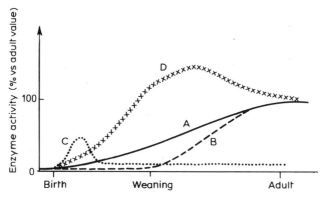

Figure 4.5 Developmental patterns for phase I metabolism.

In the rat, type A development is seen for many aromatic and aliphatic hydroxylation reactions e.g. aniline 4-hydroxylation. Type B development is shown for some *N*-demethylation reactions but in the case of hydroxylation of methylbenzanthracene, type B development is followed for a time but then activity falls to a very low level. Type C development is seen for the hydroxylation of 4-methylcoumarin.

In the rat, the sex differences (see next section) in drug metabolism exhibited by the adult confuse the developmental profile. Consider the 16α-hydroxylase acting on androst-4-ene-3, 17-dione (Figure 4.6). The enzyme activity develops according to type B in both the male and the female but at 30 days of age (puberty in the female) the activity in the female begins to disappear and by 40 days of age is undetectable, thus giving the sex differences seen in the adult period.

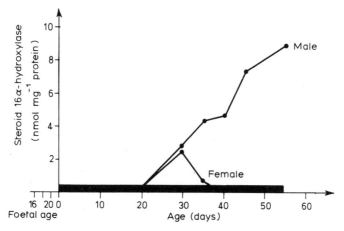

Figure 4.6 The development of the steroid 16α-hydroxylase in male and female rat liver (From Sternberg, A. (1976) *J. Endocr.*, **68** 265–72. Used with the permission of the author and publisher.)

In man and primates a somewhat different developmental profile is seen with measurable levels of activity in mid-term foetuses, indicating an earlier start to the process of development in primates. Indeed, some metabolic routes appear to be fully developed in foetal liver (e.g. the *N*-demethylation of codeine) whereas others are not present (e.g. *O*-demethylation of codeine) (Figure 4.7). It is, however, still quite clear that the foetus and neonate are, in general, less able to metabolise drugs than the adult.

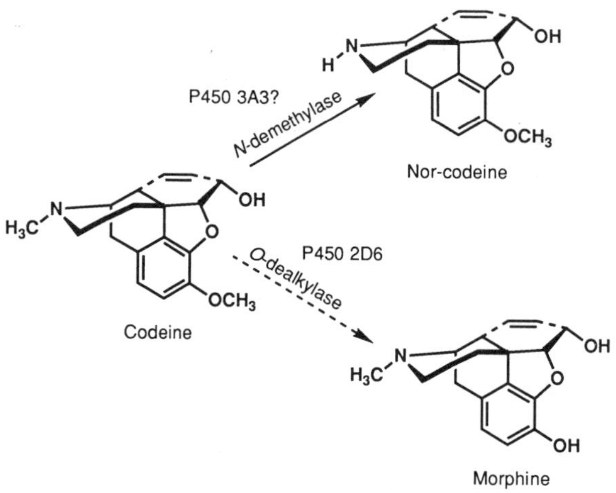

Figure 4.7 Two different metabolic routes for codeine.

In ageing animals and man, a further change in drug metabolism is seen. In rats a marked fall in overall drug metabolising capacity is seen, e.g. for testosterone hydroxylation. These changes are, however, associated with the sex differences in drug metabolism seen in the rat (see next section). There is evidence that the decline in drug metabolism in rats is also strain dependent. In man, it has been generally accepted that old age leads to a diminished capacity to clear drugs but evidence for a clear decline in drug metabolism is lacking. The apparent slower clearance in the elderly may be due in part to smaller active liver mass, decreased liver blood flow and altered plasma binding of drugs. An age-related decrease in drug metabolism is, thus, not a proven general fact.

4.4.2 Control of development of phase I metabolism

What are the biochemical changes associated with development of drug-metabolising ability, and how are they controlled? These are two essential questions for our understanding of the ontogenesis of phase I metabolism.

Most work has been performed on the cytochrome P450-dependent oxidation of drugs and the changes noted were those associated with the components of the enzyme system, notably cytochrome P450 itself. The development of a particular metabolic pathway seems to be closely linked to the appearance of a functional cytochrome P450 isozyme associated with that particular enzyme activity. For example, the 7α-hydroxylation of testosterone is highest at 3 weeks of age and is associated with a rise in cytochrome P4502A1 (an isozyme known to perform this reaction) whereas testosterone 16α-hydroxylation is associated with isoenzyme 2C11 and both of these are found to increase in parallel in male rats. The association between drug metabolism and cytochrome P450 isoenzyme profile continues into old age with the male-specific cytochrome P450s (e.g. 2C11) decreasing leading to a marked fall in the drug-metabolising activities associated with these proteins.

The development of NADPH–cytochrome P450 reductase follows that of cytochrome P450 in most cases except that appreciable activity of this enzyme is found in newborn animals. In the rat and ferret, NADPH–cytochrome c reductase is found in the neonatal period and the cytochrome P450 reductase does not develop until later. This cytochrome c reductase activity is thought to be associated with various azo reductase activities found in the neonatal period.

Hormonal changes during development can also have a profound effect on drug metabolism. The phenomenon of 'imprinting' of drug metabolism in the rat by androgens leading to sexual differentiation of enzyme activities in the adult period is important in development. It is, in fact, thought that the rapid but transient increase in activity seen for some enzymes in the first few days after birth is due to the androgen secreted at this time in order to 'imprint' the male. The rise in enzyme activity seen after weaning (type B development) is also thought to be hormone related – the hormone in this case being progesterone delivered to the infant in the mother's milk. Progestagens are, indeed, known to inhibit drug metabolism (see Table 4.6). Growth hormone has also been shown to inhibit drug metabolism in the developing rat.

Table 4.6 The effect of reduced progesterone analogues on progesterone and coumarin metabolism in newborn rats

Progestagen added	Progesterone 16-hydroxylase	Coumarin 3-hydroxylase
None	$24.1 \pm 0.7^{\dagger}$	5.0 ± 0.3
5ß-Pregnane-3α,20α-diol	$15.7 \pm 0.7^{*}$	$3.3 \pm 0.4^{*}$
5ß-Pregnane-3α-ol-20-one	$15.5 \pm 1.0^{*}$	$2.3 \pm 0.3^{*}$
5ß-Pregnane-3,20-dione	$16.8 \pm 0.6^{*}$	$3.1 \pm 0.3^{*}$

[†]activities expressed as nmoles metabolite formed per hour per mg protein; mean ± (standard deviation)
[*]= $p < 0.05$
(From Kordish, R. and Feuer, G. (1972) *Biol. Neonate,* **20** 50–67, modified. Used with permission of S. Karger AG, Basel.)

Even with all this wealth of information, the critical question, 'What is the rate-limiting step in the development of drug-metabolising capacity?' remains, however, unanswered. The answer is best summarised by Short who stated, 'It seems most likely that after birth the monooxygenase system develops largely as a unit'. The rate-limiting factor to the development of this unit depends on the species, strain and sex of the animal and the substrate under investigation.

4.4.3 Development of phase II metabolism

The development of phase II metabolism is of considerable importance as excretion of drugs and other xenobiotics is mainly in the form of conjugates – the conjugation reactions being generally regarded as the true 'detoxification' reactions. Changes in the ability of the body to conjugate drugs therefore leads to large changes in toxicity of the drugs. The balance between phase I and phase II metabolism during development is also of great importance. This topic is further discussed in chapter 6. As with the phase I metabolism, phase II routes of metabolism are poorly represented in the foetal and neonatal animal and mainly develop perinatally.

(a) *Glucuronidation.* The most thoroughly studied of the conjugation reactions is glucuronidation and here we are indebted to Professor G. Dutton for his group's excellent work on the development of glucuronidation. This group has found that there are two different developmental types (not corresponding to the types found for phase I metabolism) as shown in Figure 4.8.

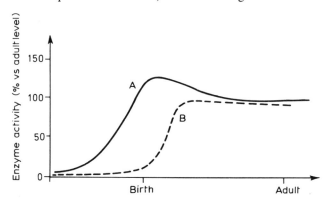

Figure 4.8 The developmental patterns of glucuronidation in the rat. Curve A is late foetal cluster (*p*-nitrophenol as substrate); B is neonatal cluster (bilirubin as substrate).

Type A development is characterised by a steadily increasing activity until birth, reaching a peak around birth and then declining slightly to adult levels, and type B development is characterised by very low activity until birth followed by a rapid rise to adult levels. Type A enzymes belong to the late foetal cluster of enzymes and metabolises predominantly exogenous compounds (e.g. *p*-nitrophenol) and type B belongs to the neonatal cluster of Greengard and metabolises mainly endogenous compounds (e.g. bilirubin). In man little glucuronidation activity is seen until after birth.

(b) *Control of development of glucuronidation.* The appearance of glucuronosyl transferase activity during development appears to be closely linked to that of the glucuronosyltransferase protein. The physiological control of development has been studied in some detail. One series of studies involved the use of chick embryos which can readily be cultured to facilitate the investigation. In this case, glucuronosyltransferase activity is negligible until hatching and then undergoes a rapid increase reaching adult level in 1–3 days. If embryonic liver is cultured its glucuronosyltransferase activity increases to adult levels spontaneously and precociously. The process of maturation involves a morphological change in the cells and protein synthesis. This precocious increase in activity in culture does not occur if the liver is cultured in the presence of the chorioallantoic membrane indicating that induction of enzyme activity can only take place after removal of the repressive influence of the embryonic environment. The nature of this repressive influence is unclear. Certain hormones were, however, shown to overcome this repressive influence such as corticosteroids (with thyroxine acting synergistically). In the chick, therefore, postnatal development is probably stimulated by corticosteroid production (and thyroxine).

In mammalian foetuses, a similar mechanism of control was shown to be in operation. Embryonic liver cultured on chorioallantoic membrane, as before, maintained its embryonic character. A pituitary graft onto the membrane stimulated glucuronosyltransferase activity to the adult level. Again corticosteroids were shown to be the natural inducers by injection of the mother with hormones and subsequent examination of the foetal liver.

This mechanism of control applies to the late foetal cluster, i.e. glucuronosyl transferase activity towards p-nitrophenol and not the neonatal cluster. There is little clear information on the changes in glucuronidation in ageing animals or man.

(c) *Other phase II reactions.* Compared to glucuronidation very little data is available on the developmental patterns of other phase II reactions (i.e. sulfation, acetylation, amino acid conjugation, methylation and glutathione conjugation). The sulfo-conjugating enzymes (sulfotransferases) are thought to be high in foetal tissue (about adult levels) and, particularly in the case of steroid sulfotransferases, develop early in gestation. This is probably a function of their role in biosynthetic and transport pathways of metabolism rather than an excretory role. Hypothalamo–pituitary factors have been implicated in the control of development of steroid sulfotransferases (see section 4.5.3). An inhibitor of phenol sulfotransferases has also been found to be present at birth accounting for the apparent fall in activity of the enzyme seen around this period.

For acetylation it was found that premature infants acetylate sulfonamides less well than full-term infants but this latter group are still below the activity of adults. In the rabbit, acetylation of isoniazid is low at 6 days, rises steadily to 14 days and then surges to adult levels between 21 and 28 days. In contrast, in the cow, N-acetylation of sulfamethoxazole is higher in the calf than the adult.

Amino acid conjugation and methylation are similar to acetylation being low in foetal and neonatal tissues and developing steadily to adult levels.

Glutathione conjugation is of particular importance in being one of the major defence mechanisms in the body against xenobiotic electrophiles (many of which are mutagens and/or carcinogens). Early studies on the development of the enzyme responsible for glutathione conjugation (glutathione-*S*-transferase) showed a steady rise in activity from 3 days prenatally to 20 days postnatally in the rat by which time adults levels had been reached. In man an even earlier development of enzyme activity is thought to occur. Later studies have shown multiple forms of glutathione-*S*-transferase, one of these, glutathione-*S*-transferase B (now referred to as GST 2-2 but originally known as ligandin), having been particularly well studied. Ligandin is absent in foetal animals and man but subsequently appears in the perinatal period and increases to reach adult levels in the first few weeks of life. Induction, by exogenous or endogenous compounds, of ligandin can also occur *in utero* particularly if other drug-metabolising enzymes are lacking (e.g. Gunn rats – see section 4.3).

In summary, phase II metabolism is generally low or absent in foetal animals, develops perinatally reaching adult levels early in life and does not seem to alter in any consistent way in old age. The multiplicity of the various enzymes involved should be remembered when studying these reactions in terms of development as the different forms of the enzyme may develop at different times and different rates.

Age-related changes are seen by the clinician to be of major importance as special dosage schedules for infants are used which are unrelated to the dose for an adult on a weight basis. The reduced metabolic activity of the older patients may also be important but this is of less general applicability.

4.5 Hormonal control of drug metabolism

Hormones play a central role in the control of drug metabolism as can be seen from the sections on age and sex differences in drug metabolism, and, in particular, the hormones of the pituitary and adrenal gland and the sex organs are involved in the developmental control and sexual dimorphism. In this section it is intended to expand this idea to include all endocrine organs and to further examine the role of the pituitary, adrenal and sex glands and consider the thyroid and pancreas in terms of their effects on drug metabolism. The effects of pregnancy (as a major disturbance in the hormonal balance of the female body) on drug metabolism will also be discussed.

4.5.1 Pituitary gland

The pituitary gland controls the release of hormones from the other endocrine organs (except in the case of the pancreas where other influences are more important) and thus any effects exerted by the endocrine organs will be mimicked by the pituitary gland. Direct effects of pituitary hormones have also been seen, however, as noted in section 4.4. Other direct effects on hepatic drug metabolism are seen with adrenocorticotrophic hormone (ACTH), luteinising hormone (LH) and follicle stimulating hormone (FSH) and prolactin. The pituitary gland, therefore, occupies a central role in the hormonal control of drug metabolism and the individual effects of this organ will be discussed under the various endocrine glands that it controls.

4.5.2 Sex glands

Sex glands in this context refer to the endocrine glands, the testes (in the male) and the ovaries (in the female). The effect of these organs on drug metabolism are, as would be expected, mainly related to sex differences.

Sex differences in drug actions were first noted by Nicholas and Barron in 1932 who saw that female rats required only half the dose of barbiturate needed by male rats to induce sleep. Later studies indicated that this was due to the reduced capacity of the female to metabolise the barbiturates. Such sex differences in drug metabolism have now been shown for a wide range of substrates including the endogenous sex steroids. Sex differences in drug metabolism have also been noted in the mouse for ethylmorphine and steroid metabolism and in man for antipyrine, diazepam and steroid metabolism although not to such a marked extent as in the rat. In general the sex differences seen in the mouse are the opposite of those seen in the rat whereas man shows a similar sex-differentiated pattern to the rat. Recently the goat has been shown to exhibit the opposite sex differences to those found in the rat. Sex differences in the rat tend to follow a general pattern of the male metabolising faster than the female particularly with regard to phase I metabolism but there are exceptions such as the 3-hydroxylation of lignocaine.

In phase II metabolism, there are marked sex differences in glucuronidation (e.g. of 1-naphthol), sulfation (e.g. of steroids) and glutathione conjugation.

4.5.3 Mechanism of control of sex differences

In 1958 it was proposed that androgens were the regulators of the sex differences. Thus the presence or absence of androgen in the perinatal period determines whether an animal is male or female with respect to drug metabolism – a process known as 'imprinting' (for review see Skett and Gustafsson, 1979). Although this still holds true, the mechanism by which perinatal androgens exert this effect is now well established and it is accepted that there is no direct effect of the androgen on the liver. The perinatal androgen 'imprints' a pattern of growth hormone secretion from the pituitary gland and it is this male or female pattern of growth hormone secretion that gives the sex differences in drug metabolism.

With respect to cytochrome P450-dependent drug oxidation, the differing patterns of growth hormone (GH) are known to cause the induction or repression of particular isoenzymes of cytochrome P450. For instance the female pattern of GH (a continuous low level of hormone) gives a reduction in cytochrome

P4502C11 and an increase in 2C12 by altering the transcription of the particular gene. This alteration leads to the female type of metabolism – a decreased 16α-hydroxylase (associated with isoenzyme 2C11) and increased 15β-hydroxylase activity (associated with isoenzyme 2C12) (Figure 4.9). Sex differences in drug metabolism are of great importance when dealing with rats, mice and some farm animals (e.g. goats) but seem to be of less importance in a clinical context.

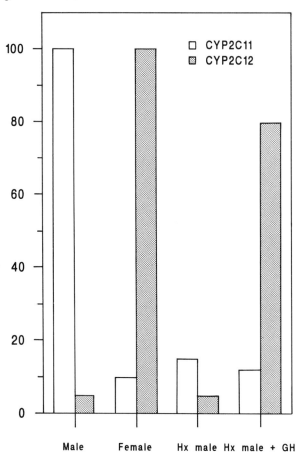

Figure 4.9 The effect is continuous growth hormone treatment on the expression of CYP2C11 and CYP2C12 genes. Hx = hypophysectomised

The adrenal glands have already been discussed in terms of glucocorticoid control of development of drug metabolism (see section 4.4). The adrenal glands are, however, also thought to be involved in the regulation of drug metabolism in the adult period. Adrenalectomy has been shown to reduce the phase I microsomal metabolism of a number of xenobiotics, whereas glucocorticoid replacement therapy can reverse the effect of adrenalectomy (see Figure 4.10).

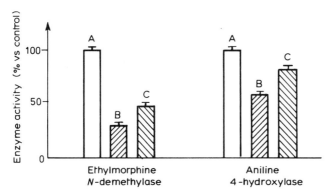

Figure 4.10 The effect of adrenalectomy and corticosteroid replacement therapy on the hepatic metabolism of ethylmorphine and aniline. A is control; B, results from adrenalectomy; C, adrenalectomy followed by corticosterone treatment. (From Furner, R.L. and Stitzel, R.E. (1968) *Biochemical Pharm.*, **17** 121–7. Used with permission of Pergamon Press.)

Glucocorticoids have, however, been shown to mimic or potentiate the action of adrenalectomy in a number of instances. This apparent paradox in glucocorticoid action was resolved by Tredger who showed that the natural, short-acting glucocorticoids are inhibitory to drug metabolism whereas the synthetic potent analogues (which are not so readily metabolised) are stimulatory (act as enzyme inducers). Few effects of adrenal hormones are seen on phase II metabolism except as regards development (see above) but again synthetic glucocorticoids (e.g. dexamethasone) can induce some phenol sulfotransferase activities.

4.5.4 Thyroid glands

The thyroid glands are known to have some influence on drug metabolism. The effect of thyroidectomy in the rat depends on the substrate being studied and on the sex of the animal used (see Table 4.7). In a recent study of the phase I metabolism of lignocaine, it was shown that there was an increase in the N-deethylation and 3-hydroxylation in both male and female animals whereas

Table 4.7 Sex dependency of the effect of thyroidectomy on hepatic drug metabolism

Enzyme activity	Effect of thyroidectomy	
	Male animals	Female animals
Alcohol oxidation	(Not determined)	Increase
Cytochrome P450	Increase	Increase
Ethylmorphine N-demethylase	Decrease	Decrease
Benzo[a]pyrene hydroxylase	Decrease	Decrease
Aniline 4-hydroxylase	Decrease	Decrease
5ß-Reductase	(No change)	Increase
11ß-Hydroxysteroid dehydrogenase	Decrease	Increase

(Data from various sources; see further reading section in chapter 5.)

imipramine and diazepam metabolism were unaffected in the male. Imipramine metabolism was enhanced in the female. The effects noted in the earlier studies could be reversed by L-thyroxine treatment.

In humans, the thyroid gland has also been implicated in the control of drug metabolism. For the limited number of substrates used (antipyrine, paracetamol and aspirin), thyroidectomy always decreases their apparent metabolism. Further work may reveal a substrate dependence in effect as seen in the rat.

The mechanism of thyroid control of drug metabolism is unclear and may involve changes in cytochrome P450 although not all changes in enzyme activity are correlated with changes in cytochrome P450. Other changes that have been reported are an increase in haem oxygenase (which degrades cytochrome P450) and changes in inducibility in thyroidectomised animals. The multiplicity of cytochrome P450 should be remembered here as the thyroid hormones may change the proportion of different isoenzymes without necessarily changing the overall amount.

Phase II metabolism can also be affected by thyroidectomy – the glucuronidation of 1-naphthol is significantly lower in thyroidectomised rats of both sexes (Table 4.8). Sulfation and gamma-glutamyltranspeptidase activities are also thyroid-dependent. Thus the thyroid glands may play a role in the hormonal control of drug metabolism and, in the rat, may be involved in the sexual differentiation of drug metabolism.

Table 4.8 The effect of thyroidectomy (TX) on glucuronidation of 1-naphthol in liver cubes

Animal	1-Naphthol glucuronide formed $(\text{min}^{-1}\text{g}^{-1}\text{ liver})^{\dagger}$
Control male	1.70 ± 0.17
TX male	$1.27 \pm 0.12^*$
Control female	0.59 ± 0.08
TX female	$0.34 \pm 0.03^*$

†Results expressed as mean $\pm$ (standard deviation)
$^* = p < 0.05$

4.5.5 Pancreas

The pancreas produces and secretes one hormone of particular relevance to the control of drug metabolism, i.e. insulin. This is produced by the β-cells of the endocrine pancreas. Diabetes mellitus (a reduction in the amount or action of insulin caused by genetic abnormalities or chemically induced by means of streptozotocin administration) causes marked changes in hepatic phase I and II metabolism (see Table 4.9).

Phase I metabolism in the liver, exemplified by diazepam and lignocaine hydroxylation and N-dealkylation, shows a marked decrease in activity (except lidocaine 3-hydroxylation) in diabetic rats whereas enzyme activities in the intestine rise. As usual in the rat, the sex of the animal must be taken into

Table 4.9 The effect of streptozotocin (STZ)-induced diabetes on liver weight, blood glucose and drug metabolism in the male rat

	Control	STZ-treated	
Liver (% body weight)	3.58 ± 0.28[†]	4.32 ± 0.47	**
Blood glucose (mM)	8.67 ± 0.68	32.13 ± 2.54	***
Cytochrome P450 (nmoles mg^{-1})	0.56 ± 0.06	0.54 ± 0.08	n.s.
Diazepam 3-hydroxylase (pmoles min^{-1} g^{-1} protein)	60.3 ± 21.4	35.6 ± 4.8	*
Diazepam N-demethylase (pmoles min^{-1} g^{-1} protein)	32.4 ± 7.6	19.4 ± 5.1	*
Lignocaine 3-hydroxylase (pmoles min^{-1} g^{-1} protein)	35 ± 6	31 ± 16	n.s.
Lignocaine N-de-ethylase (pmoles min^{-1} g^{-1} protein)	317 ± 118	182 ± 65	*
1-Naphthol glucuronidation (nmoles product min^{-1} g^{-1} liver)	1.42 ± 0.22	1.57 ± 0.15	n.s.

[†]mean ± S.D. (of at least 4 values)
* = $p < 0.05$; ** = $p < 0.01$; *** = $p < 0.001$; n.s. = not significant, $p < 0.05$

consideration – all of the effects noted are only seen in the male. Replacement therapy with insulin can reverse the effects of diabetes caused by streptozotocin (see Figure 4.11). It is accepted that the effect of insulin is direct on the liver in some cases and in others the effect is secondary to the metabolic changes induced by diabetes (i.e. ketone production inducing cytochrome P4502E1). The diabetes-inducible cytochrome P450 is now recognised to be isoenzyme 2E1 which is also induced by acetone.

It would appear that thyroid, pituitary and adrenal hormones (except adrenal androgens) and insulin can act directly on the liver, whereas androgens and oestrogens exert their effects on the liver by interaction with the hypothalamo–hypophyseal axis, modifying the release of pituitary hormones.

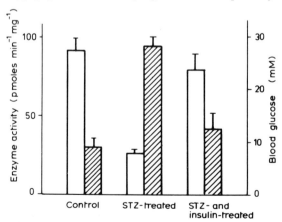

Figure 4.11 The effect of streptozotocin (STZ) and insulin treatment on blood glucose levels and the N-de-ethylation of lignocaine in the rat liver. Plain block-diagrams represent enzyme activity; hatched blocks, blood glucose.

The hormonal control of drug metabolism is, as can be seen from the above summary, quite complex and is made more so by the numerous interactions of the hormones involved (e.g. GH and insulin have been shown to be mutually antagonistic.) No one hormone can be considered in isolation. Hormonal control is considered of major importance when examining drug metabolism in rodents and some farm species but is little considered in clinical practice.

4.5.6 Pregnancy

Pregnancy is a natural condition when the hormonal balance of the female body is grossly altered. The oestrous (menstrual) cycle ceases and there are large changes in blood levels of peptide and steroid hormones. It therefore seems fitting to discuss the effects of pregnancy on drug metabolism in this section dealing with hormonal control.

The study of drug metabolism during pregnancy in the human is rather difficult due to the obvious ethical considerations of administering drugs to a pregnant woman. Most of the work, therefore has been done in animal models. In the rat, pregnancy causes a general decrease in drug metabolism, e.g. 3-hydroxylation of coumarin, but a more complex change in the metabolism of the endogenous progestagen, progesterone (Table 4.10). These changes are thought to be due to progesterone or its metabolites which are found in blood in high concentrations during pregnancy. This is the same phenomenon seen in suckling infants (see section 4.4) where progestins in the mother's milk are thought to inhibit drug metabolism in the young animal in certain cases.

Table 4.10 The effect of pregnancy on the metabolism of coumarin and progesterone in the rat

	Non-pregnant	Pregnant
Coumarin 3-hydroxylase	18.61 ± 1.92	$10.28 \pm 1.05^*$
Progesterone 16α-hydroxylase	6.68 ± 0.15	$4.63 \pm 0.33^*$
Progesterone 5α-reductase	15.38 ± 0.26	$21.86 \pm 0.47^*$

Results expressed as nmoles product $h^{-1} g^{-1}$ protein; mean $\pm$ (standard deviation)
$^* = p < 0.05$
(From Kordish, R. and Feuer, G. (1972) *Biol. Neonate*, **20** 58-67, modified. Used with permission of S. Karger AG, Basel.)

4.6 The effects of disease on drug metabolism

Many disease states have been shown to affect the way in which the body clears drugs and these are listed in Table 4.11. The major effects are seen with diseases affecting the liver. This is hardly surprising as the liver is quantitatively the most important site of drug biotransformation. Other diseases, however, such as infections and endocrine disorders are also important when looking at drug metabolism. In this section each disease will be looked at in turn and then a

Table 4.11 Disease states that affect drug metabolism

Cirrhosis of the liver
Alcoholic liver disease
Cholestatic jaundice
Liver carcinoma
Endocrine disorders
Diabetes mellitus
Hypo- and hyperthyroidism
Acromegaly
Pituitary dwarfism
Infections
Bacterial
Viral
Malaria
Inflammation

general summary included to draw together the various aspects of disease influences on drug metabolism. It will be appreciated that the majority of the data is clinical as diseases of man are the most widely studied.

4.6.1 Cirrhosis

In cirrhosis, parts of the liver are replaced by fibrous tissue and the number of functional hepatocytes is reduced. It is therefore not unreasonable that drug metabolism is impaired in this condition and, indeed, the oxidative metabolism of chlordiazepoxide to its primary metabolite, desmethylchlordiazepoxide is slower in cirrhotic patients. This appears to be true also for the conversion of diazepam to desmethyldiazepam. Oxazepam and lorazepam metabolism, however, which is purely glucuronidation is not affected by cirrhosis. The N-dealkylation of lignocaine is grossly affected by cirrhosis as is the oxidation of propranolol with a much longer half-life for each drug. The same increase in elimination half-life is seen for theophylline and tolbutamide (an oral hypo-glycaemic). The problem of equating plasma half-life with metabolism is evident here as both lignocaine and propranolol are highly extracted drugs and, thus, the blood flow through the liver rather than the rate of metabolism is important (see chapter 7).

Various drugs which are normally metabolised by the liver are not affected with respect to their metabolism by cirrhosis. Morphine, for example is converted to its glucuronide by the liver and this conversion is unaffected by cirrhosis. In one instance the activation of a prodrug is impaired by cirrhosis. The conversion of prednisone (the prodrug) to prednisolone (the active drug) is slower in cirrhotic patients.

One other aspect of cirrhosis should also be considered and that is enzyme induction by drugs and other xenobiotics. It is well known that many drugs can increase the rate at which they and other drugs are metabolised (see chapter 3). The cirrhotic condition can greatly diminish the degree of increase in drug metabolism. For example, phenobarbitone pretreatment of normal subjects markedly increases the metabolism of antipyrine whereas similar pretreatment of cirrhotic patients has little effect. Glutethimide can, however, induce antipyrine metabolism in cirrhotic patients. This apparent paradox can be explained in terms of the multiplicity of drug-metabolising enzymes, the differing degrees of cirrhosis and the different inducing agents used. The effect of cirrhosis on enzyme induction, therefore, remains unclear. Table 4.12 summarises the effect of cirrhosis on drug metabolism. It is noted that cirrhosis appears to depress phase I but have no effect on glucuronidation.

Table 4.12 The effect of liver cirrhosis on drug metabolism

Drugs affected	(Metabolic route)	Drugs not affected	(Metabolic route)
Chlordiazepoxide	(N-Demethylation)	Oxazepam	(Glucuronidation)
Diazepam	(N-Demethylation)	Lorazepam	(Glucuronidation)
Barbiturates	(Oxidation)	Morphine	(Glucuronidation)
Antipyrine	(Oxidation)	Paracetamol	(Glucuronidation)
Glutethimide	(Oxidation)		
Methadone	(Oxidation)		
Salicylates	(Glycine conjugation)		

(Data from various sources; see further reading section in chapter 5.)

4.6.2 Alcoholic liver disease

Chronic alcohol administration can lead to a condition similar to that of cirrhosis with large portions of the liver replaced by fibrous masses following the death of the parenchymal cells. Before this stage is reached, however, alcohol adminis- tration can markedly affect drug metabolism in different ways. The stages of alcohol's effects on drug metabolism are summarised in Figure 4.12.

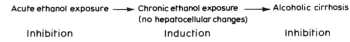

Figure 4.12 The stages in the development of the effect of ethanol on hepatic drug metabolism.

Acute ethanol exposure in general decreases drug metabolism such that drugs metabolised primarily by phase I routes e.g. chlordiazepoxide, diazepam, aminopyrine, pentobarbitone and chlorpromazine or phase II routes e.g. lorazepam, p-nitrophenol, harmol and paracetamol exhibit longer half-lives if administered with ethanol. The inhibition of phase I metabolism is thought to be due to ethanol binding to cytochrome P450 (the liver actually has a cytochrome P450-dependent ethanol oxidising system – cytochrome P4502E1) in a competi- tive manner. Inhibition of electron flow from the reductase to cytochrome P450 has also been seen. Ethanol seems to inhibit the metabolism of type II binding substrates more than type I binding substrates. The alteration of the NADP/NADPH ratio and the disturbance of the lipid environment have also been put forward as possible explanations of the effects of ethanol on phase I metabolism. A number of workers have suggested a mediating role of the adrenal gland in the effects of ethanol.

The inhibition of phase II metabolism is not due to inhibition of the enzymes involved. In the case of glucuronidation, ethanol is thought to increase the NADH/NAD ratio (via oxidation of ethanol by alcohol dehydrogenase). This in turn inhibits the production of the co-factor for glucuronidation, UDP–glucuronic acid (which requires NAD) (Figure 4.13). In one reaction, acute ethanol administration has been shown to increase activity and that is the acetylation of sulfadimidine. No explanation for this effect has been given.

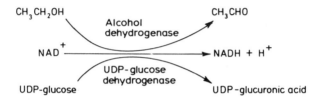

Figure 4.13 The interaction of ethanol with UDPGA production.

Chronic ethanol exposure in the absence of pathological change in the liver is usually associated with enhanced drug metabolism. Ethanol is classed as a microsomal enzyme inducer of a type different to both phenobarbitone and the polycyclic hydrocarbons (see chapter 3). It has been shown to induce phase I and II metabolism. In terms of induction of cytochrome P450, ethanol is thought to cause an increase in the amount of isoenzyme 2E1 (the isoenzyme also induced by acetone and in diabetes) and this leads to the marked increase in aniline 4-hydroxylase seen after ethanol exposure. Once the extent of alcoholic liver disease has become extensive, a pattern of effects similar to cirrhosis is seen such that metabolism of diazepam, paracetamol and lignocaine is reduced.

4.6.3 Viral hepatitis

Little is known of the effects of viral hepatitis but what information is available suggests that this condition causes a decrease in hepatic drug metabolism. Chlordiazepoxide clearance is decreased in viral hepatitis as is the clearance of meperidine (pethidine). Clearance of lignocaine is unaffected by viral hepatitis whereas tolbutamide exhibits an enhanced clearance in this condition (see discussion of drug clearance in chapter 7).

4.6.4 Hepatoma

A hepatoma is a cancerous growth derived from the liver parenchymal cells. The drug metabolising capacity of the tumour cells, however, is very much less than the corresponding normal cells. This is a typical loss of differentiated function in dedifferentiated cells. The loss of differentiated function is noted for the metabolism of aniline to 4-aminophenol. The level of aniline metabolism in the tumours was similar to that in foetal and regenerating liver. The faster growing (i.e. less differentiated) the tumour the less drug metabolism was evident. This was shown particularly well with the 5α-reduction of testosterone (Table 4.13). Metabolism of oestrogens, methadone, benzphetamine and 4-nitroanisole are also found at much reduced levels in hepatoma tissue.

Table 4.13 The steroid 5α-reductase activity of various rat hepatomas

Hepatoma (code no.)		5α-Reductase activity (% vs control liver)
44		3.6
38B		2.6
7795	Growth rate increasing	2.0
5123A		1.5
7288C		1.0
7777		0.6
42A		0.2

(From Houglum, J. E. *et al.* (1974) *Cancer Res.*, **34** 938–41. Used with permission of the authors and Cancer Research Inc.)

One interesting point emerged from these studies, which was that the unaffected liver tissue of the animal with the hepatoma also showed a reduced capacity to metabolise drugs. The decreases were not as dramatic as those of the hepatoma itself but the presence of a dedifferentiated hepatoma could reduce hepatic drug metabolism by 20%. This has been challenged by Sultatos and Vessell who showed enhanced drug metabolism in liver tissue surrounding a hepatoma. The answer to this paradox lies, say the authors, in the fact that previous studies have used intramuscularly implanted hepatomas whereas they used intrahepatic hepatomas. This enhancement of drug metabolism in tumour adjacent tissue would seem to extend to man (Table 4.14).

Table 4.14 Drug metabolism in heptaoma tissue and surrounding normal liver tissue

Tissue studied	Ethylmorphine N-demethylase (% vs control tissue)	Aniline hydroxylase (% vs control tissue)
Normal liver	100	100
Tumour	70	27
Tumour-adjacent liver	250	290
Far-removed liver	100	100

(From Sultatos, L. G. and Vessell, E. S. (1980) *P.N.A.S.*, **77** 600-3. Used with the permission of the authors.)

The changes in drug metabolising capacity seen in hepatoma lines and liver adjacent to hepatomas are related to changes in cytochrome P450 levels – markedly decreased in hepatoma tissue but elevated in histologically normal liver tissue close to a tumour. Little difference appears to exist between the drug metabolising system of the tumour and normal tissue, each can be induced and inhibited similarly and, thus, the only difference lies in the amount of enzyme present.

4.6.5 Summary of effects of liver diseases on drug metabolism

As has been seen, diseases of various types generally decrease the liver's ability to metabolise drugs (with the notable exception of chronic ethanol exposure). The possible reasons for this decreased capacity are listed below:

(1) decreased enzyme activity in liver

(2) altered hepatic blood flow (intra/extrahepatic shunting)

(3) hypoalbuminaemia (leading to lower plasma binding of drugs)

Of these reasons only (1) is really to be classed as a change in metabolism of the drug but the other two can lead to apparent changes in metabolism and, thus, must be considered.

Two theories have been put forward to explain the poor metabolism in cirrhotic patients. One, the 'sick cell' theory maintains that blood flow through the liver is normal but the cells are deficient in drug metabolising enzymes, whereas theory two, the 'intact hepatocyte' theory, says that the cells are normal but do not receive the normal blood flow due to shunting of blood past some parts of the liver (to get round the fibrous masses). Both theories have some evidence in favour of them such as reduced cytochrome P450 levels and drug metabolising enzyme activity in cirrhotic rats ('sick cell' theory) and increased intrahepatic shunting (nine times normal) in cirrhotic animals ('intact hepatocyte' theory) and it is probable that both theories are correct and vary in importance depending on the stage of cirrhosis and substrate, animal etc. being studied.

4.6.6 Non-hepatic diseases

Other non-hepatic diseases should also be considered in terms of influencing drug metabolism and these particularly include the hormonal diseases such as hyperthyroidism; pituitary insufficiency (dwarfism); adrenal insufficiency; pituitary, thyroid or adrenal tumours, diabetes, and the genetic abnormalities of sexual development. All of the above mentioned diseases states have been shown to influence drug metabolism (most of which have been discussed to a greater or lesser extent in section 4.5).

More recently it has become obvious that general infectious diseases can affect drug metabolism. For instance, *Listeria monocytogenes* infection can dramatically reduce aminopyrine *N*-demethylase activity (to <10% of control) within 2 days and this is accompanied by a similar drop in cytochrome P450 content. Haem oxygenase activity rises during this period perhaps indicating that cytochrome P450 degradation is to blame for the fall in enzyme content. A similar effect is seen with malarial or viral infections and with treatment with endotoxin. The common feature in all cases is an activation of the host defence mechanisms in the body and it has been suggested that interferons may be the common link in inhibiting drug metabolism. Other candidates are the cytokines and nitric oxide produced by immunocompetent cells of the liver. The health of the patient/animal can thus play a major role in drug metabolising capacity of the liver of that patient/animal and together with age probably represents the major consideration when deciding the dose of drug to be given to a patient or, indeed, whether a drug should be given at all.

This chapter has shown how the physiological and pathological make-up of the animal can influence the way in which it metabolises drugs. In the next chapter it is intended to discuss the other major controlling influences on drug metabolism: the external factors. Further reading for this chapter will be found after chapter 5.

5 Factors affecting drug metabolism: external factors

5.1 Introduction

In the previous chapter, the physiological and pathological factors affecting drug metabolism and how these factors vary in importance was discussed. There are, however, factors from outside the body that can also have a profound influence on drug metabolism. The body can be exposed to these factors by design (e.g. alcohol, tobacco smoke, and substances taken as food) or by accident (air, water and food contaminants or pollutants). The first group will be referred to as dietary factors and the second group as environmental factors. The substances to be examined under each heading are listed in Table 5.1.

Table 5.1

Dietary factors	Environmental factors
Protein	Petroleum products
Fat	Pyrolysis products
Carbohydrate	Heavy metals
Vitamins	Insecticides, herbicides
Trace elements	Industrial pollutants
Pyrolysis products	
Tobacco smoke	
Alcohol	

5.2 Dietary factors

In discussing dietary factors, two major groups of chemicals can be distinguished; the macronutrients (e.g. proteins, carbohydrates and fats, making up the bulk of the diet) and micronutrients (vitamins and minerals, essential in small quantities). Under dietary factors can also be placed alcohol (which provides a large number of calories) and the components of tobacco smoke. Although the latter is not strictly a dietary factor, it is taken intentionally and has similar effects to some of the other non-nutrients in the diet. It should be remembered that also taken in the diet are many other non-nutrients such as food colourings, flavourings, antioxidants etc. The effects of these components on the diet have been little studied and will not be considered in detail here.

5.2.1 Macronutrients

(a) *Proteins*. The normal proportion of protein in an animal's diet is about 20% – animals kept on a diet containing this amount of protein show normal development of drug-metabolising enzymes. If, however, rats are fed on a 5% protein (casein) diet then oxidative drug-metabolising capacity decreases (Table 5.2). The decrease in drug metabolism is partially due to decreases in overall microsomal protein and partially to specific effects on the enzymes still remaining. Work by Campbell *et al.* using isolated mixed-function oxidase components (cytochrome P450, reductase and phospholipid) in cross-over experiments, has indicated that it is a fault in the cytochrome P450 and not the reductase or lipid component that is responsible for the decrease in drug metabolism. It was suggested that the interaction of the cytochrome P450 with the reductase was affected in protein restriction.

Table 5.2 The effect of feeding a 5% and 20% casein diet on the hepatic ethylmorphine *N*-demethylase activity in the rat

	Enzyme activity (nmoles HCHO per 100g bw per 10 min)
Control (20% casein)	10.5
5% Casein (4 days)	6.0
5% Casein (8 days)	< 1.0

A correlation with this *in vitro* effect has been found *in vivo*, where a low protein diet delayed the clearance of pentobarbitone and theophylline from rats. In many other cases, however, little correlation has been seen between the effects of protein on microsomal metabolism of a drug and the effect of the drug *in vivo*. One example of this is the hepatotoxicity of aflatoxin, the toxicity of which depends on phase I metabolism forming an epoxide. Both phenobarbitone treatment (an inducer of phase I metabolism) and low protein diet (an inhibitor of phase I metabolism) decrease production of the epoxide and thus reduce the hepatotoxicity of aflatoxin. A number of possible explanations for this have been put forward such that the metabolism measured *in vitro* at saturating substrate concentrations does not necessarily reflect the *in vivo* metabolism at lower concentrations, or that the rate-limiting step for epoxide appearance/hepatotoxicity may not be epoxide formation – it may be epoxide disappearance, for instance. These possibilities must be taken into account when dealing with correlations of *in vitro* and *in vivo* data (for further discussion of this point see chapter 7).

A similar effect of protein restriction is seen in man with decreases in aminopyrine and theophylline metabolism. There is no correlation, however, between this effect and the appearance of symptoms of protein deficiency and it has been postulated that the effect on drug metabolism of protein restriction in man is hormonal in origin. The effect of protein deficiency on phase II drug metabolism is more complex with some activities decreasing e.g. acetaminophen (paracetamol) glucuronidation while others increase e.g. 4-nitrophenol glucuronidation.

(b) *Fats*. Lipids are required by the drug metabolising enzymes as membrane components and, possibly, for specific interactions and certain lipid components can also act as inhibitors of drug metabolism (e.g. steroids, discussed in chapter 4). How would a fat-deficient diet, therefore, affect drug metabolism?

It is seen that diets deficient in the essential fatty acids, notably linoleic acid, caused a reduction in the metabolism of ethylmorphine and hexobarbitone in the liver, and that subsequent addition of corn oil (containing linoleic acid) to the diet could reverse this effect. It is linoleic acid and arachidonic acid that seem to be particularly important in the control of drug metabolism. Treatment with corn oil or polyunsaturated fatty acids, for instance, increases microsomal content of these fatty acids and also increases drug metabolising capacity whereas replacement with saturated fats (e.g. stearic acid) does not have this effect. The effects may be different for different tissues – for example, a high-fat diet can decrease arylhydrocarbon hydroxylase in the lung while increasing the same activity in the kidney and having no effect in the liver.

Various explanations of these effects have been put forward such as the theory that essential fatty acids are needed for the interaction of substrate with the active site of cytochrome P450, the essential fatty acids in this case being incorporated into phospholipids. No consistent effects of deprivation of, or supplementation with, essential fatty acids on substrate binding to cytochrome P450 (either for type I or II substrates) has been seen. An effect mediated via a direct effect on the amount of cytochrome P450 has also been postulated, as deficiencies in essential fatty acids lead to decreased concentrations of cytochrome P450 in some instances (see Figure 5.1).

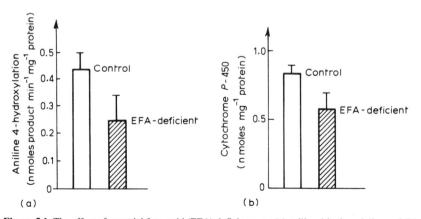

Figure 5.1 The effect of essential fatty acid (EFA) deficiency on (a) aniline 4-hydroxylation and (b) cytochrome P450 levels in liver. (From Kaschnitz, R. (1970) *Hoppe-Seyler's Z. Physiol Chem.*, **351** 771–4. Used with permission of the author and Walter de Gruyter and Co.)

(c) *Carbohydrates.* Carbohydrates seem to have few effects on drug metabolism although high intake of glucose, particularly, can inhibit barbiturate metabolism and, thus, lengthen the sleeping time caused by the drug. Glucose excess has also been shown to decrease hepatic cytochrome P450 content and to lower biphenyl-4-hydroxylase activity. It has been suggested that carbohydrate manipulations are effective by more diverse effects on intermediary metabolism and hormone balance, and not by a direct effect on the liver.

Although examples have been given of the effects of protein, fat and carbohydrate on drug metabolism, it is clear from the literature that the individual influence of these macronutrients is difficult to assess as each influences the use of the other and, thus, an effect of one component may be due to changes it caused in another. Indeed, if isocaloric replacement is used then a high fat/low carbohydrate diet will be replaced by a low fat/high carbohydrate diet (to maintain the same number of calories) and, thus, the effect seen could be due to either change.

This may be further illustrated by looking at one particular aspect of diet, starvation. Starvation of female rats causes marked rises in some enzyme activities (contrast this with the effect of isocaloric protein deficiency) while having little effect on other activities (Table 5.3) while in male rats there is a marked reduction in aminopyrine *N*-demethylation and an increase in aniline 4-hydroxylation. It would appear that starvation can actually induce the synthesis of some microsomal proteins in contrast to the marked loss of protein from the liver as a whole. The effects of starvation in the male rat can be directly related to the change in cytochrome P450 isoenzyme profile – cytochrome P4502C11 falls (thus the decrease in aminopyrine metabolism) and 2E1 rises (thus the increase in aniline metabolism). The rise in cytochrome P4502E1 is most likely a result of breakdown of fatty tissue releasing free fatty acids which are partially converted to ketone bodies (e.g. acetone) which are known to induce this isoenzyme (see effect of diabetes in chapter 4) (Figure 5.2). It is interesting to note that over-feeding of rats (a good model of human obesity) also causes an increase in cytochrome P4502E1 for the same reason, i.e. excess free fatty acids in the blood.

Table 5.3 The effect of starvation on drug metabolism in rats

Enzyme	Change (%) after starvation
Aminopyrine *N*-demethylase	+114
4-Nitroanisole *O*-demethylase	+90
Aniline 4-hydroxylation	+94
Zoxazolamine hydroxylation	+15
Dichlorophenolindophenol reductase	+7

(Data from various sources: see further reading section in chapter 5.)

It is clear, therefore, that changes in macronutrients can markedly effect the drug metabolising capacity of the liver and other tissues. Apart from the above mentioned macronutrients there are many other components of the diet that can

affect drug metabolism. The most noticeable of these are the micronutrients, vitamins and minerals.

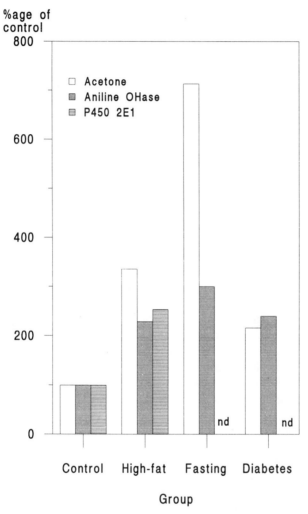

Figure 5.2 Effect of high-fat, fasting and diabetes mellitus on plasma acetone levels, hepatic aniline
4-hydroxylase activity and hepatic mRNA for cytochrome P450 2E1 in rats. nd = not determined.
Data taken from Yun *et al.* (1992) *Mol. Pharmacol.*, **41** 474–9.

5.2.2 Micronutrients

(a) *Vitamins.* Vitamins are an essential part of the diet and are needed for the
synthesis of proteins and lipids, both of which are vital components of the
drug-metabolising enzyme system. It is, therefore, not surprising that changes in

vitamin levels, particularly deficiencies, cause changes in drug-metabolising capacity. The vitamins indicated to be involved in drug metabolism are listed in Table 5.4.

Table 5.4 Vitamins affecting drug metabolism

Vitamin A
Vitamin B group
Thiamine (B_1)
Riboflavin (B_2)
Vitamin C
Vitamin E
Vitamin K

(i) *Vitamin A.* Vitamin A deficiency was found to decrease some pathways of drug metabolism. For example, it was seen that rats fed a vitamin A-free diet had lower levels than the control, of aniline 4-hydroxylase and aminopyrine N-demethylase. This was shown to be related to reduced cytochrome P450 levels. In other cases, e.g. the N-oxidation of pyridine, vitamin A deficiency has been shown to have no effect. Vitamin A deficiency has, therefore, enzyme-selective effects on drug metabolism.

(ii) *Thiamine (vitamin B_1).* Thiamine deficiency has been shown to increase the metabolism of aniline and reduce hexobarbitone metabolism whereas excess thiamine inhibits aniline and ethylmorphine metabolism. The effect of thiamine is related to changes in the microsomal cytochromes (P450 and b_5) and NADPH–cytochrome P450 reductase levels. The effects were not similar to starvation although it was suggested that the effects of thiamine were mediated via a reduction in blood glucose. More recently thiamine has been found to change the type of cytochrome P450 present – an increase in isoenzyme 2E1 and reduction in 2C11 – and this could account for the effects seen.

(iii) *Riboflavin (vitamin B_2).* Riboflavin is an essential component in the flavoprotein NADPH–cytochrome P450 reductase, which is itself a component of the mixed-function oxidase system. A deficiency of riboflavin, therefore, would be expected to reduce NADPH–cytochrome P450 reductase content and thus decrease drug-metabolising capacity. This is seen for azo reduction of 4-dimethylaminoazobenzene in rats deficient in vitamin B_2 whereas aminopyrine N-demethylase shows an increase.

The degree of riboflavin deficiency may, however, complicate the interpretation of the data. Opposite effects of mild, short-term and severe, long-term deficiency of this vitamin on drug metabolism have been reported. Soon after the start of a riboflavin-deficient diet, a marked decrease in NADPH–cytochrome P450 reductase is seen together with an increase in cytochrome P450. This leads to an overall increase in aniline 4-hydroxylase and aminopyrine N-demethylase activity. Later in the treatment, however, the levels of cytochrome P450 fall sharply leading to lower levels of all enzyme activities.

(iv) *Vitamin C*. Of the animal species studied in terms of drug metabolism, only man, monkey and guinea-pig show a nutritional requirement for vitamin C and, thus, only these animals have been used in the study of vitamin C's effects on drug metabolism.

Vitamin C deficiency has been well studied following the early observation that guinea-pigs deficient in the vitamin were more sensitive to the effects of pentobarbitone and procaine. This increased sensitivity is caused by a marked reduction in drug-metabolising capacity. The reasons for this are not completely clear although reduced levels of cytochrome P450 have been detected in vitamin C deficient animals. Specifically, cytochrome P4501A2 and 2E1 (but not isoenzymes 2B1 or 3A1) are reduced leading to the expected decrease in aniline 4-hydroxylase but not testosterone 6β-hydroxylase (Figure 5.3). There is

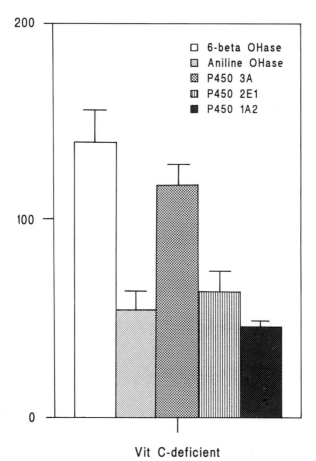

Figure 5.3 The effect of vitamin C deficiency on aniline 4-hydroxylase and testosterone 6-hydroxylase activity and specific forms of cytochrome P450 in the guinea-pig. Data taken from Kanazana *et al.* (1991) *Mol. Pharmacol.*, **39** 456–60.

evidence to suggest that the deficiency of vitamin C may interfere with haem biosynthesis and, thus, affect cytochrome P450 levels. Abnormal binding spectra have also been seen in vitamin C deficient guinea-pigs – the binding spectra could be returned to normal using ascorbyl palmitate (the fatty acid derivative of vitamin C). It may, thus, be that vitamin C is involved in the maintenance of the membrane structure of the endoplasmic reticulum.

(v) *Vitamin E.* Deficiencies of vitamin E reduce drug metabolising capacity when assayed with a variety of substrates but, again, as with the other vitamin deficiencies no definite biochemical reasons can be put forward. Two interesting theories have been advanced. The first states that vitamin E is required for haem biosynthesis notably for the function of the enzyme δ-aminolevulinic acid dehydratase, and, indeed, microsomal cytochrome P450 does fall during vitamin E deficiency. The second theory is based on the proposed role of vitamin E in the body as an inhibitor of the oxidation of selenium-containing proteins (selenium can act instead of sulfur in some instances, a selenide group replacing the sulfhydryl group) and the need for such a protein in drug metabolism. Evidence for this theory comes from the observation that phenobarbitone induction of drug metabolism is accompanied by a large increase in selenium incorporation, an effect which is inhibited by vitamin E deficiency. Phenobarbitone, however, affects many more enzymes than those involved in drug metabolism, and the effect noted above may be related to one of those.

(vi) *Vitamin K.* Vitamin K deficiency is reported to cause a decrease in a number of enzymes associated with drug metabolism such as the microsomal oxidation and reduction reactions and the glutathione conjugating and hydrolysing reactions of the cytosol. This generalised effect of vitamin K deficiency would seem to rule out a specific mechanism of action.

Vitamins of the A, B, C, E and K class are, therefore, not only dietary requirements for good health but also for the maintenance of normal levels of drug metabolism. Both deficiencies, and, in some cases, excesses, of these vitamins can cause marked alterations in the way in which the body handles drugs. The significance of this to clinical practice in the malnourished, for example, is obvious.

(b) *Minerals.* Minerals are the elements needed in the diet to maintain good health and normal physiological function. Those which have been shown to affect drug metabolism are iron, calcium, magnesium, zinc, copper, selenium and iodine. The overall effects of mineral deficiency are shown in Table 5.5. As is seen, most mineral deficiencies lead to a fall in drug metabolism.

Iron deficiency is an exception to the general rule in that it causes an increase in drug metabolising capacity (see Table 5.5). Excess iron in the diet can also inhibit drug metabolism. This is an unusual finding considering that iron is an essential component of the haem moiety of cytochrome P450 and, thus, would

Table 5.5 The effects of mineral deficiencies on hepatic drug metabolism

Mineral	Effect of deficiency on drug metabolism	Enzymes affected
Calcium	Decrease	Aminopyrine N-demethylase
	Decrease	Nitroreductase
	Decrease	Hexobarbitone oxidation
Magnesium	Decrease	Aniline 4-hydroxylation
	Decrease	Aminopyrine N-demethylase
	No change	Nitroreductase
	No change	Pentobarbitone oxidation
	Decrease	Cytochrome P450
Iron	Increase	Hexobarbitone oxidation
	Increase	Aminopyrine N-demethylation
	Increase	Cytochrome b_5
	No change	Cytochrome P450
	Increase/no change	Aniline 4-hydroxylation
	No change	Nitroreductase
	No change	Glucuronyltransferase
Potassium	No change	Aniline 4-hydroxylation
	No change	Aminopyrine N-demethylation
	No change	Nitroreductase
Copper	Decrease	Aniline 4-hydroxylation
	Increase	Benzo[a]pyrene hydroxylation
	Decrease	Hexobarbitone oxidation
	Decrease	Zoxazolamine 6-hydroxylation
Zinc	Decrease	Aminopyrine N-demethylase
	Decrease	Pentobarbitone oxidation
	Decrease	Cytochrome P450
Selenium	No change	Ethylmorphine N-demethylase
	No change	Biphenyl 4-hydroxylase
	No change	Pentobarbitone oxidation
Iodine	Increase	Aminopyrine N-demethylase
	Increase	Hexobarbitone oxidation
	Increase	Benzo[a]pyrene hydroxylation
	Increase	Aniline 4-hydroxylation
	No change	Glucuronyltransferase

(Data from various sources; see further reading section in chapter 5.)

be expected to be essential for cytochrome P450 synthesis. Cytochrome P450 levels are, however, unchanged in iron deficiency. Iron levels in liver are inversely correlated to NADPH-dependent lipid peroxidation. As increased lipid peroxidation has been associated with decreased drug metabolism, this may offer an explanation of the effects of iron. Iron deficiency limits the degree of lipid peroxidation and thus allows more expression of the drug-metabolising enzymes. The active form of iron may be ferritin as ferritin added directly to microsomal incubations can inhibit aminopyrine and aniline metabolism. Iron-deficient diets markedly decrease intestinal drug metabolism, and this may be of greater pharmacological and toxicological importance considering the protective role of the intestinal enzymes, particularly against the procarcinogenic polycyclic hydrocarbons. This latter effect is associated with a fall in the levels of cytochrome P450 in this tissue.

Calcium and magnesium deficiency are associated with a decrease in drug metabolism, particularly phase I cytochrome P450-dependent metabolism such as aniline 4-hydroxylation and aminopyrine N-demethylation and, in the case of magnesium, drug glucuronidation. The effects of calcium deficiency take longer to develop than those of magnesium deficiency (40 days as opposed to 10 days). Magnesium deficiency, often found in conjunction with calcium deficiency, gives a specific effect and is not related to decreased food intake or starvation effects. Various explanations for the effect of magnesium deficiency have been put forward. Decreases in NADPH–cytochrome P450 reductase have been correlated to a reduced ability to metabolise drugs and decreased liver magnesium levels. In many studies, however, no decrease in liver magnesium levels is evident and alternative explanations are needed. One such explanation is found in the interaction of magnesium, thyroid hormones and phospholipids. Thyroid hormone levels are depressed in magnesium-depleted animals, a change that can lead to decreased drug metabolism (see chapter 4). Magnesium-depleted diets also markedly reduce microsomal content of lysophosphatidylcholine and, to a lesser extent, phosphatidylcholine – an effect also associated with decreased drug-metabolising capacity. The possibility that magnesium affects drug metabolism via thyroid hormones which act through an effect on phospholipid metabolism must be considered.

The effects of copper deficiency on drug metabolism are variable (see Table 5.5) and no consensus is evident on the mechanism of these effects. Alterations in NADPH–cytochrome P450 reductase or binding of substrate to cytochrome P450 have been put forward as possible mechanisms, but these do not explain all of the effects seen. One interesting effect of copper deficiency on drug metabolism is the toxicity of parathion. Parathion is normally metabolised to the toxic compound, paraoxon, or to the relatively non-toxic 4-nitrophenol. In copper-deficient mice, parathion is found to be more toxic than in normal mice due to a reduced ability to produce the non-toxic 4-nitrophenol, thus allowing more of the substance to be converted to paraoxon. It is interesting to note that excess copper has the same effect as copper deficiency, i.e. a reduced ability to metabolise drugs in some cases. Thus an optimum level of dietary copper exists for the maintenance of drug metabolism in the body.

Zinc deficiency leads to reduced drug metabolism for some substrates (e.g. benzo[a]pyrene hydroxylation and aminopyrine N-demethylation) but no effects on others (e.g. aniline and zoxazolamine hydroxylation). The effects were related to reduced cytochrome P450 levels. There are also marked changes in phase II metabolism with falls in glutathione-S-transferase and UDP–glucuronosyltransferase activities. Zinc-deficient diets lead to extreme poor health in the animals and the effects seen may be a function of this malnutrition rather than a specific effect of zinc.

Selenium, as an essential trace element, is linked to vitamin E and the effects of both on drug metabolism are closely linked (see section 5.2.2). No direct effects of selenium deficiency on drug metabolism have been seen but a role for dietary selenium in the biosynthesis of microsomal components has been suggested. Selenium deficiency impairs the ability of the liver to respond to phenobarbitone treatment. In the presence of selenium a 3.65-fold induction is seen but this falls to 2.64-fold in selenium-deficient animals. As with copper, an optimal level of selenium in the diet exists, with excessive selenium intake also being inhibitory to drug metabolism. The biochemical reasons behind the effects of selenium are unclear with some, but not all, of the effects being related to vitamin E.

It can thus be seen that a deficiency (or, to a lesser extent an excess) of many micronutrients can have noticeable effects on drug metabolism. The whole subject of the interaction of dietary components and drug metabolism can become extremely complex even if one only examines the nutritional elements in the diet and the effects can overlap and involve other control mechanisms such as the hormones. A summary of the effects of macro- and micro-nutrients is given in Figure 5.4.

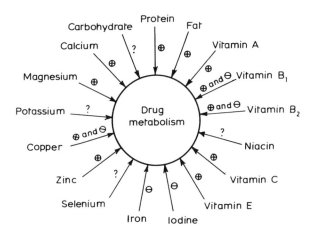

Figure 5.4 The effects of dietary nutrients on drug metabolism: a summary. Key: ⊕ = an increase in drug metabolism; ⊖ = a decrease in drug metabolism.

The importance of nutritional factors on drug metabolism is greatest in conditions of deficiency and, thus, in cases of malnutrition. As this is particularly prevalent in Third World societies, it is here that these effects are most often encountered but where funding is deficient to study and counteract the effects.

5.2.3 Non-nutrients

When dealing with the effects of diet on drug metabolism, it must be remembered that food contains not only nutritional factors (discussed above) but also other chemical substances, and any examination of diet-related effects on drug metabolism should include studies on these substances. The most notable group of these substances naturally occurring in food which affect drug metabolism are the pyrolysis products – chemicals formed by the cooking (literally burning) of the food.

The pyrolysis products that are formed in meat and fish, particularly when fried or charcoal-broiled, have been isolated as breakdown products of amino acids, mainly tryptophan. The structures of some of them are shown in Figure 5.5. All these compounds are known inducers of cytochrome P4501A1 (aryl hydrocarbon hydroxylase) and are also potential mutagens/carcinogens. It is found that feeding charcoal-broiled beef to rats induces the metabolism of phenacetin in the intestines thus lowering bioavailability of the drug. A fall is also seen in plasma concentration of phenacetin in humans fed on a charcoal-broiled beef diet, and it seems to be related to metabolism of the phenacetin. Further work has indicated that it is benzo[a]pyrene (a polycyclic hydrocarbon inducer of cytochrome P450; see chapter 3) in the charcoal-broiled beef that causes the effects seen. The metabolism of antipyrine and theophylline is also increased by the same treatment.

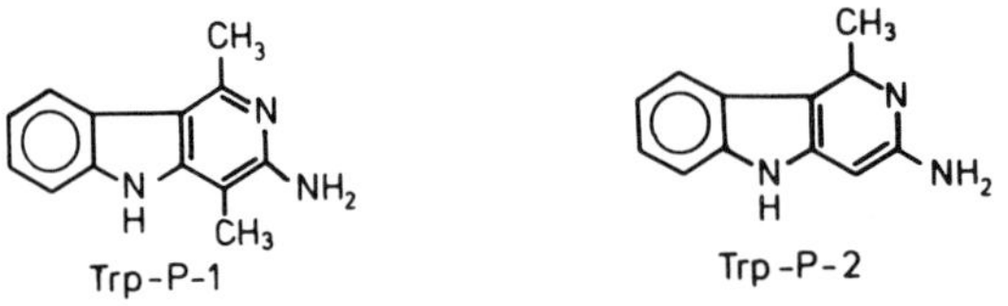

Figure 5.5 Tryptophan pyrolysis products found in fried or charcoal-broiled meat and fish.

One other group of compounds which could also be considered in this category are the substances found in cabbages and Brussels sprouts (*Brassica*). These compounds are of the indole type (Figure 5.6) and are also seen to be enzyme inducers. The chemical similarity of these indoles to the tryptophan pyrolysis products is noticeable. Dietary Brussels sprouts and cabbage induce the hydroxylation of benzo[a]pyrene and hexobarbitone, the *O*-dealkylation of phenacetin (see above) and 7-ethoxycoumarin in the rat. Other vegetables not containing indoles did not induce drug metabolism. Studies in humans have shown a similar induction of caffeine metabolism following short-term dietary supplementation with *Brassica* vegetables. It was suggested that the induction of cytochrome P4501A2 may be responsible for the alterations in metabolism seen.

Thus, even non-nutrient components of food can have marked effects on drug metabolism. It is likely that many more non-nutrient components of the diet (such as colourings, flavourings, food additives) can act as inducers or inhibitors of drug metabolism and that this is a common phenomenon.

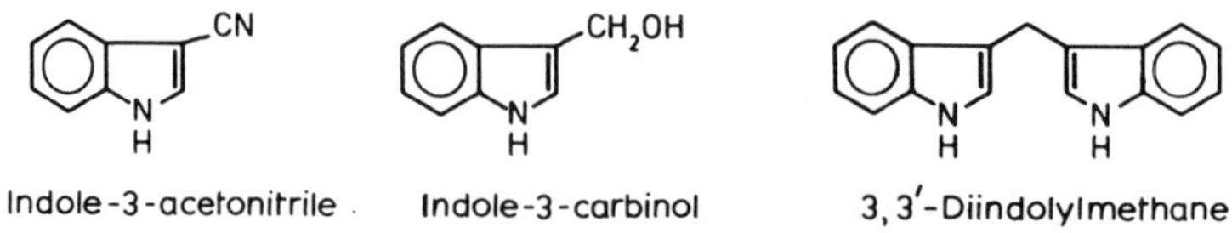

Figure 5.6 Indoles found in cabbage and Brussels sprouts.

5.2.4 Tobacco smoking

One other 'dietary' component can be considered, tobacco smoke. Although not strictly a food component, tobacco smoke is inhaled deliberately and, thus, is a self-inflicted effector of drug metabolism. Tobacco smoking can be thought of as a different way of ingesting pyrolysis products (from the burning of the plant materials in tobacco) with the lungs the first site of interaction rather than the intestine as in the case of charcoal-broiled meat. The most common effect of tobacco smoking is an increase in biotransformation of drugs – an effect very similar to that seen for ingestion of charcoal-broiled meat. Indeed, there is a common factor, the polycyclic hydrocarbon, benzo[*a*]pyrene. This substance is found in both charcoal-broiled meat and tobacco smoke. A marked effect on the plasma phenacetin level can be seen following tobacco smoking (cf. effect of charcoal-broiled meat on phenacetin plasma levels) (Figure 5.7). The lower plasma level of phenacetin was due to increased metabolism either by the intestinal mucosa or 'first-pass' through the liver.

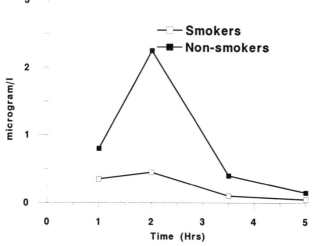

Figure 5.7 Mean plasma concentrations of phenacetin as a function of time in smokers and non-smokers. (Data from Pantuck, E.J.*et al.* (1972) *Science* **175** 1248–50.)

Another well-studied marker of drug metabolism is antipyrine, the metabolism of which is directly related to its rate of excretion. Using antipyrine as a substrate, smoking was found to increase drug clearance and thus, by inference, the rate of metabolism of antipyrine. Stopping smoking returns the rate of metabolism of antipyrine to the pre-smoking level. The metabolism of a number of other drugs are affected by smoking whereas some have shown no change in metabolism following smoking; a summary of these is shown in Table 5.6. Thus tobacco smoking selectively induces the metabolism of some drugs. Tobacco smoke contains at least 3000 different chemicals, some of which are known enzyme inducers (such as the polycyclic hydrocarbons discussed above) and some known enzyme inhibitors (e.g. carbon monoxide, hydrogen cyanide). From the results obtained it is the inductive effects of tobacco smoke that are prevalent. Animal experiments have indicated that the great majority, if not all, of the effects of tobacco smoking can be mimicked by treatment with benzo[a]pyrene (see chapter 3). Thus, it seems likely that the major effects of tobacco smoking are due to induction of drug metabolism by benzo[a]pyrene and other such compounds. Marijuana smoking produces identical effects to tobacco smoking and cannot be looked upon as a 'safer' habit in this respect.

Table 5.6 The effect of tobacco smoking on the metabolism of drugs

Affected (increased)	Not affected
Nicotine	Diazepam
Theophylline	Phenytoin
Imipramine	Warfarin
Pentazocine	Nortriptyline

A summary of the effects of the non-nutrient compounds of the diet on drug metabolism is given in Figure 5.8. It should be remembered that there are many more dietary non-nutrients such as colourants, anti-oxidants, flavourings which could also influence drug metabolism. Space limitations, however, restrict our coverage of this extensive subject.

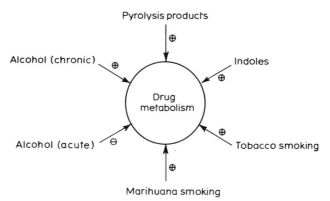

Figure 5.8 The influence of dietary non-nutrients on drug metabolism: a summary. Key: ⊕ = an increase in drug metabolism; ⊖ = a decrease in drug metabolism.

5.3 Environmental factors

Environmental factors are those influences in our surroundings that can affect drug metabolism; no conscious act is required to be influenced by them (cf. dietary factors) but the effects on drug metabolism can be profound. The environment is replete with substances which can affect drug metabolism and reviewers have different views concerning what constitutes an environmental factor. Many include dietary factors in this category and one should not be confused by these differences in nomenclature. It should also be realised that there are a large number of environmental chemicals that could potentially affect drug metabolism; the representative examples of a number of groups of compounds discussed here are only a small part of this. Those chemicals to be considered in this section are:

Heavy metals – lead, mercury, cadmium

Industrial pollutants – tetrachlorodibenzodioxin (TCDD), solvents, polychlorinated biphenyls (PCBS)

Insecticides and herbicides – DDT, parathion, mirex

5.3.1 Heavy metals

Exposure of the human population to heavy metals can be related to occupation (cadmium from zinc smelting), diet (such as cadmium in vegetables) or other phenomena (e.g. lead in exhaust from petrol-driven vehicles or in water from lead pipes). Most exposure is low-level and long-term and so cumulative exposure becomes important. These facts are rarely taken into account when examining heavy metal effects on drug metabolism in experimental animals.

Chronic exposure of rats to lead in the diet has little effect on drug-metabolising capacity but does induce cytochrome P450 levels. The increased level of cytochrome P450 indicates that lead induces a form of enzyme that does not metabolise any of the substrates so far tested – different substrates may show induction of drug-metabolising capacity. Acute lead toxicity in rats, however, is associated with reduced drug-metabolising capacity. The situation found in human subjects was similar but only young children exhibited the inhibition of drug metabolism during acute lead toxicity. No measurement of cytochrome P450 in humans was performed; thus, the possible induction of this enzyme by chronic lead exposure is still open to investigation. Two possible explanations for the effect of acute lead exposure on drug metabolism have been put forward. If lead is added to incubations of microsomes the activity of NADPH–cytochrome P450 reductase is inhibited and this could lead to inhibition of drug metabolism with certain substrates. Lead has also been shown to inhibit one of the enzymes involved in the synthesis of haem, δ-aminolevulinic acid dehydratase, and thus could inhibit the production of the haem moiety in cytochrome P450.

Little work has been done on mercury's effects on drug metabolism; what has been done has used excessively high doses of this toxic metal. Inorganic forms of mercury (Hg^{2+}) seem to induce drug metabolism whereas organic mercury (methylmercury) inhibits drug metabolism after chronic administration. No explanations for the effects of mercury were found.

The great majority of the work published on the interaction of heavy metals with drug metabolism has been done with cadmium. This is an industrial pollutant in the manufacture of a number of metals including zinc, and is a dietary pollutant in vegetables grown in cadmium-rich soil. High intake of cadmium has been shown to be associated with inhibition of drug-metabolising enzymes. In the rat, however, an interesting sexual dimorphism of the effect has been seen (Table 5.7). The male rat responds to cadmium treatment with marked inhibition of all enzyme activities studied and a concomitant decrease in cytochrome P450 levels. The female rat, on the other hand, shows no reduction in cytochrome P450 levels and, indeed, marked induction of diazepam metabolism. A hormonal control of cadmium sensitivity similar to that of drug metabolism in general (see chapter 4) was found to operate, i.e. removal of androgens from the male by castration removed their sensitivity to cadmium.

Table 5.7 The effect of cadmium on hepatic drug metabolism in male and female rats

Enzyme	Change (%) in enzyme activities caused by cadmium	
	Male	Female
Diazepam 3-hydroxylase	−58	+65
Diazepam N-demethylase	−55	+66
Imipramine 2-hydroxylase	−33	+9
Imipramine N-demethylase	−55	−4
Imipramine N-oxidase	−60	+7
Cytochrome P450	−25	+3

Cadmium was shown to have many effects on the various components of the drug metabolising enzyme system. Cytochrome P450 and cytochrome b_5 levels were reduced, and cytochrome P450 could be converted to the inactive cytochrome P420 *in vitro*. The former effect seems to be due to cadmium's ability to induce haem oxygenase activity (the enzyme that breaks down the cytochromes P450 and b_5). The fact that only males respond to cadmium with marked inhibition of drug metabolism suggests that the cadmium-sensitive cytochrome P450 (or b_5) is sex related. The alternative explanation that

Table 5.8 The effect of cadmium and testosterone treatment on hepatic drug metabolism in the male rat

Parameter	+Cd (% vs control)	+Cd +testosterone (% vs control)
Cytochrome P450	82	71
Diazepam 3-hydroxylase	75	72
Diazepam N-demethylase	64	66
Lignocaine 3-hydroxylase	292	229
Lignocaine N-de-ethylase	69	53
Plasma testosterone	17	78

cadmium exerts its effects by reducing androgen levels does not hold, as androgen-replacement therapy cannot reverse the effects of cadmium although it is known that cadmium causes massive testicular damage and does drastically reduce plasma testosterone levels (Table 5.8).

So cadmium not only reduces plasma testosterone levels but also makes the liver non-responsive to androgens. Little work has been done on the inducing ability of cadmium in the female rat although it has been suggested that the female is less sensitive to the toxic effects of cadmium by virtue of having a cadmium-binding protein which takes up the metal and prevents it being toxic.

Heavy metals can, therefore, induce and/or inhibit drug metabolism depending on the species and sex of animal and substrate studied. The relevance of this animal data to the environmentally encountered low-level, long-term exposure is debatable and much more work is needed to ascertain the effects of environmental exposure to these metals.

5.3.2 Industrial pollutants

There are literally thousands of industrial pollutants that, in experimental animals, have been shown to affect drug metabolism; the toxicological literature is full of such examples (see chapter 6). Three important and well-studied industrial pollutants will be discussed in detail to illustrate the general principles; these are: 2,3,7,8 – tetrachlorodibenzo-*p*-dioxin (TCDD), industrial solvents of the benzene and chlorinated hydrocarbon types, and polychlorinated biphenyls (PCBs).

(a) *TCDD*. TCDD is a polycyclic compound (Figure 5.9) with a rigid planar structure. It is a precursor for a number of herbicides and was a contaminant of the toxin released in the Seveso incident in Italy, causing widespread chloracne and fears for the future welfare of the population exposed to the chemical. TCDD causes marked induction of the metabolism of polycyclic hydrocarbons and of the enzymes, UDP–glucuronosyltransferase, δ-aminolevulinic acid synthetase and ligandin; it thus can affect both phase I and II metabolism. The mechanism of action of TCDD in inducing aryl hydrocarbon hydroxylase has been particularly studied. It appears that TCDD has a specific high-affinity, low-capacity binding site in the liver cytosol (a classical receptor similar to that for the steroid hormones). Once bound to the receptor, TCDD is taken to the nucleus where it interacts with DNA and, thus, gives its induction effects. This is very similar to the activation of the 'Ah locus' and is very probably the same system (see chapter 3) leading to the induction of cytochrome P4501A1 amongst other effects.

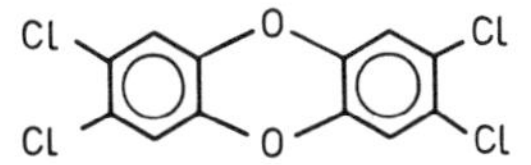

2,3,7,8 -Tetrachlorodibenzo-*p*-dioxin (TCDD)

Figure 5.9 The structure of TCDD.

(b) *Solvents.* Solvents are in very widespread use in industry (and in the home). Serious concern is now being expressed about their effects on the body. The two groups of solvents of most interest in the study of drug metabolism are the benzene derivatives (benzene, toluene and the xylenes) and the chlorinated hydrocarbons (chloroform, trichloroethylene, dichloromethane).

The aromatic hydrocarbons (Figure 5.10) have been shown to induce cytochrome P450-dependent enzymes in the liver but have little effect on conjugation with glucuronic acid except after long-term exposure when induction is also seen. As human exposure to these solvents is mainly by inhalation, experiments in animals tend to be inhalation experiments as well. Levels of solvent around the maximum allowed in industrial atmospheres are used so that an extrapolation of the data to man can be attempted; species differences have, however, to be taken into account here.

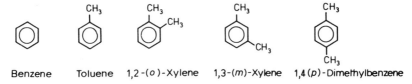

Benzene   Toluene   1,2-(o)-Xylene   1,3-(m)-Xylene   1,4(p)-Dimethylbenzene

Figure 5.10 The structures of some aromatic hydrocarbons.

Xylene has also been shown to be an inducer of cytochrome P450 when administered by inhalation. Use of the individual components of the xylene mixture indicates that *p*-xylene (1,4-dimethylbenzene) was less active than the other isomers. The increases in ethoxyresorufin *O*-deethylase, n-hexane and benzo[*a*]pyrene hydroxylase activities were matched by elevated cytochrome P450 levels (Table 5.9). Drug-metabolising activity was also induced in the kidney of these animals but, in the lung, xylene caused an inhibition of some enzymes. The overall effect on the body, however, was an increase in drug-metabolising capacity by induction of cytochrome P450 and, possibly, NADPH–cytochrome P450 reductase activity. The induction was similar to that found for phenobarbitone (see chapter 3).

The aromatic hydrocarbons, therefore, seem to be phenobarbitone-like inducers of drug metabolism and are active by inhalation thus indicating that the

Table 5.9 The effects of xylene and xylene isomers on hepatic drug metabolism in the rat

	Cytochrome P450	7-Ethoxyresorufin *O*-de-ethylase	n-Hexane 2-oxidation	Benzo[*a*]pyrene 4,5-hydroxylation
Xylene	190*	350*	480*	1000*
o-Xylene	175*	420*	820*	620*
m-Xylene	180*	370*	650*	1200*
p-Xylene	130*	150	450	450*

Results expressed as % vs control
$^* = p < 0.05$
(Data from Toftgård, R. and Nilsen, O. (1982) *Toxicology*, **23** 197-212. Used with permission of the authors and Elsevier Biomedical Press B.V.)

workers in industries using such solvents (e.g. paint industry) may have induced drug metabolism as a result of occupational solvent exposure.

The chlorinated hydrocarbons, in contrast to the aromatic hydrocarbons discussed above, do not always show induction of drug metabolism. For example, trichloroethylene (the solvent often used in dry cleaning and fatty stain removal), when given chronically to rats, causes an increase in NADPH–cytochrome P450 reductase but a decrease in cytochrome P450 with concomitant increase in aniline 4-hydroxylation and decrease in ethylmorphine N-demethylase. An increase in 4-nitrophenol glucuronidation was also seen. Some of these effects can be explained in terms of a direct effect of trichloro-ethylene on the liver enzymes. It is a 'suicide substrate' of cytochrome P450, i.e. it is metabolised by cytochrome P450 to an intermediate that destroys the enzyme. Trichloroethylene also competitively inhibits the metabolism of ethyl-morphine when added into microsomal incubations and activates glucuronosyltransferase activity in vitro. The increase in aniline 4-hydroxylation is thought to be due to induction of specific forms of cytochrome P450, whereas overall cytochrome P450 levels fall. Trichloroethylene is, therefore, an unusual compound inthat it simultaneously activates, inhibits, induces and destroys various drug-metabolising enzyme activities.

Chloroform elicits similar effects to trichloroethylene particularly with regard to the destruction of cytochrome P450, but dichloromethane, a close relative of chloroform, when administered to rats by inhalation only caused induction of drug metabolism. There seemed to be a dose-dependent induction of a number of enzyme activities, notably biphenyl 2-hydroxylation. Chlorinated hydrocar-bons can, thus, give induction of drug metabolism as the aromatic hydrocarbons, but can also cause destruction of cytochrome P450 by acting as suicide sub-strates. The ease of exposure to solvents (trichloroethylene is the solvent used for dry-cleaning fluids; toluene and xylene are the solvents in some adhesives) means that many people are subjected to the effects noted above, and this should be considered as a serious environmental problem.

(c) *Polychlorinated biphenyls (PCBs)*. The polychlorinated biphenyls (PCBs) are a large group of compounds used in various manufacturing industries. Structurally the compounds can be split into two distinct groups, the planar and non-planar types (Figure 5.11). The 3,4,5-chloro-derivatives are planar whereas steric hindrance keeps the rings in the 2,4,6-chloro-derivatives at right angles

3, 3', 4, 4', 5, 5'-Hexachlorobiphenyl
(a)

2, 2', 4, 4', 6, 6'-Hexachlorobiphenyl
(b)

Figure 5.11 The structures of (a) planar and (b) non-planar polychlorinated biphenyls.

to each other. These two groups of compound have different effects on drug metabolism. The planar PCBs induce hepatic drug metabolism similar to the polycyclic hydrocarbons whereas the non-planar PCBs exhibit induction of drug metabolism of the phenobarbitone type.

Mixtures of PCBs (called Clophen A-50 or Arochlor-1254) induced cytochrome P450, NADPH–cytochrome P450 reductase, 4-nitroanisole O-demethylase, epoxide hydratase and UDP–glucuronosyltransferase activities in rats within 1 week of the start of treatment. The overall induction pattern is typical of a mixed type of induction (probably due to both planar and non-planar isomers being present in the mixture). The induction of cytochrome P4501A1 is particularly well established for Arochlor-1254 and appears to work via interaction with the Ah-receptor. The point of interest is that a single dose of PCBs can maintain the induced level of enzymes for at least 1 month indicating that these substances persist for long periods of time in the body.

5.3.3 Pesticides

Pesticides of various types are prevalent environmental contaminants in air, water and food. Again, there are many different chemical types of herbicides, insecticides, etc. and only a few will be discussed here with respect to their effects on drug metabolism. The compounds to be discussed are mirex, kepone, malathion, parathion and DDT.

Mirex and kepone are structurally similar insecticides. The effects of these compounds on drug-metabolising capacity of rats is shown in Table 5.10. There is an indication that both of these compounds are specific inducing agents differing from each other and from the classical enzyme inducers, phenobarbitone and 3-methylcholanthrene.

Malathion and parathion are well-known, phosphothionate-type insecticides which are converted *in vivo* and *in vitro* to the corresponding phosphates,

Table 5.10 Effects of mirex, kepone, 3-methylcholanthrene (3-MC) and phenobarbitone (PB) on hepatic drug metabolism

Inducing agent	Cytochrome P450 (nmoles mg^{-1} protein)	Biphenyl 4-hydroxylation (nmoles product $min^{-1} mg^{-1}$ protein)	Biphenyl 2-hydroxylation (pmoles product $min^{-1} mg^{-1}$ protein)	S-Warfarin 6-hydroxylation (pmoles product $min^{-1} mg^{-1}$ protein)
Control	1.07 ± 0.01	0.54 ± 0.02	39 ± 2	0.13 ± 0.02
Mirex	$1.77 \pm 0.21^{**}$	0.56 ± 0.01	$66 \pm 1^{***}$	$0.23 \pm 0.02^{**}$
Kepone	$1.95 \pm 0.05^{**}$	0.55 ± 0.06	$56 \pm 14^{*}$	0.08 ± 0.02
3-MC	$1.98 \pm 0.17^{**}$	0.61 ± 0.03	$232 \pm 6^{***}$	$0.18 \pm 0.01^{**}$
PB				0.07 ± 0.01

Results expressed as: mean $\pm$ (standard error); $^{*} = p < 0.05$; $^{**} = p < 0.01$; $^{***} = p < 0.001$.
(From Kaminsky, L.S. *et al.* (1978) *Tox. Appl. Pharm.*, **43**, 327-38. Used with permission of Academic Press.)

malaoxon and paraoxon. These insecticides are inhibitors of drug metabolism both *in vivo* and *in vitro* probably due to competitive inhibition of the cytochrome P450-dependent reaction which also metabolises the insecticides.

DDT causes induction of many drug-metabolising enzymes but generally only affects phase I metabolism of drugs.

Pesticides can, therefore, be inducers or inhibitors of drug metabolism. Their widespread use and persistence in the environment and in the body make them potentially important in determining drug metabolism both in man and in wild and domestic animals.

5.4 Relative importance of physiological and environmental factors in determining drug-metabolising capacity in the human population

As has been seen in the last two chapters, there are numerous factors that can affect the way in which the body handles drugs, varying from the genetic make-up of the person to how much grilled fish they eat. Attempts have been made to ascertain how much of the (sometimes quite large) inter-individual variations in drug metabolism are due to genetic differences and how much to environmental factors. Two opposing views – almost diametrically opposite to each other – have been put forward. The twin and family studies discussed earlier (see chapter 4) seem to show that most, if not all, of the differences in drug metabolism in the population are due to genetic differences. Other research has indicated, by statistical analysis of family groups, that all of the inter-individual variations can be accounted for by environmental factors (alcohol, tea and coffee consumption and tobacco smoking) although the sex of the person has been included as an environmental factor.

Genetic sub-populations with respect to drug metabolism certainly exist (e.g isoniazid 'fast' and 'slow' acetylators, and debrisoquine 'poor' and 'extensive' metabolisers (indicating differences in cytochrome P4502D6)) and so a genetic component of control of drug metabolism cannot be denied. The influence of environmental factors, on top of these obvious genetic differences, then leads to the inter-individual differences seen in the general population. The different research groups probably pick up different influences by virtue of different substrates used, different experimental procedures and methods of statistical analysis. Antipyrine metabolism, for instance, may be mainly controlled by environmental factors, while debrisoquine is mainly genetically controlled.

The control of drug metabolism is, thus, an extremely complex subject with many controlling factors, some of which are interactive. A comprehensive summary of the subject is impossible but it is hoped that this chapter, together with chapter 4, has given some idea of the factors involved and has stimulated the reader into further examination of one or more aspects of the subject, to which end a further reading list is included at the end of the chapter.

Further reading

Textbooks and symposia

Calabrese, E.J. (1981) *Nutrition and environmental health. The influence of nutritional status in pollutant toxicity and carcinogenicity, Vols. I and II,* Wiley, London

Coon, M.J. *et al.* (eds) (1980) *Microsomes, drug oxidations and chemical carcinogenesis, Vols. I and II,* Academic Press, New York

Fleischer, S. and Packer, L. (eds), (1978) *Biomembranes part C, Methods in Enzymology, Vol. 52,* Academic Press, New York

Kalow, W. (ed) (1992) *Pharmacogenetics of drug metabolism.* Pergamon Press, Oxford.

Parke, D.V. and Smith, R.L. (eds), (1977) *Drug metabolism from microbe to Man,* Taylor and Francis, London

Williams, R.T. (1959) *Detoxification mechanisms,* Chapman and Hall, London

Reviews

Alvan, G. (1992) Genetic polymorphisms in drug metabolism. *J.Internal Med.,* **231** 571–3.

Alvares, A.P. *et al.* (1979) Regulation of drug metabolism in man by environmental factors. *Drug Metab. Rev.,* **9** 185–206.

Alvares, A.P. and Kappas, A. (1979) Lead and polychlorinated biphenyls: effects on heme and drug metabolism. *Drug Metab. Rev.,* **10** 91-106.

Anderson, K.E. *et al.* (1982) Nutritional influences on chemical biotransformations in humans. *Nutrition Rev.,* **40** 161–71.

Anderson, K.E. (1988) Influence of diet and nutrition on clinical pharmacokinetics. *Clin. Pharmacokinet.,* **14** 325–46.

Azri, S. and Renton, K.W. (1991) Factors involved in the depresion of hepatic mixed function oxidase during infection with Listeria monocytogenes. *Int. J.Immunopharmacol,* **13,** 197–204.

Becking, G.C. (1978) Dietary minerals and drug metabolism. In *Nutrition and drug interrelationships* (J.N. Hathcock and J. Coon), Academic Press, New York

Berthou, F. *et al.* (1992) Interspecies variation in caffeine metabolism related to cytochrome P4501A enzymes. *Xenobiotica,* **22** 671–80.

Besunder, J.B. *et al.* (1988) Principles of drug biodisposition in the neonate. *Clin. Pharmacokinet.,* **14** 189–216.

Caldwell, J. (1982) Conjugation reactions in foreign-compound metabolism: definition, consequences and species variations. *Drug Metab. Rev.,* **13** 745-78.

Campbell, T.C. (1978) Effects of dietary protein on drug metabolism. In *Nutrition and drug interrelationships* (J.N. Hathcock and J. Coon), Academic Press, New York

Campbell, T.C. *et al.* (1979) The influence of dietary factors on drug metabolism in animals. *Drug Metab. Rev.,* **9** 173–84.

Conney, A.H. *et al.* (1971) Effects of environmental chemicals on the metabolism of drugs, carcinogens and normal body constituents in man. *Ann. N.Y. Acad. Sci.,* **179** 155–72.

Dawling, S. and Crome, P. (1989) Clinical pharmacokinetic considerations in the elderly. *Clin. Pharmacokinetic.,* **17** 236-63.

Dutton, G.J. (1978) Developmental aspects of drug conjugation, with special reference to glucuronidation. *Ann. Rev. Pharm. Tox.,* **18** 17–36.

Eichelbaum, M. and Gross, A.S. (1990) The genetic polymorphism of debrisoquine/sparteine metabolism – clinical aspects. *Pharmacol. Ther.,* **46** 377–94.

Feuer, G. (1979) Action of pregnancy and various progesterones on hepatic microsomal activities. *Drug Metab. Rev.,* **9** 147–72.

Gonzalez, F.J. and Meyer, U.A. (1991) Molecular genetics of the debrisoquine/sparteine polymorphism. *Clin. Pharmacol. Ther.,* **50** 233–8.

Gustafsson, J.Å. *et al.,* (1980) The hypothalamo-pituitary-liver axis: a new hormonal system in control of hepatic steroid and drug metabolism. *Rec. Prog. Hormone Res.,* **7** 48–91.

Hodgson, E. (1979) Comparative aspects of the distribution of cytochrome P450 dependent mono-oxygenase systems: an overview. *Drug Metab. Rev.,* **10** 15-34.

Horbach, G.J.M.J. *et al.* (1992) The effect of age on inducbility of various types of rat liver cytochrome P450. *Xenobiotica,* **22** 515–22.

Howden, C.W. *et al.* (1989) Drug metabolism in liver disease. *Pharmacol. Ther.,* **40** 439–74.

Hoyumpa, A.M. and Schenker, S. (1982) Major drug interactions: effect of liver disease, alcohol and malnutrition. *Ann. Rev. Med.,* **33** 113–50.

Hucker, H.B. (1970) Species differences in drug metabolism. *Ann. Rev. Pharm. Tox.,* **10** 99–118.

Huupponen, R. *et al.* (1991) Activity of xenobiotic metabolising liver enzymes in Zucker rats. *Res. Comm. Chem. Path. Pharmacol.,* **72** 307-14.

Idle, J.R. and Smith, R.L. (1979) Polymorphisms of oxidation at carbon centres of drugs and their clinical significance. *Drug Metab. Rev.,* **9** 301–18.

Johnson, J.A. and Burlew, B.S. (1992) Racial differences in propranolol pharmacokinetics. *Clin. Pharmacol. Ther.,* **51** 495–500.

Jusko, J.W. (1979) Influence of cigarette smoking on drug metabolism in Man. *Drug Metab. Rev.,* **9** 221–36.

Kato, R. (1977) Drug metabolism under pathological and abnormal physiological states in animals and Man. *Xenobiotica,* **7** 25–92.

Krishnaswamy, K. (1983) Drug metabolism and pharmacokinetics in malnutrition. *TIPS,* **4** 295–9.

Kroemer, H.K. and Klotz, U. (1992) Glucuronidation of drugs. *Clin. Pharmacokinet.,* **23** 292–310.

Ladona, M.G. *et al* (1991) Differential foetal development of the *O*- and *N*-demethylation of codeine and dextromethorphan in man. *Brit. J. Clin. Pharmacol.,* **32** 295–302.

Lavrijsen, K. *et al* (1992) Comparative metabolism of flunarizine in rats, dogs and man: An *in vitro* study with subcellular liver fractions and isolated hepatocytes. *Xenobiotica* **22** 815-36.

Longo, V. *et al* (1991) Drug-metabolising enzymes in liver, olfactory and respiratory epithelium of cattle. *J. Biochem. Toxicol.,* **6** 123–8.

Lou, Y.C. (1990) Differences in drug metabolism polymorphism between Orientals and Caucasians. *Drug Metab. Rev.,* **22** 451–75.

Neims, A.H. *et al* (1976) Developmental aspects of the hepatic cytochrome P450 mono-oxygenase system. *Ann. Rev. Pharm. Tox.,* **16** 427–46.

Ohmori, S. *et al.* (1991) Decrease in the specific forms of cytochrome P450 in liver microsomes of a mutant strain of rat with hyperbilirubinuria. *Res. Comm. Chem. Path. Pharmacol.,* **72** 243–53.

Omaye, S.T. and Turnbull, J.D. (1980) Effect of ascorbic acid on heme metabolism in hepatic microsomes. *Life Sci.,* **27** 441–9.

Prescott, L.F. (1975) Pathological and physiological factors affecting drug absorption, distribution, elimination and response in Man. In *Handbook of experimental pharmacology, Vol. 27* (J.R. Gillette and J.R. Mitchell), Springer, Berlin

Rikans, L.E. (1989) Hepatic drug metabolism in female Fischer rats as a function of age. *Drug Metab. Disp.,* **17** 114-6.

Scavone, J.M. *et al.* (1990) Differential effect of cigarette smoking on antipyrine oxidation and acetaminophen conjugation. *Pharmacol.,* **40** 77–84.

Schenkman, J.B. *et al.* (1989) Physiological and pathophysiological alterations in rat hepatic cytochrome P450. *Drug Metab. Rev.,* **20** 557–84.

Schmucker, D.L. *et al.* (1990) Effect of age and gender on *in vitro* properties of human liver microsomal monooxygenases. *Clin. Pharmacol. Ther.,* **48** 365–74.

Scott, A.K. *et al.* (1988) Oxazepam elimination in patients with diabetes mellitus. *Brit. J. Clin. Pharm.,* **26** 224P.

Sim, E. and Hickman, D. (1991) Polymorphism in human N-acetyltransferase – the case of the missing allele. *TIPS,* **12** 211–3.

Skett, P. and Gustafsson, J.Å. (1979) Imprinting of enzyme systems of xenobiotic and steroid metabolism. *Rev. Biochem. Tox.,* **1** 27–52.

Skett, P. (1988) Biochemical basis of sex differences in drug metabolism. *Pharmacol. Ther.,* **38** 269–304.

Smith, D.A. (1991) Species differences in metabolism and pharmacokinetics: are we close to an understanding? *Drug Metab. Rev.,* **23** 355.

Srivastava, P. *et al.* (1991) Effect of *Plasmodium berghei* infection and chloroquine on the hepatic drug metabolising system of mice. *Int. J. Parasitol.,* **4** 463–6.

Vessell, E.S. (1975) Genetically determined variations in drug disposition and response in Man. In *Handbook of experimental pharmacology, Vol. 27* (J.R. Gillette and J.R. Mitchell), Springer, Berlin

Vestal, R.E. (1989) Aging and determinants of hepatic drug clearance. *Hepatology,* **9** 331–4.

Walker, C.H. (1978) Species differences in microsomal mono-oxygenase activity and their relationship to biological half-lives. *Drug Metab. Rev.,* **7** 295–324.

Walker, C.H. (1980) Species variations in some hepatic microsomal enzymes that metabolise xenobiotics. *Progress in Drug Metab.*, **5** 113–64.

Wilkinson, G.R. and Schenker, S. (1975) Drug disposition and liver disease. *Drug Metab. Rev.*, **4** 139–76.

Williams, R.T. (1978) Nutrients in drug detoxification reactions. In *Nutrition and drug interrelationships* (J.N. Hathcock and J. Coon), Academic Press, New York

Weinshilboum, R. (1989) Methyltransferase pharmacogenetics. *Pharmacol. Ther.*, **43** 77–90.

Woodhouse, K. (1992) Drugs and the Liver. III. Ageing of the liver and the metabolism of drugs. *Biopharmaceut. Drug Dispos.*, **13** 311– 20.

6 Pharmacological and toxicological aspects of drug metabolism

6.1 Introduction

In general, the intensity and duration of drug action is proportional to the concentration of the drug at the site of action and the length of time it remains there. Therefore any factor that effectively alters the drug concentration at the active site will result in a changed pharmacological response to the drug. As indicated in previous chapters, the processes of drug metabolism result in biotransformation of the drug to metabolites that are chemically different from the parent drug and would therefore be expected to have an altered affinity for the drug receptor. Thus the processes of drug metabolism change the structure of the drug and essentially result in the production of a different chemical that often is not recognised by the relevant receptor system, and hence results in little or no pharmacological response. In this case, drug metabolism results in *pharmacological deactivation*. In contrast to the above, many drugs are pharmacologically inert and absolutely require metabolism to express their pharmacological effect. Therefore in this case, the process of drug metabolism results in *pharmacological activation*.

The above simplified picture is somewhat confounded by the fact that drug metabolites can also elicit additional biological responses that are unrelated to the pharmacological properties of the parent compound. For example, drug metabolism may result in a *change* of the pharmacological properties of the drug, enabling metabolites to interact with other receptor systems. In addition, many toxicological responses to drugs and chemicals can be rationalised by the unique biological toxicity of metabolites not shared by the parent compound, and is therefore an example of *toxicological activation*.

From the above discussion it is clear that the processes of drug metabolism have to be considered as a 'double-edged sword' in that, depending on the specific drug or chemical in question, a change in the pharmacology or toxicology of the drug may arise. Accordingly, it is the purpose of this chapter to consider this concept in more detail by examining the pharmacological and toxicological aspects of drug metabolism.

6.2 Pharmacological aspects of drug metabolism

The metabolism of a drug may alter the drug's pharmacological properties in one of several ways:

- Pharmacological deactivation
- Pharmacological activation
- Change in type of pharmacological response
- No change in pharmacological activity
- Change in drug uptake (absorption)
- Change in drug distribution
- Enterohepatic circulation

6.2.1 Pharmacological deactivation

The concept of specific enzyme systems existing for the deactivation or detoxication of drugs is not novel. For example, many chemicals or metabolites that are produced during normal intermediary metabolism are potentially toxic to the organism and enzyme systems are present that facilitate their inactivation. This is clearly seen in the efficient detoxication of hydrogen peroxide (arising from oxidative metabolism of endogenous substrates) by enzymes such as catalase. In a similar manner, many therapeutically used drugs and other xenobiotics are inactivated by the phase I enzymes of drug metabolism due to the substantially reduced pharmacological activity of the metabolite as compared to the parent drug (Figure 6.1).

An interesting and specific example of the above concept is the cytochrome P450-dependent pharmacological inactivation of the anticoagulant drug, warfarin. In man, the major route of warfarin biotransformation is the hepatic P4502C9-dependent hydroxylation of the parent compound at the 7-position (Figure 6.2). Since there is a narrow margin of clinical safety for this drug, (i.e. a low therapeutic index), then it follows that the levels and activity of this cytochrome P4502C9 isoform crucially influence both the pharmacology and toxicology of this drug. As a related issue, it should be noted that warfarin can be metabolised at various positions in the molecule by different cytochrome P450 isoenzymes, further emphasising the importance of the tissue *complement* of cytochrome P450 isoenzymes in dictating the clinical response to drugs. As a further refinement of cytochrome P450 selectivity in drug biotransformation, warfarin exists in racemic (R)+ and (S)– forms, each racemate exhibiting a different preference for regioselectivity of hydroxylation by the cytochrome P450 isoforms.

It should be pointed out that the phase II conjugating enzymes play a very important role in the pharmacological inactivation of drugs and further inactivation of their phase I metabolites. Although a few exceptions are known, the majority of drug conjugates are pharmacologically less active than the parent compound. This effect is achieved by both gross chemical modification of the drug thereby decreasing receptor affinity and by enhancement of excretion and

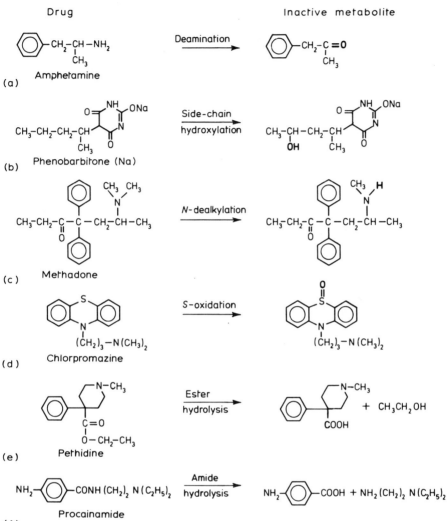

Figure 6.1 Role of phase I enzymes in the pharmacological inactivation of drugs.

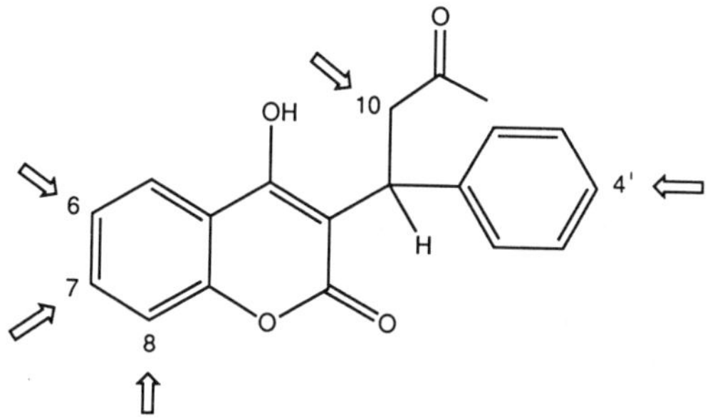

Figure 6.2 Structure of the anticoagulant warfarin and sites of metabolic hydroxylation by the cytochrome P450s.

removal from the body. It is quite clear that if drug clearance from the body is enhanced by phase II conjugation, then the duration of action is curtailed.

The widely used analgesic drug paracetamol also serves as an example of phase II metabolism resulting in pharmacological inactivation of the parent drug. As shown in Figure 6.3, paracetamol undergoes glutathione, glucuronide and sulfate conjugation and the resulting phase II conjugates are pharmacologically inactive. Furthermore, many drugs are pharmacologically deactivated by simultaneous phase I and phase II metabolic attack at different positions in the molecule as is observed in the metabolic inactivation of the betablocker, propranolol (Figure 6.4).

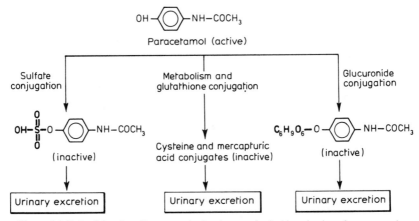

Figure 6.3 Role of the phase II enzymes in the pharmacological inactivation of paracetamol.

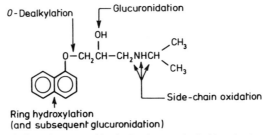

Figure 6.4 Metabolic pathways resulting in the pharmacological inactivation of propranolol.

6.2.2 Pharmacological activation

In contrast to the concepts discussed above, many drugs and chemicals require metabolic activation before they can exert their pharmacological action. This process of metabolic activation is usually associated with the phase I enzymes. Many of these parent drugs are essentially devoid of pharmacological activity and this has led to the development of the so-called 'pro-drugs'. A classical example of pro-drug activation by metabolism was the early use of the dye prontosil in the 1930s to treat bacterial infections. *In vitro* studies clearly showed that prontosil itself was inactive and required metabolic azo reduction to liberate the pharmacologically active component, sulfanilamide (Figure 6.5).

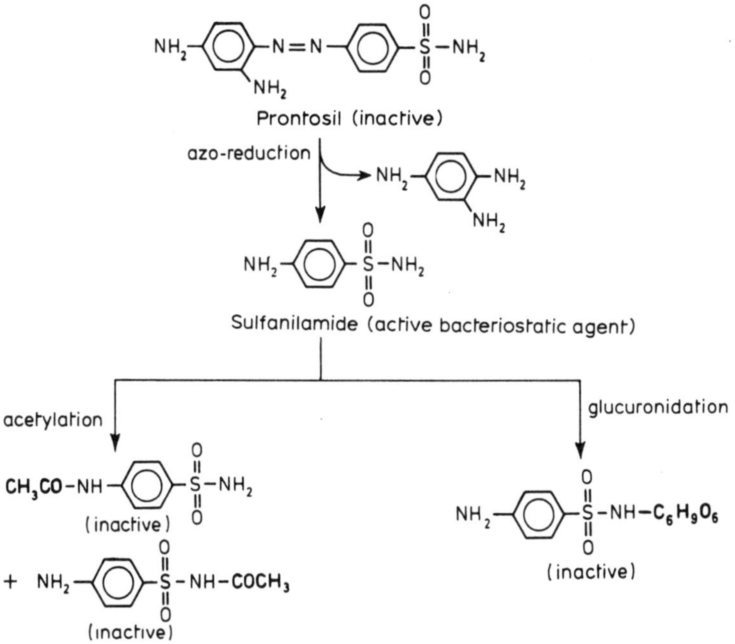

Figure 6.5 Role of metabolism in the pharmacological activation of prontosil and the pharmacological inactivation of its major metabolite sulfanilamide.

It should be noted that the active sulfanilamide is subsequently metabolically inactivated by *N*-acetylation at both nitrogen atoms and by *N*-glucuronidation at the amide nitrogen. Accordingly, it is clear that the therapeutic effectiveness of this class of drugs is strongly influenced by the prevailing tissue balance of the azo reductase on the one hand and the *N*-acetylase and glucuronidation enzymes on the other.

The above concept of pro-drug activation has been used to target drugs to their specific site of action. For example, the drug levodopa is metabolically activated in the neurone to dopamine, but the drug is given as the levodopa precursor due to its more facile uptake into the neurone. Dopamine does not cross the blood–brain barrier. Therefore, L-dopa is given as a precursor as it does cross the blood–brain barrier.

Another example of biotransformation resulting in pharmacological activation is in the clinical usage of mercaptopurine, a chemotherapeutic agent used in the treatment of patients with leukaemia. The clinical usefulness of mercaptopurine is limited by its rapid biotransformation by xanthine oxidase to the inactive metabolite, 6-thiouric acid. Because of this extensive metabolism, the drug has to be given in high doses thereby predisposing the liver and other tissues to cellular damage and hence toxicity. The above clinical limitations can be largely overcome by administering mercaptopurine as its cysteine conjugate where advantage is taken of the fact that the anionic form of the pro-drug conjugate is selectively taken up by the renal organic anion transport system. The conjugate is subsequently cleaved by the kidney β-lyase enzyme system (Figure 6.6), thus creating a clinical use for the cysteine conjugate in the treatment of kidney tumours.

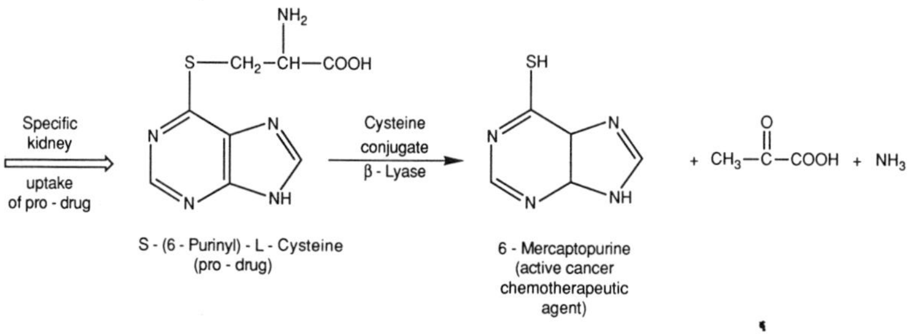

Figure 6.6 Kidney uptake and pharmacological activation of the pro-drug S-(6-purinyl)-L-cysteine.

There are many other examples of drugs whose metabolism results in pharmacological activation and some of these are given in Table 6.1.

Table 6.1 Drug metabolism reactions resulting in pharmacological activation

Pro-drug	Clinical use	Metabolic conversion	Active drug/metabolite
Azathioprine	Immunosuppressant	Thio-ether hydrolysis	Mercaptopurine
Chloral hydrate	Sedative/hypnotic	Reduction	Trichloroethanol
Clofibrate	Hypolipidaemic	Ester hydrolysis	Clofibric acid
Cyclophosphamide	Anti-tumour/ immunosuppressant	Hydroxylation	4-Hydroxy-cyclophosphamide (precursor to other active metabolites)
Disulphiram	Alcohol withdrawal	Dithiol reduction	Diethylthiocarbamic acid
Glyceryl triacetate	Antifungal	Ester hydrolysis	Acetic acid
Methyldopa	Antihypertensive	Decarboxylation and hydroxylation	α-methylnoradrenaline
Prednisone	Anti-inflammatory	Keto reduction	Prednisolone
Primaquine	Antimalarial	Demethylation and oxidation	Primaquine quinone
Primidone	Anti-epileptic	Oxidation	Phenobarbitone
Proguanil	Antimalarial	Cyclization	Cycloguanil
Prontosil	Antibiotic	Azo-reduction	Sulfanilamide
Succinylsulfathiazole	Antibiotic	Amide hydrolysis	Sulfathiazole

6.2.3 Change in type of pharmacological response

In addition to modulating pharmacological responses in either a positive or negative manner as described above, the process of drug metabolism can also result in a *change* in the pharmacology of the parent compound. For example, iproniazid was formerly used as an anti-depressant, but has subsequently been removed from the market because it caused severe liver toxicity. Iproniazid is metabolised by *N*-dealkylation resulting in the formation of the metabolite isoniazid which has pronounced anti-tubercular activity, a pharmacological activity not associated with the parent drug. Another example of this phenomenon is seen in the metabolism of the tricyclic anti-depressant drug imipramine. This drug undergoes an enzymatic *N*-demethylation reaction resulting in the formation of desmethylimipramine, a compound that is substantially more potent than the parent drug as an inhibitor of the neuronal uptake of noradrenaline but less potent for the uptake of 5HT.

A third example of the ability of drug metabolism to result in a change in pharmacological response is seen in the metabolism of diazepam (Valium), a benzodiazepine chiefly used as a tranquilliser. The drug undergoes *N*-demethylation and subsequent ring hydroxylation yielding oxazepam as a metabolite, the metabolite having pronounced anti-convulsant properties. The metabolic pathways involved in the above reactions are summarised in Figure 6.7.

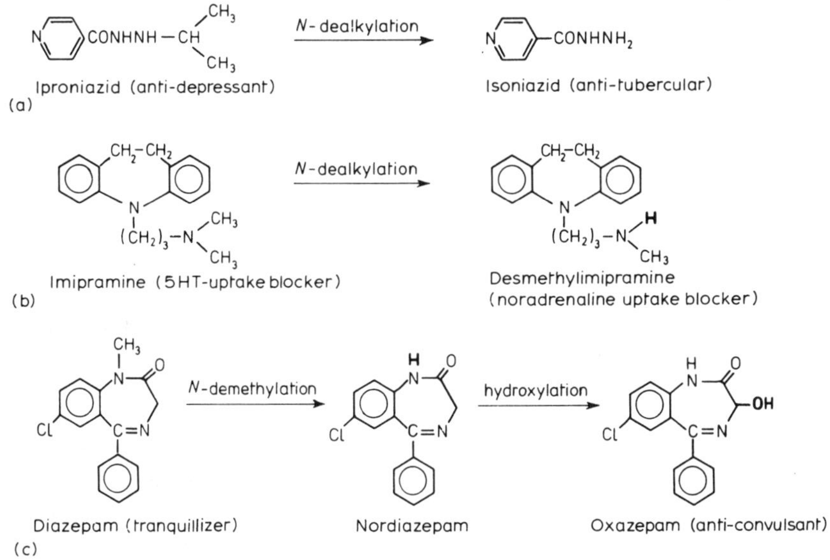

Figure 6.7 Drug metabolism resulting in a change in the type of pharmacological activity.

6.2.4 No change in pharmacological activity

Several drugs are metabolised to compounds that have the same or similar pharmacological activity. An example of this type is the *N*-deethylation of the local anaesthetic lignocaine. The *N*-deethylated metabolite (monoethylglycylxylidine) is as active as the parent compound and it would appear that metabolism serves no useful immediate purpose here. However, it should be emphasised that metabolism may prime the substrate for subsequent phase II reactions and indirectly facilitate drug execretion and hence termination of pharmacological activity.

6.2.5 Change in drug uptake

Changes in drug uptake by metabolism may be seen after the oral administration of drugs and is dependent on the enzymes at the site of uptake, for example, the gastrointestinal tract. In most cases, drug metabolism at the site of uptake inhibits drug absorption as seen in the formation of sulfate conjugates of phenolic drugs after oral administration. As shown in Figure 6.8, isoprenaline sulfation and isoniazid acetylation by enzymes in the intestinal wall and gut flora, result in more polar metabolites. The polar metabolites are less readily absorbed across the gut wall as compared to the parent drug and are consequently preferentially excreted in the faeces.

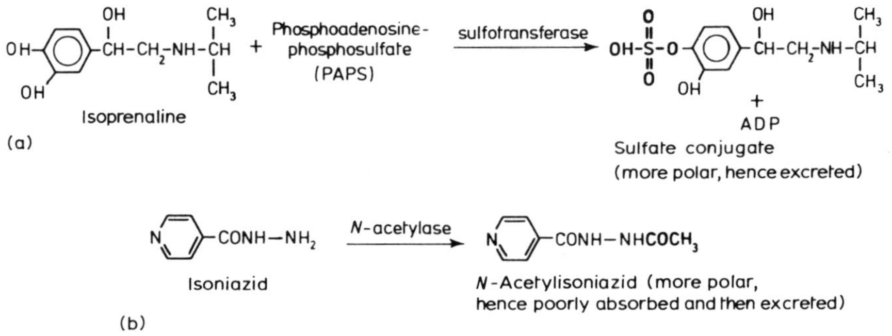

Figure 6.8 The role of drug metabolism in modifying drug uptake

It is interesting to note that in certain cases the metabolism of a drug at the uptake site is an important factor in determining the most effective route of administration. For instance, in the example of the anti-asthmatic drug, isoprenaline, given above, it is clear that oral administration is not an effective means of getting the drug to its site of action (lung) because of extensive gut metabolism. To get over this problem, isoprenaline may be given sublingually and absorbed through the buccal mucosa. Unfortunately, the circulating drug is rapidly inactivated (again by metabolism) in the liver. Isoprenaline is best administered via aerosol inhalation – in this way, the inactivating metabolic pathways are by-passed and the drug directly reaches the lungs in sufficiently high concentration to be pharmacologically active.

In contrast to the above, gut metabolism can be used to advantage as in the oral administration of the 4-amino substituted sulfonamide antibiotics such as succinylsulfathiazole. This drug is poorly absorbed through the gut wall and is readily hydrolysed by gut enzymes to the active sulfathiazole. This local hydrolysis in the gut ensures high, effective antibiotic concentrations, and is therefore very useful in the treatment of gut infections.

6.2.6 Change in drug distribution

Drug distribution to the various tissues in the body (and hence the site of action), is dependent on several factors including the lipid solubility of the drug. A highly lipophilic drug will be localised in highest concentrations in tissues with high fat content such as adipose tissues and the brain. As metabolism causes drugs to be less lipid soluble in most cases, metabolism will then alter drug distribution away from the high-fat tissues and into the high water tissues such as blood and the kidney.

A good example of the above concept is the distribution of the narcotic analgesic morphine. Morphine is highly lipophilic and is not readily excreted because it is quickly absorbed into lipid-rich tissues including the brain. However, morphine undergoes phase II conjugation with glucuronic acid in the liver, forming the morphine-3-glucuronide metabolite. This metabolite is water-soluble and does not readily enter the brain and the conjugate is then readily excreted. Thus hepatic metabolism in this instance precludes the access of morphine to the brain and thereby diminishes the pharmacological response by redistribution away from the site of action.

The lipophilicity of drugs can also radically influence the rate of onset of drug action. For example, diamorphine (diacetylmorphine or as it is better known, heroin) enters the brain much more rapidly than morphine because of its higher lipophilicity, and therefore has a more rapid onset of action. Once in the brain, the diamorphine is rapidly metabolised to morphine, whereupon the pharmacological effects (primarily analgesia) are observed.

6.2.7 Enterohepatic circulation

The specific route of drug excretion is largely influenced by its molecular weight. Drugs having a molecular weight of under approximately 300 are largely excreted in urine, whereas drugs with a higher molecular weight are mainly excreted in the bile and hence into the intestine. Once in the intestine, a drug glucuronide conjugate has two possible fates. It can either be excreted in the faeces or additionally, the glucuronide conjugate can be hydrolysed back to the parent drug by the action of the enzyme β-glucuronidase which is present in gut bacteria. The free, de-conjugated drug is then absorbed through the gut wall and re-enters the liver via the hepatic portal vein. The free drug can then be re-conjugated with glucuronic acid, secreted into the bile and then intestine and the cyclic process starts again. This cycling of drug is known as the entero-hepatic circulation and is outlined in Figure 6.9.

The above recirculation of drugs can take place for several cycles and the overall result is that the drug is retained in the body and has a substantially increased half-life. Provided that the drug concentration is maintained high enough at the site of action, it is quite clear that this metabolism-based cycle can result in a prolongation of pharmacological activity, as is seen in the example given for chloramphenicol (Figure 6.9). The eventual excretion of the drug then arises from the faecal excretion of drug–conjugate that escapes hydrolysis in the intestine during each turn of the cycle and by other metabolic pathways.

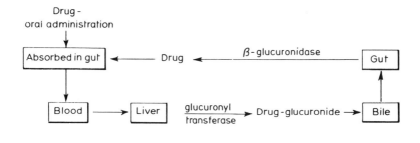

Figure 6.9 Enterohepatic circulation of drugs.

It would appear that drugs get trapped in this cycle by accident rather than design. It is well known that conjugates of endogenous compounds such as steroids, bile salts and bilirubin undergo the same enterohepatic circulation, and therefore drugs are 'ensnared' in a normal physiological process.

In conclusion, drug metabolism can profoundly alter the uptake, distribution and pharmacological action of a particular drug as well as direct its excretion pattern. In addition, drug metabolism is of major importance in determining the method of administration and on deciding the correct dose and frequency of drug delivery. In fact, apart from the inherent pharmacological activity of the drug itself, the metabolism of a drug is probably the most important considera-tion to be made in drug design and therapeutics.

6.3 Toxicological aspects of xenobiotic metabolism

As discussed above for the pharmacological properties of drugs and their metabolites, drug metabolism can result in either a decreased or increased toxi-city of the parent compound, depending, of course, on the inherent biological potencies (toxicities) of the drug and its metabolite(s).

6.3.1 Metabolism resulting in increased toxicity

As summarised in Table 6.2, many examples are known where the hepatic metabolism of drugs and chemicals results in an increased toxicity of the parent

Table 6.2 Metabolism resulting in increased toxicity of drugs and chemicals

Compound	Metabolic pathway	Toxicity
2-Acetylaminofluorene	N-Hydroxylation and sulfation	Hepatocarcinogenesis
Benzene	Epoxidation (and other pathways leading to ring opening)	Aplastic anaemia/leukaemia
Cyclophosphamide	Hydroxylation (and rearrangement)	Teratogenesis
Halothane	Defluorination	Hepatitis
Isoniazid	Acetylation and hydrolysis	Hepatic necrosis
Methoxyflurane	Defluorination	Nephrotoxicity

compound. The enzymes responsible for this metabolic toxification are mainly the phase I enzymes. Although some examples have been documented on the participation of phase II reactions, these latter enzymes are more often associated with detoxication reactions (see next section). This concept of metabolic toxification can be amply demonstrated by considering the following specific examples of toxic reactions to drugs and chemicals.

(a) *Carcinogenesis.* As discussed previously, the polycyclic aromatic hydrocarbons represent a ubiquitous group of environmental chemicals that are well documented in causing cancer in many mammalian species. The parent compounds are relatively innocuous and chemically inert, but their metabolites are biologically active and are potent carcinogens. The polycyclic aromatic hydrocarbons are metabolised by the cytochromes P450 and epoxide hydrolase forming the electrophilic diol-epoxide metabolites which are then capable of covalent binding to nucleic acids and hence the initiation of chemical carcinogenesis.

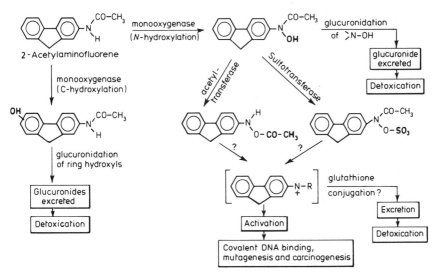

Figure 6.10 Metabolic activation and inactivation of the hepatocarcinogen 2-acetylaminofluorene. (Adapted from T.M. Guenthner and F. Oesch, *Trends in Pharmacol. Sci.*, May 1981, pp. 129–32.)

Another example of the role of metabolic activation in chemical carcinogenesis is the metabolism of the compound 2-acetylaminofluorene. This synthetic compound was originally intended for use as an insecticide and during routine safety studies prior to introduction to the market, it was discovered that it was an extremely potent hepatocarcinogen. Further studies on this carcinogen have amply documented the fact that both phase I and phase II enzymes are involved in the bioactivation of this carcinogen (Figure 6.10). The importance of the drug metabolising enzymes in many types of chemical carcinogenesis cannot be overemphasised and in addition to the above examples, many other chemicals (including the aflatoxins, aromatic amines and nitrosamines) are dependent on metabolism for expression of their carcinogenicity. As a caveat to the above general description, it must be borne in mind that metabolism alone is not the sole determinant of carcinogenicity of drugs and chemicals – many other factors are important for expression of carcinogenicity including promotion and genetic predisposition. However, this is a large and complex area outside the scope of this discussion.

(b) *Teratogenesis.* Several drugs and chemicals are known to interfere with the processes of embryo development and if given at the critical stage of organogenesis can result in malformations of the embryo (teratogenesis). The anti-tumour drug cyclophosphamide is a well-documented teratogen and several studies have shown that the metabolites of cyclophosphamide are much more teratogenic than the parent compound. As shown in Figure 6.11, cyclophosphamide undergoes cytochrome P450-dependent hydroxylation at the 4-position and this hydroxylated metabolite serves as the precursor for the toxic metabolites acrolein and phosphoramide mustard.

Although it is not known with any degree of certainty which of these two metabolites of cyclophosphamide is the major teratogen, it is quite clear that metabolism is a prerequisite for the expression of cyclophosphamide teratogenicity.

(c) *Pulmonary toxicity.* 4-Ipomeanol, a furan derivative found on mouldy sweet potatoes, produces a characteristic pulmonary toxicity in several mammalian species (necrosis of the non-ciliated bronchiolar epithelial or Clara cells). Current evidence suggests that 4-ipomeanol is metabolised by a specific pulmonary cytochrome P450, resulting in the formation of a highly biological reactive intermediate. This intermediate covalently binds to critical macromolecular targets in the Clara cell resulting in the observed necrosis in this cell type. It is interesting to note that 4-ipomeanol is selectively toxic to the lung and is relatively non-toxic to the liver, an organ very rich in xenobiotic metabolising enzymes. This apparent contradiction is rationalised by the observation that the liver lacks the appropriate isoenzyme of cytochrome P450 necessary for activation or that the liver is well-endowed with the detoxifying phase II enzymes that remove the reactive intermediate.

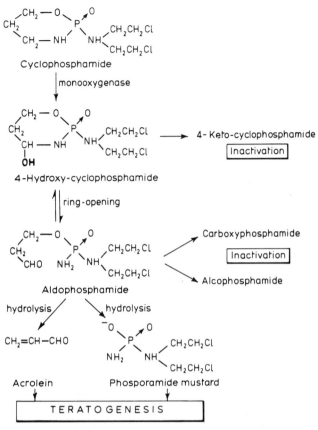

Figure 6.11 Metabolic activation of the teratogen, cyclophosphamide (Adapted from Nau *et al.*, *Mutation Research*, **95** 105–18 1982).

The herbicide paraquat is a very toxic compound as witnessed by the many accidental deaths in humans, particularly young children. Paraquat appears to 'hijack' the specific pulmonary uptake mechanism for polyamines, thus concentrating this chemical in the lung. The resultant pulmonary toxicity of paraquat is therefore due to a combination of several factors including specific pulmonary uptake, redox cycling and generation of toxic oxygen metabolites and perturbation of redox homeostasis in this tissue.

The above discussion emphasises the importance of metabolism in producing toxic metabolites. Furthermore, it is clear that the presence (or absence) of phase I and phase II enzymes is an important determinant of selective organ toxicity of drugs and chemicals.

(d) *Hepatic toxicity.* Many of the drugs and chemicals shown in Table 6.2 are toxic to the liver, resulting in hepatic necrosis. A well documented example of a hepatotoxin is paracetamol, which in high doses produces hepatic necrosis, in both experimental animals and man. Again, as in the previous examples, paracetamol requires metabolic activation for expression of its toxicity. This is thought to occur by an initial *N*-hydroxylation reaction catalysed by the hepatic mixed function oxidase enzymes (Figure 6.13) and subsequent chemical rearrangement of the hydroxylamine producing a reactive electrophile which then covalently binds to hepatic macromolecules as a prelude to liver necrosis. It must be emphasised that the reactive intermediate(s) of paracetamol may be enzymatically detoxified by conjugation with glutathione (catalysed by the glutathione-*S*-transferases), a concept that will be more fully developed later in this chapter.

(e) *Nephrotoxicity.* Many drugs exhibit a selective toxicity to the kidney, including antibiotics such as the sulfonamides. A major route of sulfonamide metabolism is by acetylation of the 4-amino group in the molecule, a pathway that results in pharmacological inactivation. However, an occasional toxic effect of the sulfonamides is crystalluria, a condition caused by precipitation of the less soluble acetylated sulfonamide metabolite in the tubular urine, especially when the urine is acidic.

In addition, the kidney has significant amounts of the mixed function oxidase system enzymes and prostaglandin endoperoxide synthetase, two enzyme systems that have the potential to metabolically activate innocuous drugs and chemicals to toxic metabolites. Although our knowledge of the kidney metabolism of xenobiotics is not as fully developed as the equivalent system in the liver, it is becoming clearer that the kidney can also activate drugs. For example, paracetamol can be metabolised both by mixed function oxidation and by co-oxidation in the presence of arachidonic acid and prostaglandin endoperoxide synthetase. Both of these pathways result in the production of toxic metabolites that bind to critical, cellular macromolecules and ultimately result in necrosis of the kidney tissue in a similar fashion to the liver as described above. In addition many urinary bladder carcinogens such as benzidine and many nephrotoxic chlorinated hydrocarbons (including chloroform, carbon tetrachloride and trichloroethylene) require metabolic activation as a necessary prelude to the expression of their nephrotoxicity.

The kidney is apparently susceptible to the toxicity of drugs and chemicals that are metabolised by conjugation with glutathione and subsequent metabolic processing to renal toxins. Toxic compounds in this class include halogenated alkenes used in the chemical industry, including hexachlorobutadiene, perchloroethylene and trichloroethylene. As discussed previously, the glutathione adduct of these xenobiotics is metabolised to the corresponding cysteine conjugate, which as an organic anion, is selectively taken up and concentrated in the P_3 segment of the proximal convoluted tubule, coincident with the kidney localisation of the β-lyase enzyme which further metabolises the compound to necrotic, mutagenic and carcinogenic metabolites (Figure 6.12). However, it

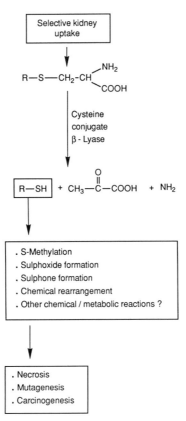

Figure 6.12 Selective kidney uptake and cysteine conjugate β-lyase dependent bioactivation of xenobiotics. R represents a xenobiotic substrate.

must be borne in mind that predisposition to the nephrotoxicity of compounds metabolised via this pathway depends on many factors, with the overall balance of activating/deactivating enzymes playing a major role.

6.3.2 Metabolism resulting in decreased toxicity

From the above discussion, it is clear that many phase I reactions result in the production of toxic metabolites of xenobiotics. However, this phenomenon must not be considered in isolation as many of the toxic phase I metabolites are substrates of phase II enzymes, the resultant conjugate, in general, being considerably less toxic than the initial metabolite. For example, paracetamol is activated by the mixed function oxidase system but in low doses, the reactive metabolite (Figure 6.13) is conjugated with cellular glutathione and safely excreted as thiol conjugates. This protective influence of the phase II enzymes is clearly seen in experimental animals depleted of cellular glutathione by compounds such as diethyl maleate. Such glutathione-depleted animals are then

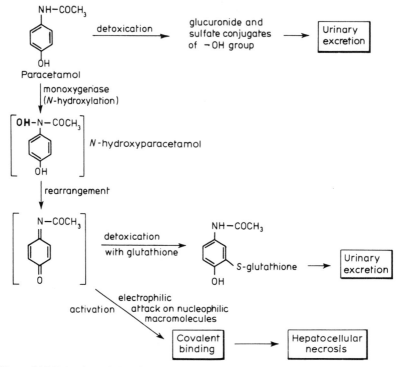

Figure 6.13 Role of metabolism in toxicological activation of paracetamol (modified from B. G. Lake and S. D. Gangolli, in *Concepts in Drug Metabolism*, P. Jenner and B. Testa, eds., pp 166–218, Marcel Dekker, New York, 1981).

rendered more susceptible to paracetamol hepatotoxicity, whereas the animals are protected against the toxicity of this analgesic by glutathione supplementation.

Another example of phase II metabolism resulting in decreased toxicity is seen in glucuronidation reactions when comparing the LD_{50} values of various compounds in species that have different abilities to form glucuronide conjugates. Whereas the rabbit is competent at glucuronidation, the cat is well known to be defective in this phase II pathway, resulting in an increases susceptibility to various compounds, as demonstrated by substantially lower LD_{50} values (Table 6.3).

6.4 Balance of toxifying and detoxifying pathways

If a drug can be metabolised either to a toxic metabolite or inactivated by metabolism, what then determines the ultimate toxicological response to the drug? An obvious answer to this question is that there is a balance of activating and deactivating enzymes, as is exemplified with the hepatocarcinogen 2-acetylaminofluorene. With reference to Figure 6.10 two main routes of metabolism exist. The first is cytochrome P450-dependent monooxygenation

Table 6.3 Role of glucuronic acid conjugation in the toxicity of xenobiotics in the rabbit and cat

Compound	LD$_{50}$ (mg/kg)	
	Rabbit	Cat
Phenol	250	80
Paracetamol	1200	250

Adapted from Caldwell, J. (1980) in *Concepts in Drug Metabolism, Part A* (P. Jenner and B. Testa), Marcel Dekker, New York.

of the fluorenyl ring system and subsequent glucuronidation (detoxification) and the second is cytochrome P450-dependent monooxygenation of the amide nitrogen and subsequent sulfation of the hydroxylamine (activation). In the first instance, it is thought that different isoenzymes of cytochrome P450 catalyse the above two initial oxidation reactions and therefore the relative amounts and activities of these isoenzymes will determine, in part, the ultimate biological response. In addition, Figure 6.10 shows that sulfate esterification of the *N*-hydroxy metabolite is a key metabolic step in the activation of this compound to a carcinogen. Thus it is clear that the concentration and activity of the cytoplasmic sulfotransferase enzymes are a major determinant of the hepatic toxicity of 2-acetylaminofluorene. Accordingly, species such as the guinea-pig which have low hepatic sulfotransferase activity, are resistant to 2-acetylamino-fluorene-induced hepatic cancer.

As shown in Figure 6.14, the phase I metabolism of the anti-psychotic/seda-tive drug chlorpromazine is complex, consisting of ring hydroxylation, *N*-demethylation, *S*-oxidation and *N*-oxidation reactions occurring in the microsomal fraction of the hepatocyte. In fact the metabolism of this drug is even more complex when the phase II glucuronidation and sulfation reactions are taken into account, resulting in the excretion of approximately 20–30 different metabolites in human urine. At present, although the pharmacological and toxicological potencies of these various metabolites have not all been definitively characterised, it is likely that the metabolites have different potencies and the metabolism of this drug is another illustration of the importance of the balance of metabolic pathways in determining the ultimate biological responses.

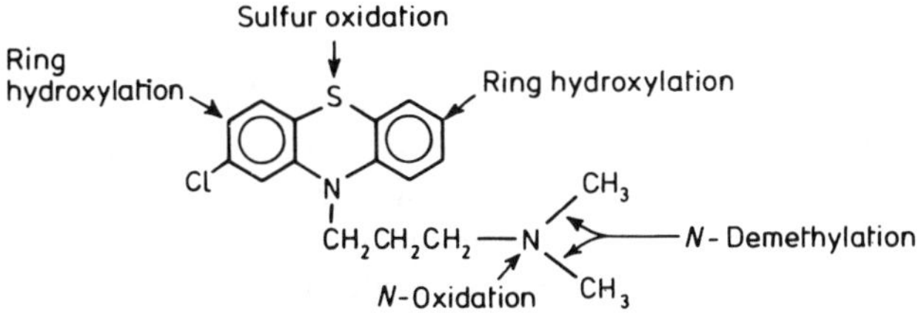

Figure 6.14 Multiple phase I metabolic pathways for chlorpromazine.

The metabolism of the organic compound bromobenzene serves as another excellent example of the importance of the balance between toxifying and detoxifying enzymes. Bromobenzene is hepatotoxic and in sufficiently high doses may result in the expression of hepatic necrosis in experimental animals fed this compound. Many studies have shown that bromobenzene requires metabolic activation to express its hepatotoxicity, but it must be emphasised that other detoxifying metabolic pathways exist (Figure 6.15). Initially, bromobenzene is metabolised to the key reactive metabolite bromobenzene-3, 4-epoxide by the cytochrome P450-dependent mixed function oxidase system. This reaction is preferentially catalysed by a phenobarbitone-induced isoenzyme of cytochrome P450 whereas epoxidation of bromobenzene is directed towards the 2–3 position by a polycyclic aromatic hydrocarbon-induced variant of the haemoprotein (cytochrome P4501A1). The prevailing balance of these cytochrome P450 isoenzymes is an important determinant of bromobenzene toxicity as the 3–4 epoxide is considerably more toxic to the liver cell than the 2–3 epoxide. Once formed, the 3–4 epoxide may undergo several different fates (Figure 6.15). The epoxide

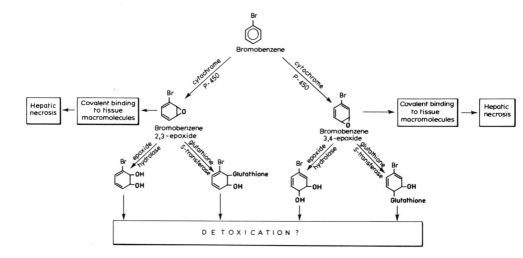

Figure 6.15 Metabolic activation and inactivation of the hepatotoxin, bromobenzene.

may be inactivated by diol formation (catalysed by the enzyme epoxide hydrolase), glutathione conjugation (catalysed by the glutathione-S-transferases) or covalently bind to critical tissue macromolecules, the presumed chemico-biological interaction that initiates cellular necrosis. It has also been postulated that the hepatotoxicity of bromobenzene is associated with the cellular depletion of glutathione (as a direct result of metabolism) and hence the attendant potential toxicity associated with substantial changes in cellular glutathione homeostasis. Although the precise mechanism(s) of bromobenzene-induced hepatic toxicity have yet to be elucidated, it should be clear from the above dicsussion that the balance of the metabolising enzymes and the availability of glutathione is an important determinant of toxicity.

One important feature of the phase II reactions is that they are quite frequently capacity limited by the availability of the endogenous compound required for conjugation with the parent drug or its phase I metabolite (Table 6.4).

Table 6.4 Capacities of conjugation reactions

Capacity	Reaction
High	Glucuronidation
Medium	Amino acid conjugation
Low	Sulfation and glutathione conjugation
Variable	Acetylation

Adapted from Caldwell, J. (1980) in *Concepts in Drug Metabolism, Part A* (P. Jenner and B. Testa), Marcel Dekker, New York.

This capacity-limited phenomenon is readily understood because many of the endogenous conjugating molecules such as glucuronic acid, sulfate and glutathione are additionally required for the metabolism and conjugation of endogenous substrates such as steroids and bile acids. Accordingly, when the body is challenged with high doses of drugs, higher than normal levels of conjugating molecules are required for metabolism. If the synthesis of the endogenous conjugating compounds is limited in any way then a predictable result of drug therapy in high doses would be the inability to conjugate the drug in question. In the majority of cases, where phase II conjugation reactions result in detoxification, failure to conjugate the drug would then result in an overt expression of drug-induced toxicity (Table 6.5).

A good example of the capacity-limited conjugation of drugs is seen with aspirin excretion in man. As shown in Figure 6.16, aspirin can be conjugated

Table 6.5 Detoxication failure due to saturation of conjugation reactions

Compound	Species	Saturatable reaction	Nature of toxicity
Paracetamol, bromobenzene	Several	Glutathione conjugation	Hepatocellular necrosis
Chloramphenicol	Human neonate	Glucuronidation	Agranulocytosis
Benzoic acid	Cat	Glycine conjugation	Death
Phenol	Cat	Sulfation	Death

Adapted from Caldwell, J. (1980) in *Concepts in Drug Metabolism, Part A* (P. Jenner and B. Testa), Marcel Dekker, New York.

with either the amino acid glycine or with glucuronic acid. At low doses of aspirin, glycine conjugation is the main metabolic pathway. However, on increasing the aspirin dose, the glycine conjugating system becomes readily saturated and conjugation switches to glucuronide formation. At the top doses of aspirin, the glucuronidation system also becomes saturated, and salicylic acid becomes a major excretory product.

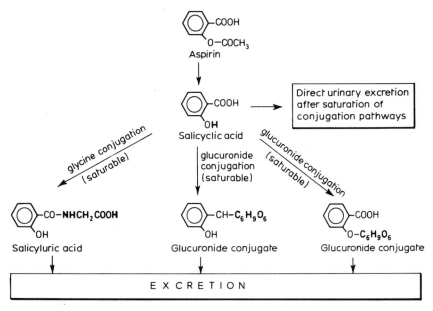

Figure 6.16 Capacity-limited metabolism of aspirin.

6.5 Assessment of human drug-metabolising enzymes in pharmacology and toxicology

Most of the examples described so far in the pharmacological and toxicological aspects of drug metabolism relate to the use of purified animal enzymes or tissues preparations. Because of practical and ethical reasons, it is obviously much more difficult to gather the same amount of sophisticated biological information on human drug-metabolising enzymes. However, with the advent of rapid advances in molecular biology and biotechnology, many of the human enzymes have been cloned and expressed in heterologous cell-based systems, thereby allowing a more facile and incisive approach to assessing human activation/ deactivation potential (Figure 6.17). Whereas there are many refinements and pitfalls associated with this type of approach, it offers excellent potential for exciting developments in understanding human enzymology.

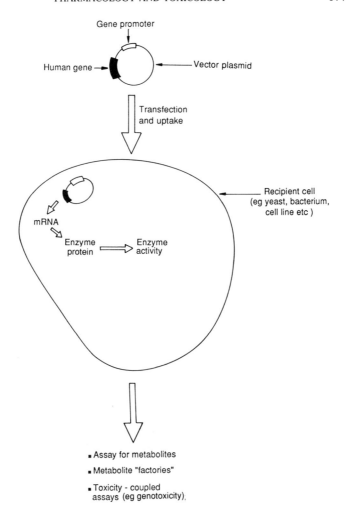

Figure 6.17 Assessment of human drug-metabolising enzymes.

6.6 Conclusions

The classical viewpoint of drug metabolism being a detoxifying pathway is now no longer entirely true. Although many examples are known where metabolism results in decreased pharmacological and toxicological responses, it must be emphasised that activation reactions have also been amply verified. This chapter has focused on specific examples of activation and inactivation and emphasis has been placed on the critical role played by the balance of the drug-metabolising enzymes in determining the ultimate biological response(s) to the drug. Accordingly, this chapter should be considered as 'integrative' i.e.

consolidating the previous chapters that were descriptive of metabolic pathways and factors affecting metabolism with the responses of organisms to foreign compounds.

Further reading

Textbooks and symposia

Arinc, E. *et al.* (1989) *Molecular Aspects of Monooxygenases and Bioactivation of Toxic Compounds*, NATO ASI Series A, Life Sciences Volume 202, Plenum, New York

Hawkins, D. R. (1988, 1989, 1991 and 1992) *A Survey of the Biotransformations of Drugs and Chemicals in Animals, Volumes 1-4*, Royal Society of Chemistry, Cambridge.

Hodgson, E. and Levi, P. E. (1993) *Introduction to Biochemical Toxicology*, 2nd Edition, Appleton and Lange, East Norwalk.

Kalow, W. (1992) *Pharmacogenetics of Drug Metabolism*, Pergamon, New York.

Klein-Szanto *et al.* (1991) *Comparative Molecular Carcinogenesis*, Wiley–Liss, New York.

Roloff, M. W. (1987) *Human Risk Assessment*, Taylor and Francis, London.

Volans, G. N. *et al.* (1990) *Basic Science in Toxicology* (Fifth International Congress of Toxicology), Taylor and Francis, London.

Reviews and original articles

Anders, M. W. *et al.* (1992) Glutathione-dependent toxicity. *Xenobiotica*, **22** 1135–45.

Bock, K. W. (1991) Roles of UDP-glucuronosyl transferases in chemical carcinogensis. *Critical Reviews in Biochemistry and Molecular Biology*, **26** 129–50.

Caccia, S. and Garattini, S. (1992) Pharmacokinetic and pharmacodynamic significance of antidepressant drug metabolites. *Pharmacological Research*, **26** 317–29.

Davidson, I. W. F. and Beliles, R. P. (1991) Consideration of the target organ toxicity of trichloroethylene in terms of metabolite toxicity and pharmacokinetics. *Drug Metabolism Reviews*, **23** 493–599.

Dekant, W. *et al.* (1990) Bioactivation of hexachlorobutadiene by glutathione conjugation. *Food and Chemical Toxicology*, **28** 285–93.

Fawthrop, D. J. *et al.* (1991). Mechanisms of cell death. *Archives of Toxicology*, **65** 437–44.

Green, T. *et al.* (1990 Perchloroethylene-induced rat kidney tumours: an investigation of the mechanisms involved and their relevance to humans. *Toxicology and Applied Pharmacology*, **103** 77–89.

Guengerich, F. P. (1991) Oxidation of toxic and carcinogenic chemicals by human cytochrome P450 enzymes. *Chemical Research in Toxciology*, **4** 391–407.

Guengerich, F. P. (1992) Metabolic activation of carcinogens. *Pharmacology and Therapeutics*, **54** 17–61.

Hodgson, E. and Levi, P. E. (1992) The role of the flavin-containing monooxygenase (EC 1.14.13.8) in the metabolism and mode of action of agricultural chemicals. *Xenobiotica*, **22** 1175–83.

Koob, M. and Dekant, W. (1991) Bioactivation of xenobiotics by formation of toxic glutathione conjugates. *Chemico-Biological Interactions*, **77** 107–36.

Langenbach, R. *et al.* (1992) Recombinant DNA approaches for the development of metabolic systems used in *in vitro* toxicology. *Mutation Research*, **277** 251–75.

Maret, G. *et al.* (1990) The MPTP Story: MAO activates tetrahydropyridine derivatives to toxins causing Parkinsonism. *Drug Metabolism Reviews*, **22** 291–332.

MacFarlane, M. *et al.* (1989) Cysteine conjugate β-lyase of rat kidney cytosol: characterisation, immunocytochemical localisation and correlation with hexachlorobutadiene nephrotoxicity. *Toxicology and Applied Pharmacology*, **98** 185–97.

Nash, J. A. *et al.* (1984) The metabolism and disposition of hexachloro-1, 3-butadiene in the rat and its relevance to nephrotoxicity. *Toxicology and Applied Pharmacology*, **73** 124–37.

Nelson, S. D. and Pearson, P. G. (1990) Covalent and noncovalent interactions in acute lethal cell injury caused by chemicals. *Annual Review of Pharamacology and Toxicology*, **30** 169–95.

Recknagel, R. O. *et al.* (1989) Mechanisms of carbon tetrachloride toxicity. *Pharmacology and Therapeutics*, **43** 139–54.

Rettie, A. E. *et al.* (1992) Hydroxylation of warfarin by human cDNA-expressed cytochrome P450: a role for P4502C9 in the etiology of (S)-warfarin-drug interactions. *Chemical Research in Toxicology*, **5** 54–9.

Tarloff, J. B. *et al.* (1990) Xenobiotic transformation by the kidney: pharmacological and toxicological aspects. In *Progress in Drug Metabolism, Volume 12* (C. G. Gibson), Taylor and Francis, London.

Vermeulen, N. P. E. (1988) Toxicity-related stereoselective biotransformation. In *Metabolism of Xenobiotics* (J. W. Gorrod *et al.*), Taylor and Francis, London.

Vos, R. M. E. and Van Bladeren, P. J. (1990) Glutathione *S*-transferases in relation to their role in the biotransformation of xenobiotics. *Chemico-Biological Interactions*, **75** 241–65.

Walker, R. J. and Duggin, C. G. (1992) Cellular mechanisms of drug nephrotoxicity. In *The Kidney: Physiology and Pathophysiology*, 2nd Edition (D. W. Seldin and G. Giebisch), Raven Press, New York, pp 3571–95.

Yost, G. S. *et al.* (1989) Mechanisms of lung injury by systemically administered chemicals. *Toxicology and Applied Pharmacology*, **101** 179–95.

7 Pharmacokinetics and the clinical relevance of drug metabolism

7.1 Introduction

The two most important parameters of a drug are its intensity and duration of action and these are related to the concentration of drug at its site of action and the time during which the effective concentration of drug remains there. It is often difficult to assess the concentration of a drug at its actual site of action but, fortunately, the concentration of drug in the blood plasma is most often a good measure of this. Measurement of plasma concentration of drugs and how these change is, therefore, an important exercise in determining drug action. One of the main contributors to the change in active drug concentration in plasma is the metabolism of the drug. Remember that metabolism may create or destroy an active drug molecule and, thus, can increase or decrease its action (see chapter 6). The theoretical and mathematical interpretations of tissue drug concentration data is termed *Pharmacokinetics*.

Drug metabolism in man is more difficult to study than in animals, due to the practical and ethical constraints on experimentation. There is only limited access to tissue samples (see discussion of methods later in chapter) and it is very difficult to find a reasonably homogeneous group of patients on which to perform the studies. Different approaches to the study of drug metabolism have to be adopted in man as routine procedures, the most usual of which is the measurement of drug concentrations in blood plasma over an extended time period. Other biological fluids (such as urine) may also be used and these methods are discussed later.

Pharmacokinetics is particularly important from a clinical view because of the relationship between the intensity and duration of action of a drug and the concentration of drug present at the active site and how long an effective concentration is found there respectively. The ability to calculate the concentration of drug in the plasma at a particular time point can be vital in assessing the dose and frequency of dosing of a drug of low therapeutic index, e.g. anticoagulants, cardiac glycosides, anti-cancer drugs (see examples later). The ability to correlate *in vivo* pharmacokinetic and metabolic data with *in vitro* metabolic data is also important. Does increased drug metabolism have any effect on clearance of drugs from the body? This question is examined in detail later.

Pharmacokinetics will be considered mainly from a physiological point of view but mathematical equations will be given where they assist in the understanding of the principles (no derivations of equations will be given; these can be found in any standard textbook on pharmacokinetics and are of little relevance here). The special relevance of the hepatic drug metabolising capacity to pharmacokinetics will be highlighted. The methods of obtaining clinical data related to drug metabolism will also be discussed and the correlation of *in vivo* and *in vitro* data considered. Finally, specific examples of the clinical relevance of drug metabolism will be given with a discussion of the wider implications such as induction/inhibition of drug metabolism in drug interactions and the effects of disease states on pharmacokinetic parameters.

7.2 Pharmacokinetics

Pharmacokinetics (literally the movement of drugs) is the study of the uptake, distribution and clearance (by excretion/metabolism) of drugs with respect to time. In practice this means measuring the concentration of drug in various tissues and body fluids over a period of time. The processes involved in the determination of pharmacokinetic patterns are illustrated in Figure 7.1. In order to interpret pharmacokinetic data, it is necessary to set up certain models of the body so that mathematical equations describing the movement of the drugs can be formulated. Here we will briefly describe two simple, well-used models to illustrate how this may be done.

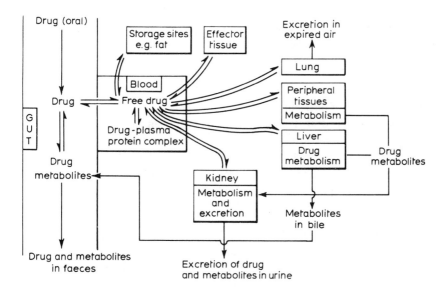

Figure 7.1 Processes involved in the determination of pharmacokinetic parameters.

7.2.1 The one-compartment model

It can be appreciated that the movement of drug between different compartments of the body (blood, adipose tissue, liver, etc.) is a complex, dynamic process and not readily amenable to direct analysis. It is therefore assumed, as a first approximation in this model, that all body compartments are in rapid equilibrium with a central compartment (normally equated with the blood), and that the concentration of drug is constant throughout, i.e. the body is considered as a single compartment through which the drug equilibrates instantaneously. The actual correlation of pharmacokinetic compartments with real anatomical tissues or organs is rather complex and, at times, impossible; this should be borne in mind during these discussions (for further discussion of this point see later in this chapter). Using the approximation discussed above a pharmacokinetic model can be constructed where the areas in the body that the drug reaches are represented by a single compartment (Figure 7.2). This is the *one-compartment model*.

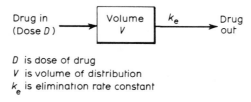

D is dose of drug
V is volume of distribution
k_e is elimination rate constant

Figure 7.2 The one-compartment model.

It is assumed that the drug is injected directly into this compartment (e.g. intravenous injection) and distributes itself instantaneously through the compartment. Thus the concentration of drug at time 0 (C_0) can be calculated or, conversely if C_0 is known V can be calculated.

$$C_0 = D/V \text{ or } V = D/C_0 \qquad (7.1)$$

where V is volume of distribution and D is dose of drug.

Clearance of the drug from the compartment then takes place at a rate determined by the elimination rate constant (k_e). For most drugs this clearance is directly related to the concentration of drug, ie. a plot of log drug concentration versus time yields a straight line (referred to as first order kinetics) (Figure 7.3). This means that the time taken for a decrease in drug concentration to half the original value (wherever on the curve the original value is taken) will always be the same. This time is referred to as the half-life ($t_{1/2}$) for the drug. The actual form of such a semi-log plot for real data is more often similar to that shown in Figure 7.4. The deviation of the actual and theoretical curves at the start is due to distribution of the drug taking a finite time (not instantaneous as the model demands) therefore the sampled (plasma) compartment has a higher concentration of drug than the body as a whole.

We thus have various parameters that can be measured or calculated for a first-order, one-compartment model:

V = volume of distribution
C_0 = concentration of drug at time 0
C_t = concentration of drug at various times
$t_{1/2}$ = half-life of elimination
k_e = elimination rate constant
D = dose of drug given.

The elimination rate constant (k_e) is defined as the rate of change of drug concentration at unit initial drug concentration (or mathematically as below)

$$dC/dT = -k_e C_0 \qquad (7.2)$$

Using this equation and measurements of plasma drug concentrations at various times the elimination rate constant can be calculated. The elimination rate constant is a composite figure encompassing all methods of elimination (excretion of urine, faeces, expired air, sweat, etc., biotransformation and sequestration in tissues not sampled). It is almost impossible to separate it into its components and this is important when discussing the correlations between *in vivo* and *in vitro* measures of drug metabolism (see later in this chapter).

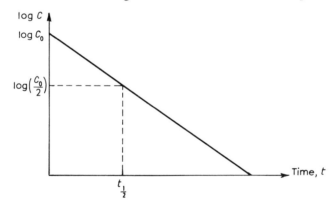

Figure 7.3 Theoretical curve for change in plasma drug concentration in the one-compartment model.

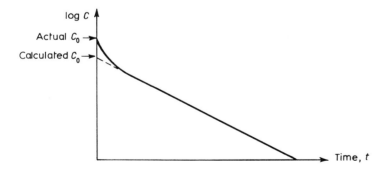

Figure 7.4 Experimental curve for change in plasma concentration of a drug approximating to the one-compartment model.

If the equation above is expressed in another form

$$\log C = \log C_0 - k_e t \log e \tag{7.3}$$

then a relationship between k_e and $t_{1/2}$ can be seen

$$\log[C/C_0] = -k_e t \log e \tag{7.4}$$

where e = the exponential function ($\log e = 0.434$)

At $t_{1/2}$, $C = C_0/2$

Thus $\log t_{1/2} = -0.301 = -0.434 \, k_e t$ and

$$k_e = \frac{0.693}{t_{1/2}} \tag{7.5}$$

So the elimination rate constant is inversely proportional to the half-life of the drug. This is quite logical, as the faster the clearance of the drug (greater k_e) the faster one half of the drug will be cleared and therefore the shorter the half-life.

So overall the rate at which a drug is cleared from the body is dependent on a complex elimination rate constant, the dose of drug and the body volume through which the drug is distributed

$$dC/dT = k_e D/V \tag{7.6}$$

The volume of distribution of a drug is also a complex 'constant'. In physiological terms it is sometimes difficult to equate calculated volumes of distribution with actual body compartments. The drug may only enter the blood plasma and have a small volume of distribution, or it may enter the extracellular fluid or even permeate all cells (total body water), thus giving a large volume of distribution – more often, the calculated volume of distribution lies somewhere in between. In certain circumstances a volume of distribution greater than the body volume can be obtained. This is a function of the way in which volume of distribution is calculated from a measurement of plasma concentration of drug. The plasma concentration of drug may be very low due to sequestration of drug in, say, adipose tissue; therefore, the volume of distribution according to equation 7.1 will seem to be very large whereas in reality it is small (only distributed in adipose tissue).

The simple model of the body as a single compartment can yield some useful information on the movement and the intensity and duration of action of drugs within the body and lead to the calculation of some important parameters of drug action (e.g. volume of distribution, half-life and elimination rate constant). The problems with the interpretation of these parameters should, however, be remembered.

7.2.2 The two-compartment model

The one-compartment model discussed above assumes that elimination can occur from all compartments and that the drug can enter all areas of the body equally easily but a glance at Figure 7.1 shows that this is not always valid; many peripheral tissues cannot excrete directly and excretion takes place mainly from the blood (via urine, faeces). A refinement can be added to account for this in the form of an outer, non-excreting compartment (Figure 7.5). This is called the *two-compartment model*, where the two compartments are kinetically distinguishable.

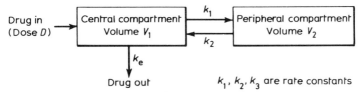

Figure 7.5 The two-compartment model.

Such a model is more complex to analyse and gives a plot of log drug concentration in the central compartment, i.e. blood plasma versus time as shown in Figure 7.6. There are two distinct slopes, the first (steeper) slope being primarily related to distribution of drug from the central to the peripheral compartment, and the second (shallower) slope to the elimination of drug from the central compartment. The second half-life $(t_{1/2})$ is the true half-life of elimination defined earlier. This theoretical slope more closely follows the actual experimental plots found for many drugs and thus can be considered a more realistic model.

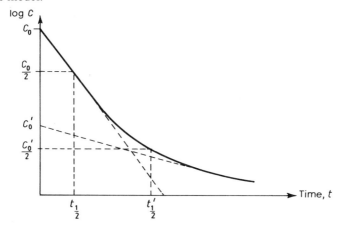

Figure 7.6 Theoretical curve for the change in plasma drug concentration in the two-compartment model.

The central compartment in this model is generally equated with the blood plasma and other non-fatty highly perfused tissues and the peripheral compartment with other tissues (Table 7.1). Which of the groups are included in the central and which in the peripheral compartment depends on the drug in question.

Table 7.1 Tissue groupings for pharmacokinetic assessment

Description of group	Tissues
Plasma	Plasma
Highly perfused non-fat	Blood cells
	Heart
	Lung
	Liver
	Kidney
	Glands
Poorly perfused non-fat	Muscle
	Skin
Fatty tissues	Adipose tissue
	Bone marrow
Negligible perfusion	Bone
	Teeth
	Cartilage
	Hair

As can be imagined, mathematical analysis of a two-compartment model is more complex than that of a one-compartment model and, although all parameters calculated from the one-compartment model can also be calculated from this model, one further parameter is necessary to understand the analysis, i.e. area under the concentration times curves (AUC). This is exactly what its name suggests, the area under the curve when plasma drug concentration is plotted against time (Figure 7.7). The area under the curve is a measure of the total body

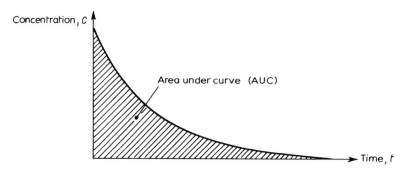

Figure 7.7 The area under the concentration–time curve.

load of drug (i.e. its bioavailability) and is therefore an indirect indication of the therapeutic value of the drug. Provided clearance of the drug remains constant, changes in AUC relate to changes in bioavailability of the drug (for instance by giving the drug via different routes). The AUC can be measured experimentally and used to calculate the clearance of drug from the body as below. Clearance is defined as the volume of the central compartment which is cleared of drug in unit time, and thus is a measure of the efficiency with which a drug is eliminated from the body via all routes.

$$\text{Clearance} = D/\text{AUC} \tag{7.7}$$

where D is the dose of drug given

Clearance can also be expressed in terms of the elimination rate constant.

$$\text{Clearance} = k_e.v_1 \tag{7.8}$$

where k_e is the elimination rate constant and v_1 is volume of the central compartment.

Clearance is a very important concept in pharmacokinetics and therapeutics, as we will see later.

A number of problems are inherent in the two-compartment model. One problem is the fact that the concentration of drug in the central compartment is no longer related solely to drug elimination but also to movement of drug between the central and peripheral compartments. It depends on the relative rate constants (k_1, k_2, and k_e) whether movement of drug or elimination is the most important and, thus, analysis of changes in drug concentration becomes more complex. A second problem is more pharmacological, and relates to the position of the receptor for the drug. The action of the drug will be related to the concentration of drug in the same compartment as the receptor. Thus, analysis of drug concentrations in both compartments is strictly necessary to evaluate the relevance of pharmacokinetic data to clinical use of the drug using a two-compartment model. The difficulty of assigning anatomical regions to the various compartments makes this somewhat difficult.

7.2.3 Kinetic order of reaction

One final theoretical consideration to be discussed is the kinetic order of reaction. All of the theory so far discussed assumes that the elimination of drug is directly related to its concentration (i.e. the elimination is first order). If, however, the processes of elimination are saturated (normally at high drug concentration), elimination rate is independent of drug concentration (i.e. zero-order kinetics) and drug is being cleared as fast as possible. In this case a plot of drug concentration versus time is linear. This can be seen very well with higher doses of aspirin (Figure 7.8). At first, salicylate concentration falls linearly with time until a certain concentration is reached and sub-saturation is reached, when first-order kinetics reappear. In exceptional circumstances, involving two or more substances in metabolism or excretion, multi-order kinetics can be seen but such instances are rare.

7.2.4 Clinical application of pharmacokinetics

In clinical practice it is unusual to give a drug as a single intravenous dose. It is more usual to give multiple doses by a method other than intravenous injection. Consideration of multiple drug dosing and other forms of administration is therefore in order.

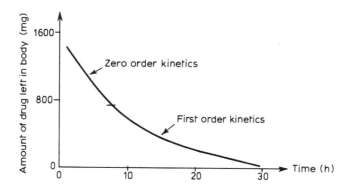

Figure 7.8 Clearance of acetylsalicylic acid in man. (Taken from Levy, G. (1965) *J. Pharm. Sci*, **54** 959. Used with permission of the copyright owner.)

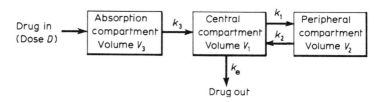

Figure 7.9 Modification of one- and two-compartment models to include the absorption compartment.

Let us first examine a drug administered in a way that does not give direct entry into the central compartment (e.g. oral administration) and which therefore involves absorption of the drug. In these cases the drug first enters another compartment, the absorption compartment. This is an extension of the one- or two-compartment models outlined above (Figure 7.9). The drug is subsequently distributed to the central compartment (and in the case of the two-compartment model to the peripheral compartment) and excreted. It can be seen that absorption could still be proceeding as distribution and elimination starts, and this gives the log dose response curves as shown in Figure 7.10 (a) for the one-compartment and (b) for the two-compartment model. For the one-compartment model both the absorption rate constant (k_a) and the elimination rate constant (k_e) can be calculated by extrapolation of the respective curves and by using the equations given earlier. In the two-compartment model, however, absorption, distribution and elimination are proceeding simultaneously and the early phase of the curve cannot be analysed satisfactorily. Further complications arise in oral dosing as the rate of dissolution of the drug must also be taken into account. Pharmacokinetic data from orally administered drugs are, therefore, sometimes very difficult to interpret.

Most drugs are administered for an extended period of time and it is of great interest to the clinician to know what dose and at what dosage interval to give a

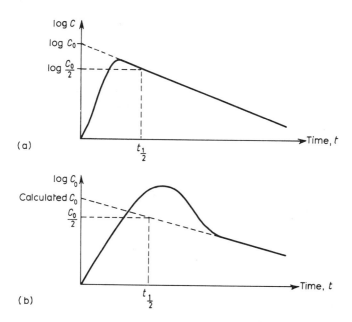

(a)

(b)

Figure 7.10 Theoretical curve for change in plasma drug concentration in the modified (a) one- and (b) two-compartment models.

drug in order to achieve an effective drug concentration at its site of action. A consideration of the kinetics of multiple dosing is thus of interest. The effect of multiple dosing depends on the relationship between the half-life of the drug and the frequency of dosing. If the dosing interval is much longer than the half-life then the dose will be effectively cleared before the next is given and each dose can be considered as entirely separate. If, however, the dosage interval is about $t_{1/2}$ or less, then accumulation of drug occurs until a steady-state concentration is reached (Figure 7.11). The steady-state concentration of drug is dependent on the dose of drug given, the fraction of drug absorbed, the half-life of the drug, the volume of distribution and the dose interval.

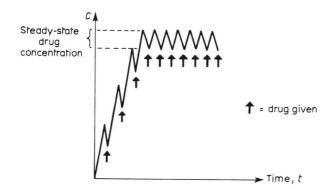

Figure 7.11 Theoretical curve for change in plasma drug concentration on multiple dosing.

$$C = \frac{1.44 \, t_{1/2} \, FD}{Vi} \qquad (7.9)$$

where C is steady state concentration, $t_{1/2}$ is half-life, F is fraction of drug absorbed, D is dose of drug, V is volume of distribution and, i is dose interval. Factors affecting drug half-life, absorption and volume of distribution thus affect the steady-state concentration of drug during multiple dosing (see earlier for discussion of these parameters).

7.2.5 Hepatic drug clearance

One of the major methods of removing drug from the central compartment is hepatic drug metabolism, i.e. removal by conversion to a metabolite. The ability of the liver to remove drug from the blood is related to only two variables, i.e. the intrinsic hepatic clearance (Cl_{int}) and the hepatic blood flow (B)

$$\text{Hepatic clearance} = B.(Cl_{int}/(B + Cl_{int})) = B.R_e \qquad (7.10)$$

Intrinsic clearance is the maximum ability of the liver to extract drug in the absence of blood flow restrictions. The term $(Cl_{int}/(B + Cl_{int}))$ in equation 7.10 is referred to as the extraction ratio (R_e).

When intrinsic clearance (Cl_{int}) is very much greater than hepatic blood flow then the extraction ratio approaches 1.0 and hepatic clearance is dependent only on blood flow, i.e. the liver extracts all of the drug presented to it. Thus the more blood passing through the liver the more drug will be extracted. On the other hand, if Cl_{int} is very much less than blood flow, then hepatic clearance is dependent only on Cl_{int}, i.e. the liver extracts as much drug as it can from whatever blood flow is presented. These two extremes are called flow-limited and metabolism-limited extraction, respectively. The characteristics of the two conditions are summarised in Table 7.2. Intermediate values of extraction ratio (0.2–0.8) give hepatic clearance rates that are dependent on both blood flow and hepatic intrinsic clearance to varying extents. It is obvious, therefore, that hepatic clearance of drugs may not only be related to the ability of the liver to metabolise drugs but may also be dependent on factors affecting the hepatic blood flow, such as changes in cardiac output and redistribution of blood flow (e.g. during exercise or stress).

7.2.6 Pharmacokinetics: a summary

The first part of this chapter gives a very brief overview of pharmacokinetics as it relates to drug metabolism. It is not designed as a formal introduction to the

Table 7.2 Comparison of flow- and metabolism-limited hepatic clearance

	Flow-limited	Metabolism-limited
Clearance related to	Blood flow	Intrinsic clearance
Extraction ratio	> 0.8	< 0.2
Examples	Lignocaine, propranolol	Antipyrine

subject as a whole but it is hoped that it has indicated the physiological correlation of the pharmacokinetic parameters and that it has shown the relevance of pharmacokinetic analysis to clinical practice. The usefulness of this approach must, however, be tempered by the inability of a purely mathematical analysis to completely mimic the actual behaviour of the organism, due to the complexity of the processes under study.

7.3 Methods of studying drug metabolism in man

As the ability to metabolise a particular drug may be of prime importance in determining the efficacy, duration of action and toxicity of the drug, it is of importance to be able to assess the ability of patients to metabolise drugs, especially if the drug has a low therapeutic index and needs to be present in the body at a level close to the toxic threshold (e.g. cardiac glycosides). Many methods have been developed to try and measure drug-metabolising capacity in man and, in this section, a number of methods will be outlined and the relevance of the method briefly discussed together with the problems of interpreting the results obtained. The methods are listed in Table 7.3.

7.3.1 In vivo *clearance*

In examining *in vivo* clearance as a marker for drug-metabolising capacity, the measurement of clearance of the test drug or 'probe' from the blood plasma or

Table 7.3 Methods of assessing drug metabolism in man

Methods	Substrates used
In vivo clearance	Antipyrine
	Phenacetine
	Caffeine
	Theophylline
	Paracetamol
	Debrisoquine
	Sparteine
	Sulfadimidine
	Mephobarbital
	Diazepam
	Mephenytoin
	Codeine
	Isoniazid
	Warfarin
Breath analysis	Aminopyrine
	Antipyrine
	Caffeine
	Diazepam
	Erythromycin
In vitro methods	Various
Non-invasive methods	
Plasma bilirubin	
Urinary 6ß-hydroxycortisol	

other relevant body fluid is the ideal. The mathematical theories underlying the measurement of *in vivo* clearance have been discussed above, and study of the models reveals a number of criteria that must be fulfilled before clearance can be equated to drug metabolism. These are:

- The drug must be rapidly and reproducibly absorbed (preferably 100% absorbed).

- The drug should be distributed throughout total body water (i.e. equivalent to a one-compartment model).

- The drug should not bind to tissue or plasma protein (only free drug is metabolised, excreted, etc.).

- The drug should only be metabolised by the liver with a low extraction ratio (i.e. metabolism is not flow-limited).

- The drug should have negligible renal clearance (i.e. hepatic clearance is the predominant method of clearance).

If all these criteria are met then drug clearance serves as a meaningful measure of drug metabolism that is not influenced by hepatic blood flow. If urinary excretion of drug and metabolite is measured then in addition the drug and metabolite must be excreted in the urine at the same rate and other excretion pathways should be negligible.

The first model drug which came nearest to this ideal was antipyrine where the drug's half-life and clearance both give a good estimate of hepatic metabolism (indicating one-compartment kinetics). Antipyrine has a number of other advantages:

- It is easily measured in body fluids after a dose that is pharmacologically inactive.

- Salivary pharmacokinetics are similar to plasma pharmacokinetics, therefore saliva can be sampled instead of the more painful and potentially damaging venepuncture.

The disadvantages of antipyrine are relatively minor but should be considered. Antipyrine clearance does not always correlate well with metabolism (clearance) of other drugs and therefore is a poor marker for certain drug-metabolising enzyme activities. This is due to the existence of multiple forms of drug-metabolising enzymes in the human liver. The isoforms of cytochrome P450 metabolising antipyrine in man are not well characterised. Antipyrine is metabolised to at least three metabolites, and the kinetics of clearance although appearing simple are, in fact, quite complex:

Clearance (total) = Clearance (a) + Clearance (b) + Clearance (c) + Clearance (rest)

where (a) = metabolite a, (b) = metabolite b, (c) = metabolite c, and (rest) = unchanged drug + non-identified metabolites.

Total clearance is a complex term, including clearance of all metabolites and unchanged drug; a change in one or more of these parameters leads to a change in total clearance, and opposite changes in two parameters can give no apparent change in total clearance thus masking the effects. Antipyrine is also an inducer of hepatic drug metabolising enzymes and therefore repeated tests with the drug should be avoided to prevent misleading results being obtained.

Other model substrates have also been employed as markers of hepatic drug metabolism (see Table 7.3). Of these, phenacetin, caffeine and theophylline are thought to be metabolised by cytochrome P4501A2 and thus act as markers of a different isoenzyme than does antipyrine. Theophylline is, perhaps, the better of these, as phenacetin undergoes significant metabolism in the gut wall to the O-de-ethylated product, paracetamol. Caffeine has been more recently introduced but suffers the same drawback as theophylline – abstinence from caffeine-containing beverages (coffee, tea, cola) is necessary during the rest period. Probes for cytochrome P4502D6 activity are also being used e.g. debrisoquine and sparteine. Here the metabolite ratio in the urine is used as a measure of metabolism.

Mephenytoin metabolism has been correlated to the existence of cytochrome P4502C9 and this may be correlated to the ability to metabolise mephobarbital and, possibly diazepam. Cytochrome P4503A is also thought to be of importance in man and recently a test based on the probe drug, erythromycin has been reported to correlate to activity of this isoenzyme.

For phase II metabolism, paracetamol has been suggested as a probe for UDP – glucuronosyltransferase activity as has the appearance of codeine-6-glucuronide in the urine. The assessment of acetylator phenotype is more advanced with a number of test drugs being used. Caffeine, isoniazid and sulfadimidine have all been used to measure N-acetylation by urinary metabolic ratio techniques. Isoniazid N-acetylation can also be determined by saliva analysis.

A number of substrates can be used in the study of drug clearance, many of which are good indicators of hepatic drug metabolism. Critical use of this technique can yield useful information regarding the functioning of the liver in man. A further discussion of the relevance of drug clearance to hepatic drug metabolism can be found earlier in this chapter.

7.3.2 Breath analysis

This method relies on the hepatic breakdown of certain drugs via demethylation to yield carbon dioxide (CO_2) which is excreted via the lungs. Appropriate radiolabelling (with ^{14}C) of the substrate leads to $^{14}CO_2$ being excreted which can be collected and measured (Figure 7.12). The example given is aminopyrine but caffeine, antipyrine, diazepam and erythromycin have also been used. The drugs are predominantly metabolised by the hepatic mixed-function oxidise system by N-demethylation and, thus, the CO_2 breath test can be used as an indicator of the functioning of this enzyme system. Indeed the correlation

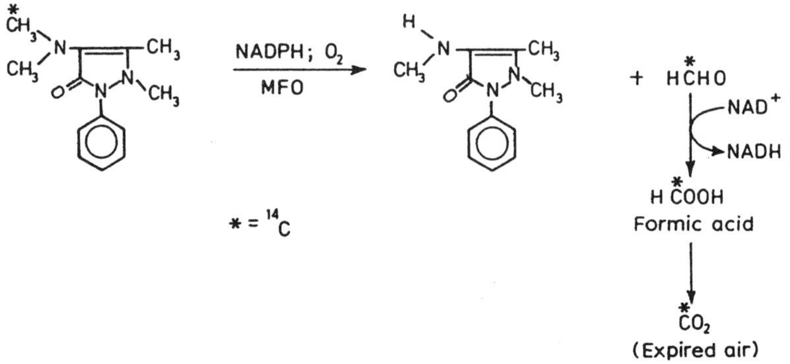

Figure 7.12 The metabolism of ^{14}C-aminopyrine showing release of $^{14}CO_2$ in expired air.

between $^{14}CO_2$ excretion and *in vivo* clearance rate for aminopyrine is good, indicating the relevance of this method. The different substrates also allow assay of different isoforms of cytochrome P450, e.g. isoform 1A2 with caffeine. The disadvantages of this method are that it is assumed that formation of formaldehyde (i.e. drug demethylation) is the rate-limiting step in the production of carbon dioxide (i.e. oxidation of formaldehyde to carbon dioxide is much more rapid than formaldehyde production); this has not been conclusively proved. The patient is also subjected to radioacitivity which is not an ideal situation; a breath test using ^{13}C (a stable non-radioactive form of carbon) is also used which circumvents this objection.

7.3.3 In vitro *methods*

It is clear that if one wishes to investigate drug metabolism in a particular tissue then the best way is to obtain a sample of that tissue and assay the activity directly. If the liver is to be examined, surgical removal of part (or all) of the liver and subjecting it to various tests of drug-metabolising ability is the ideal way of gaining information on hepatic drug metabolism. This is the method most commonly employed in animal experiments and is undeniably the most logical. A number of things have to be considered, however, before such studies are initiated in man:

- Ethical considerations

- Sampling procedures

- Assay methods

Is it ethically acceptable to take a liver sample from a healthy volunteer considering the risks involved in such a procedure? The widely held view is that it is not acceptable, and therefore most human liver material is to some extent pathological. It is only acceptable to obtain human liver biopsy if it is suspected that something is wrong with the liver and no other less stressful method of diagnosis is available. This, of course, means that one is generally dealing with more or less diseased tissue which makes interpretation of data and extrapolation to the normal human situation difficult. The only time when 'normal' liver does become available is from individuals who have died of a non-liver related cause, (e.g. during kidney or heart transplant operations (to remove organs from the donor)). This procedure raises its own ethical problems of consent to removal of organs for medical research – a topic which is not within the scope of this book.

From the practical point of view, even if a sample of liver tissue is available it may not be suitable for assay of drug-metabolising ability. Samples of liver tissue can be obtained from living patients by percutaneous needle biopsy or wedge biopsy during abdominal surgery. These methods produce fresh tissue directly from the body and are thus subject to minimum disturbance, but only small quantities (milligrams) of tissue can be taken. The size of the sample means that few tests can be performed per patient and also the relevance of the sample is suspect due to the known heterogeneity of the liver (differences in drug metabolism between the centrilobular and periportal areas of the liver). A further complication is the risk involved in obtaining the sample, e.g. infection and internal bleeding from needle biopsy and the inherent risks of major abdominal surgery in taking a wedge biopsy. Larger samples of liver can be obtained following death, e.g. at post-mortem. This method has the disadvantage that the liver starts degenerating from the moment of death even if stored cold and, thus, unless obtained relatively soon after death, the liver enzymes may not represent those found during life. Indeed a limit of 2–4 hours after death is put on the liver if it is to be of any use in the study of drug metabolism. As few post-mortem examinations are carried out this soon after death, this possible source of liver material is severely limited. One possibility that has been exploited is to remove the liver from clinically dead kidney donors during kidney transplant. From a practical viewpoint this is an excellent method as the liver is virtually normal and functional and so is almost the equivalent of a large biopsy sample. The ethical considerations of this approach are, however, questionable and have been discussed above. One disadvantage of transplant material is the often inadequate background knowledge of the donor (smoking and drinking habits, previous drug use, etc.) which might affect drug-metabolising capacity. A summary of the various sources of human liver material is given in Table 7.4.

Table 7.4 Comparison of the methods of liver sampling

Source	Amount	Ethical availability	Reliability	Background knowledge
Needle biopsy	Small	Good[†]	Fair	Good
Wedge biopsy	Small	Good[†]	Fair	Good
Post-mortem	Large	Good	Poor	Fair
Transplant	Large	Poor–fair	Good	Poor

[†]in cases of suspected liver disease; poor in other cases.

Table 7.5 Liver preparations

Whole liver (perfused)
Liver slices
Liver cubes
Isolated liver cells
Liver homogenate
Isolated liver cell sub-fractions (e.g. microsomes)

Having obtained a sample of liver one has to decide the best preparation to use to assess drug-metabolising capacity. A list of possible preparations is given in Table 7.5. The choice is between a physiological preparation (whole perfused liver) or a biochemical preparation (cellular sub-fractions) or a compromise situation (liver slices, cubes and cells). The physiological preparation can only be used if the intact liver is available; it is difficult to set up and keep running. It does, however, give the nearest approximation to the *in vivo* situation. The preparation of subcellular fractions, mainly microsomes, derived from the endoplasmic reticulum, is the easiest method but suffers from its non-physiological nature. An attempt to reach a mid-point between physiological complexity and biochemical ease has been the use of liver slices and isolated cells. Slices have the physiological cell–cell contact needed for liver function but are somewhat unsatisfactory due to excessive destruction of cells during preparation. It is probable that isolated liver cells will be regarded as the ideal compromise as they can be kept in culture for extended periods of time without losing their differentiated functions (although there is some loss of drug-metabolising enzyme capacity) and can be stored frozen and thawed as required for experimentation. The cells isolated from one human liver would be enough for many thousands of assays.

Table 7.6 Comparison of liver preparations in assessing drug metabolism

Method	Degree of difficulty	*In vivo* relevance	Reproducibility
Perfused liver	High	Good	Poor
Liver slices	Moderate	Fair	Fair
Liver cubes	Moderate	Fair	Fair
Liver cells	Moderate	Fair	Fair
Subcellular fractions	Low	Fair–poor	Good

No method of using the liver material obtained is, therefore, ideal and it depends on the nature of the problem whether a more physiological or biochemical approach is required. If changes in enzyme content are under investigation then subcellular fractions may be more appropriate; whereas if hepatotoxicity is being studied then a whole liver preparation may lead to the required results. A summary of the advantages and disadvantages of the various methods is given in Table 7.6.

In vitro assay of drug-metabolising capacity is the most direct method provided the techniques employed are relevant to the problem under study, and medical ethics are not contravened.

7.3.4 Non-invasive methods

Those methods not requiring the administration of a drug are referred to as non-invasive. They rely on changes in endogenous metabolism to give a measure of changes in drug metabolism. This is not unreasonable, as much of drug metabolism is related to endogenous compound metabolism, e.g. steroid metabolism is predominantly performed by mixed-function oxidase-like enzymes, neurotransmitters are metabolised by enzymes that also metabolise drugs, and glucuronidation is related to glucose metabolism (see chapter 1 for discussion of the inter-relationship between endogenous and xenobiotic metabolism). The non-invasive techniques that have been used are measurement of plasma glutamyltransferase (GGT), plasma bilirubin, urinary 6-hydroxycortisol and urinary D-glucaric acid. Most of these methods, however, are now considered unreliable and do not correlate well with drug metabolism as assayed using the probes described earlier. Only plasma bilirubin levels and the excretion of 6β-hydroxycortisol are still employed to any great extent and then only for specific purposes.

(a) *Plasma bilirubin.* Bilirubin is removed from plasma by conjugation to glucuronic acid in the liver and subsequent excretion. As many drugs also rely on glucuronide conjugation for their excretion, it was thought possible that plasma bilirubin levels could be used as a measure of hepatic glucuronidation (e.g. patients with a genetically low hepatic UDP–glucuronosyltransferase activity (Gilbert's Disease) have raised plasma levels of unconjugated bilirubin). No direct comparisons between plasma levels of bilirubin and conjugation of drugs (e.g. chloramphenicol, morphine and oxazepam, which are cleared mainly via glucuronidation in the liver) have been performed. The presence of multiple forms of UDP–glucuronosyltransferases in the liver may invalidate this possible approach to studying hepatic conjugation reactions.

(b) *Urinary 6β-hydroxycortisol (6β-OHC).* 6β-Hydroxycortisol is produced from cortisol primarily by the hepatic mixed-function oxidase system (cytochrome P4503A). This is normally a minor pathway in the excretion of glucocorticoids, the major pathway being via 17-hydroxycorticosteroids (17-OHCS). Therefore the proportion of glucocorticoids excreted as the 6β-hydroxy derivatives should give a measure of the activity of cytochrome P4503A. A ratio of 6β-OHC/17-OHCS is a better indicator of changes in hepatic drug metabolism in man than the simple measurement of 6β-OHC excretion. The excretion of 6β-hydroxycortisol is not, however, a general indicator of hepatic drug-metabolising capacity as metabolite ratio studies with debrisoquine (see above) do not correlate with excretion of 6β-hydroxycortisol and there is also no correlation between excretion of 6β-hydroxycortisol and antipyrine clearance. This is due to different isoenzymes in the liver responsible for debrisoquine, antipyrine and cortisol metabolism. This test should only be used in a comparison of different groups of subjects and not as a predictive test of inter-individual variations in drug metabolism. 6β-Hydroxycortisol excretion also does not seem to be of use in assessing inhibition of drug metabolism.

The non-invasive methods of assessing drug metabolism are, therefore, of limited use in certain circumstances but are not of general applicability.

7.3.5 In vivo/in vitro *correlations of drug metabolism*

In the study of human drug metabolism one problem has become topical – the relationship between drug clearance measured *in vivo* (i.e. in the whole organism) and drug metabolism measured *in vitro* (i.e. in fractions of tissues removed from the patient). This becomes relevant when it is known that the drug is predominantly cleared by hepatic metabolism. It is obviously much better to be able to check a patient's hepatic metabolism by a simple blood or urine test rather than by requiring a sample of liver tissue in which to examine the metabolism of the drug.

The measurement of urinary excretion of drugs has been shown to be a valid indicator of hepatic drug metabolism in certain circumstances, notably the metabolism of the model drugs, antipyrine, debrisoquine and sparteine. Antipyrine is metabolised by the liver to three main metabolites. All of these metabolites are also found in the urine of patients given antipyrine. A study of the relative proportions of each metabolite formed by isolated liver tissue and found in the urine showed a very good correlation. A direct comparison of the *in vivo* clearance of antipyrine metabolites with *in vitro* assessment of hepatic drug metabolism in the same patient gave good correlation for all three metabolites. In this example, therefore, *in vivo* clearance is directly related to the ability of the liver to metabolise the drug.

In order for this correlation to be true, the drug under investigation must have certain properties: (1) it must be absorbed well into the systemic circulation; (2) elimination must be first order; (3) the metabolites should be rapidly excreted in the urine without further metabolism; and (4) metabolism should be entirely in the liver. Antipyrine appears to fulfil all these criteria although (4) is very difficult to prove.

A good correlation has also been shown between *in vivo* and *in vitro* 3-hydroxylation of amylobarbitone but for many other drugs no correlation between *in vivo* and *in vitro* hepatic metabolism has been seen. One such example is the clearance of the anti-diabetes drug, tolbutamide. This drug is metabolised by hydroxylation in the liver. In the study of *in vivo* clearance of tolbutamide and its hepatic metabolism *in vitro*, no correlation was found to exist, presumably because one or more of the criteria mentioned above was not satisfied. Clearance of tolbutamide varied between 0.5 and 1.3 l h^{-1} without any detectable change in maximum hepatic metabolism of the same drug. The rate-limiting step in tolbutamide clearance is thus not related to hepatic metabolism.

In other studies, the *in vivo* clearance of antipyrine has been shown to be unrelated to the *in vitro* metabolism of the precarcinogen, benzo [*a*] pyrene. This is not surprising as the two compounds are metabolised by different isoenzymes of cytochrome P450 in the human liver.

In the study of human drug metabolism, therefore, *in vivo* clearance values may or may not be related to *in vitro* hepatic metabolism depending on the drug in question. Thus, *in vivo* measurements may be invalid in discussing *in vitro* drug metabolism, or vice versa. These provisos should be borne in mind when discussing such *in vivo* and *in vitro* data.

There are methods available, therefore, for the study of hepatic drug metabolism in man. In order to put these methods into perspective, a number of examples of their use in the study of human drug metabolism will be given. It is hoped that the following examples will highlight the relevance of the study of drug metabolism in man in deciding how best to use the drugs to obtain the required effects without any toxic reaction to the drug.

7.4 Clinical relevance of drug metabolism

As we have seen, drug metabolism is a major determinant of the change in drug concentration in the body and, thus, greatly affects the intensity and duration of action of drugs by altering the amount of the drug at its site of action. We have also seen how various methods can be used in measuring drug metabolism in man, and have discussed their relevance to hepatic drug-metabolising capacity. In this section we shall be looking at some examples of drug metabolism in a clinical context: how differences in drug metabolism – caused by genetic differences (pharmacogenetics), by induction and inhibition, and by various diseases – can affect the way in which drugs act and how the methods discussed above can be used clinically in the assessment of drug-metabolising capacity of the liver and, thus, assist the clinician in deciding if there is a link between the actions or toxicity of the drug and its metabolism.

7.4.1 Effects of disease

Hepatic metabolism of drugs can be affected by many diseases, most of which logically are diseases of the liver (see chapter 4). Early studies showed the cirrhosis of the liver caused a marked decrease in clearance of drugs from plasma but that the effects were mainly seen in phase I metabolism unless severe cirrhosis was examined. For instance, glucuronidation of lorazepam, oxazepam, morphine and paracetamol were unaffected in cirrhosis. Antipyrine clearance, however, one of the most common marker of phase I hepatic drug metabolism, was shown to be reduced in chronic liver disease. In severe, uncompensated cirrhosis more enzyme activities are seen to be affected including the glucuronidation of morphine, oxazepam and paracetamol. The difference in effect on phase I and II metabolism is, therefore more one of degree. Chronic liver diseases therefore seem to have marked substrate variation in their effects on hepatic drug metabolism. This was emphasised by later studies looking at the clearance of antipyrine, aminopyrine, diazepam and indocyanine green (ICG) in the same patients. Four groups of patients were used: controls, healthy volunteers, patients with hepatocellular diseases, and patients with hepatic carcinomas or cholestasis. Antipyrine clearance was measured employing the saliva test, aminopyrine and diazepam metabolism were measured using the breath tests, and indocyanine green was measured in plasma samples. It is known that antipyrine, aminopyrine and diazepam are cleared from the body mainly by hepatic metabolism and have a low extraction ratio (i.e. clearance is directly related to metabolism). Indocyanine green is not metabolised, and clearance is related to hepatic blood flow. Results obtained in the above study are shown in Table 7.7. It can be seen that the clearance of each drug is decreased by both

Table 7.7 Effects of liver disease on clearance of drugs in man

Patient group	Aminopyrine	Diazepam	Antipyrine	Indocyanine green (ICG)
Control	$100 \pm 21^{*}$	100 ± 21	103 ± 36	98 ± 31
Hepatocellular diseases	38 ± 21	56 ± 18	45 ± 27	44 ± 24
Hepatic carcinoma	57 ± 22	69 ± 35	62 ± 37	66 ± 24
Cholestasis	110 ± 34	120 ± 42	64 ± 14	70 ± 23

Results expressed as % vs control.
[*]mean ± (standard deviation)
(Adapted from Vessell, E.S. (1980) *Proc. Natl. Acad. Sci. U.S.A.*, **77** 600–3. Used with permission of the author.)

hepatocellular diseases and hepatic carcinoma to a similar extent for each drug, whereas in cholestasis the elimination of antipyrine and ICG was markedly depressed but that of aminopyrine and diazepam were unaltered. Complex statistical analysis of these results gave the conclusion that it is misleading to extrapolate pharmacokinetic data from one drug to another even though it is thought that both drugs are cleared by the same mechanism (e.g. aminopyrine and antipyrine are cleared predominantly by hepatic metabolism but show opposite effects on clearance in cholestasis, whereas antipyrine and ICG are cleared by different mechanisms but show the same effect in cholestasis). This study also shows the relevance of the test applied to the prediction of altered hepatic function in the various disease states studied. All tests indicate a reduction in hepatic clearance in both hepatocellular and neoplastic diseases, but the aminopyrine breath test seems to be the best at discriminating between control and diseased liver states (Table 7.8).

Table 7.8 Usefulness of clearance of various drugs in assessing liver disease

Test	Percentage outside normal range	
	Hepatocellular diseases	Hepatic neoplasia
Aminopyrine	94	67
Diazepam	31	18
Antipyrine	24	20
ICG	69	22

(Adapted from Vessell, E.S. (1980) *Proc. Natl. Acad. Sci. U.S.A.*, **77** 600–3. Used with permission of the author.)

Benzodiazepine metabolism in cirrhosis has been studied more extensively. Diazepam itself has been the subject of many studies which have shown marked changes in pharmacokinetics in liver disease. Liver diseases (hepatitis and cirrhosis) increase the half-life and decrease the clearance of diazepam. In patients without liver disease, diazepam half-life increased with multiple dosing due to accumulation of a metabolite, desmethyldiazepam which apparently inhibited diazepam clearance. In cirrhotic patients the half-life of diazepam was unaffected by repeat dosing probably due to the lower amount of metabolite formed leading to less product inhibition of the enzyme. These data suggest that diazepam will have a longer than expected effect in normal patients after multiple dosing but that this dosage regimen will have little effect on cirrhotic patients although they will already show a much more marked effect of diazepam due to the impaired metabolism. It might be argued that in normal patients a steadily decreasing dose of diazepam is necessary to maintain plasma concentrations whereas in cirrhotic patients a lower but constant dose is needed. The changes in metabolism of benzodiazepines are also linked to the increased possibility of drug induced coma in patients treated with these drugs who also have liver diseases. Impairment of psychomotor function has also been seen.

Changes in hepatic drug clearance also occur in other diseases not directly affecting the liver, such as hormonal disorders of the thyroid and pituitary (e.g. hypothyroidism, dwarfism and acromegaly) and diabetes mellitus. Thyroid hormones generally stimulate hepatic drug metabolism and, therefore, hypothyroidism leads to diminished clearance of antipyrine, paracetamol and oxazepam whereas hyperthyroidism gives increased antipyrine and oxazepam clearance. The effects of the diseases could be reversed by normalising the thyroid hormone levels. Pituitary dwarfism and acromegaly are lack of, and excess of, growth hormone, respectively. Growth hormone inhibits drug metabolism, particularly in children. Insulin, the hormone missing in some forms of diabetes mellitus, has recently been implicated as an inducer of drug metabolism and lack of this hormone, therefore, leads to reduced capacity of the liver to metabolise drugs. Such an effect has been reported for paracetamol glucuronidation in uncontrolled diabetics but not for oxazepam clearance. The effect on paracetamol metabolism was again reversed by treatment with insulin. Paradoxically, paracetamol clearance in obese patients (a condition often associated with type 2 diabetes mellitus) was increased over controls. This illustrates the difficulty of trying to decipher the effects of various changes on drug metabolism in the human population. The relevance of the effect of these diseases on drug treatment has not yet been assessed.

In one instance the relevance of the change in drug metabolism in a disease state is obvious and that is the alteration in primaquine clearance in patients suffering from malaria. This is a manifestation of a more general phenomenon of decreased drug clearance in patients with infectious diseases. It is becoming clear that viral, bacterial and parasitic infections, which activate the immune system, cause a decrease in drug metabolism (Figure 7.13). This is possibly due to the effects on cytokines such as interleukin-1 on the liver. In the case of

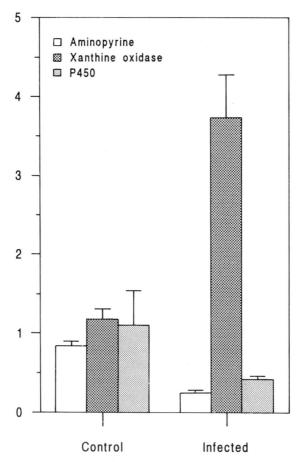

Figure 7.13 The effect of *Listeria monocytogenes* infection on aminopyrine *N*-demethylase, cytochrome P450 and xanthine oxidase in livers of mice. Data taken from Azri and Renton (1991) *Int. J. Immunopharm.*, **13** 197–204.

primaquine, this drug is activated by phase I metabolism to become a potent antimalarial agent but the immune response to the malarial parasite reduces the liver's ability to perform this activation and, thus, the disease itself reduces the effectiveness of the drug treatment of that disease.

Disease states are, thus, a major influence on the ability of the body to clear drugs from the body by metabolism and the altered drug metabolism in disease states may be of importance in the treatment of these diseases.

7.4.2 Genetic polymorphism in human drug metabolism

A genetic factor in determining the often large inter-individual variations in drug metabolism in man has been suspected for a long time since the metabolism of antipyrine in homozygous twins (identical twins) was shown to be almost the same, whereas in heterozygous (fraternal) twins there was as much variation as in the general population.

The existence of genetic control of drug metabolism has been strengthened by the discovery of a number of metabolic phenotypes (see Table 7.9). The

Table 7.9 Drug metabolism phenotypes

Group	Drugs affected
Acetylator phenotype	Sulfadimidine Isoniazid
Pseudocholinesterase phenotype	Succinyicholine
Debrisoquine 4-hydroxylation phenotype	Debrisoquine Sparteine Phenacetin Guanoxan
Mephenytoin hydroxylation phenotype	Mephenytoin Phenytoin

acetylator phenotypes, named 'slow' and 'fast' acetylators are related to toxicity of, for example, isoniazid. Isoniazid is normally cleared from the body by N-acetylation, but in the 'slow' acetylator group, the therapeutic dose of the drug is sufficient to cause marked build-up of unchanged drug and, thus, the toxic side-effects of central stimulation and peripheral neuritis. 'Fast' acetylators are, however, more susceptible to drug-induced hepatic damage. In studies using a single blood sample following oral isoniazid treatment, over half of the subjects tested showed 'slow' acetylator status, and genetic investigation revealed that control is via two autosomal alleles, R for 'fast' acetylation and r for 'slow' (R being dominant and r recessive). The high incidence of the recessive trait indicates a selective advantage for the 'slow' acetylators which is not related to drug metabolism.

The most common test for acetylator status is the acetylation of sulfadimidine which can be used to type a patient before isoniazid is given. The likely side-effects of the drug will then be known. Interaction with other drugs can also be predicted, as 'slow' acetylators develop toxicity when isoniazid and pheny-toin are given together, probably due to the higher blood levels of isoniazid inhibiting phenytoin metabolism, thus giving phenytoin toxicity. In these cases, knowing the acetylator status of the patient, toxicity can be avoided by modi-fying the dose of the drugs.

Pseudocholinesterase phenotype is characterised by a marked sensitivity to the muscle relaxant, succinylcholine, which is normally metabolised by the serum pseudocholinesterase. Succinylcholine is of particular use in conjunction with general anaesthetics, tetanic seizures and in electroconvulsive therapy because of its extremely short half-life (about 2 min). Patients with an atypical pseudo-cholinesterase, however, show a half-life of effect of the drug of about 2–3 hours. Total paralysis (including the respiratory muscles) for this length of time is obvi-ously not advisable. The atypical reaction of succinylcholine has been shown to be controlled by an autosomal recessive gene and to be related to a structurally altered pseudocholinesterase in serum. The enzyme is not absent as in some other inherited defects of metabolism but is sufficiently altered to make it unable to metabolise succinylcholine. About 1 in every 3000 individuals will have atypical pseudocholinesterase and this can be tested by inhibition studies on the serum enzyme. The rarity of the recessive trait suggests that little selective advantage can be gained from having the atypical pseudocholinesterase.

Another atypical pseudocholinesterase has also been found with a higher activity towards succinylcholine. This is a very rare occurrence and again appears to be genetically controlled. The presence of this highly active pseudocholinesterase confers succinylcholine resistance on the individual.

All early drug metabolism polymorphism was related to drug hydrolysis (succinylcholine) or drug conjugation (isoniazid and sulfonamides) and no polymorphism of drug oxidation was observed although large inter-individual differences in drug oxidations were seen. Drug oxidation polymorphism is, however, now a well-recognised phenomenon.

Debrisoquine (formerly used in the treatment of hypertension) is metabolised by the liver mixed-function oxidase system mainly to 4-hydroxydebrisoquine. The enzyme responsible is cytochrome P4502D6. Marked inter-individual variation in excretion pattern and pharmacological effect of the drug was noted with maintenance doses ranging from 20 to 400 mg/day and urinary excretion of 8–70% as unchanged drug. A good correlation between dose needed and unchanged drug excreted was seen. Investigation of the metabolite pattern in urine of volunteers given debrisoquine gave a clue to the nature of the variation (Table 7.10). One subject (no. 4) had a very low conversion of parent drug to the 4-hydroxy derivative. This subject was also very sensitive to the anti-hyper-tensive effects of debrisoquine. A larger study based on this chance finding revealed that there were, indeed, two populations of debrisoquine metabolisers, and they could be classified according to the ratio of % dose excreted as debrisoquine:% dose excreted as 4-hydroxydebrisoquine. The larger section

Table 7.10 Urinary excretion patterns of debrisoquine

Metabolite	Percentage dose excreted as metabolite			
	Subject 1	Subject 2	Subject 3	Subject 4
Debrisoquine	45	28	27	40
4-Hydroxydebrisoquine	30	37	39	2
Others	2.7	4.8	13.7	5.3

(Data from R. L. Smith, personal communication.)

of the population had a low ratio (about 1) and were termed 'extensive metabolisers' (EM); while a much smaller section, with a high ratio (about 20), were termed 'poor metabolisers' (PM). Over 90% belong to the EM group. Family studies indicated that extensive metabolism is the dominant trait. The genetic control is via a single gene pair, i.e. the offspring of a homozygous EM and a homozygous PM will all be heterozygous (Figure 7.14). All of the offspring will therefore be extensive metabolisers. Two heterozygous parents can thus produce a homozygous recessive child; this has been seen in practice (see Figure 7.15). It should be noted that heterozygous extensive metabolisers have higher ratios than homozygotes, indicating that the dominance of the extensive trait is not complete. The reason for the differences has recently been suggested to be aberrant splicing of the CYP2D6 gene controlling formation of cytochrome P4502D6.

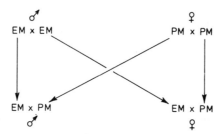

Figure 7.14 Family study of debrisoquine 4-hydroxylation. EM is extensive-metaboliser gene (dominant); PM is poor-metaboliser gene (recessive). (Data from R.L. Smith, personal communition)

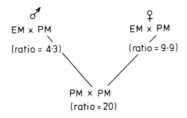

Figure 7.15 Family study of debrisoquine 4-hydroxylation showing a child with poor-metaboliser status. (Data from R.L. Smith, personal communication.)

We therefore have a drug oxidation polymorphism that can relatively easily be measured by examining the metabolite ratio of debrisoquine in urine. This would be merely of academic interest, however, if it were not for the fact that the debrisoquine polymorphism turns out to be a model for many clinically used drugs where a genetic component controlling the drug metabolism has been suspected. A list of drugs whose metabolism is associated with debrisoquine 4-hydroxylation is shown in Table 7.11. The list is expanding rapidly and debrisoquine 4-hydroxylation may be a very good model drug for a test of metabolic status. Not all genetic control of drug metabolism, however, is similar to that of debrisoquine; the metabolism of mephenytoin is also genetically regulated but is not associated with the debrisoquine polymorphism. Indeed, it is thought that another isoform of cytochrome P450 is involved, namely cytochrome P4502C9.

Table 7.11 Drugs whose metabolism is related to debrisoquine 4-hydroxylation

Nortryptiline	Metoprolol
Phenacetin	4-Methoxyamphetamine
Phenformin	Carbocysteine
Phenytoin	Bufanolol
Sparteine	Encainide
Perhexiline	Guanoxan
Metiamide	

The genetic polymorphisms discussed above could be the explanation for a number of unexplained sensitive groups of individuals, e.g. unusual sensitivity to phenytoin where sensitive individuals develop toxic side effects (e.g. nystagmus and ataxia) at much lower doses of the drug. This sensitivity was related to reduced 4-hydroxylation of phenytoin, and has now been tentatively correlated with the poor-metaboliser status of mephenytoin.

Phenacetin metabolism is thought to be related to debrisoquine metaboliser status. In some patients, phenacetin is hydroxylated rather than the usual route of de-ethylation. This unusual route of metabolism was thought to be the cause of the toxic side effects seen (methaemoglobinaemia). Impaired metabolism of phenacetin to paracetamol and subsequent conversion of the remaining phenacetin to the 2-hydroxylated products, is correlated to poor-metaboliser status for debrisoquine.

The metabolism of guanoxan is also correlated with debrisoquine 4-hydroxylation so that poor metabolisers of debrisoquine are also poor metabolisers of guanoxan (Table 7.12). Guanoxan, like debrisoquine, is used as an antihypertensive and has side effects similar to debrisoquine. Poor metabolisers are, therefore, more susceptible to the central effects and hepatotoxicity of guanoxan.

The simple debrisoquine or mephenytoin metabolite ratio test can therefore be used as a routine test for susceptibility of patients to the toxic effects of a

Table 7.12 The effect of debrisoquine phenotype on the metabolism of guanoxan

Phenotype	% dose excreted as		Ratio $\left(\dfrac{\text{parent drug}}{\text{metabolite}}\right)$
	Guanoxan	OH-guanoxan	
EM	$1.5 \pm 0.3^{\dagger}$	29 ± 5	0.06 ± 0.02
PM	48 ± 12	6.2 ± 1.4	7.8 ± 0.2

†mean $\pm$ (standard deviation)
(Data from R. L. Smith, personal communication.)

number of clinically important drugs, and it has a useful predictive value in this respect. Using these tests it has been shown that different racial groups exhibit different proportions of poor and extensive metabolisers (Table 7.13). Egyptians show the lowest incidence of debrisoquine 'poor metaboliser' status (about 1%) whereas West Africans show a high incidence (about 13%). Caucasians are intermediate between these two groups. For mephenytoin 'poor metaboliser' status, 2.7% of Caucasians and 18% of Japanese show this trait. This is a good example from the developing discipline of ethnopharmacology.

Table 7.13 Incidence of 'poor'-metaboliser (PM) phenotype in different ethnic groups

Ethnic group	Number studied	Number PM	Percentage incidence of PM
Caucasian	106	5	5
Egyptian	72	1	1.5
Nigerian	34	5	15
Ghanaian	27	3	12

(Data from R. L. Smith, personal communication.)

The existence of at least two sub-populations with markedly different drug metabolising capacities has far-reaching and important correlates, particularly where drug oxidation is concerned and especially considering the high incidence of individuals with impaired drug-oxidising capacity. From the examples given above, it becomes obvious that drugs linked to the debrisoquine or mephenytoin phenotype should be given in lower doses to PM individuals than to EM, so reducing the risk of overdose and subsequent toxic effects. It is, in fact, possible that drugs have been withdrawn from clinical use due to a high incidence of toxic side-effects, when a reduction in dosage after a debrisoquine test may have been all that was required. Phenformin, for example, has been restricted due to build-up of lactic acid (lactoacidosis) in certain individuals. Phenformin metabolism is known to be correlated to debrisoquine 4-hydroxylation but no information is available as to whether lactoacidosis is correlated to PM status. If such a correlation was found, phenformin could be re-introduced on a wider scale following a debrisoquine test of prospective recipients. Indeed, a volunteer panel of known EM/PM-status people has been used in the pharmaceutical industry to enable scientists to investigate the effect of debrisoquine metabolism status on the effects of their compounds under test.

7.4.3 Induction and inhibition of drug metabolism

In chapter 3 it was seen that the enzymes involved in drug metabolism can be induced or inhibited by a wide variety of compounds, from the drug metabolised by a particular enzyme to a food component or tobacco smoke. These effects can, of course, also be seen in man and are of great importance in determining such things as drug interactions and the effects of diet on drug metabolism. Some examples of these interactions are given below.

The use of multiple drug therapy in the treatment of many diseases has led to problems with drug interactions. Many drug interactions are the result of interference of one drug with the metabolism of another, and the subsequent increase or decrease in the clearance of the latter drug. Interaction of drugs with phenobarbitone is, perhaps, the most studied example of this phenomenon as phenobarbitone is an inducer of the metabolism of many other drugs (see chapter 3) and numerous clinical interactions with this drug are seen. Table 7.14

Table 7.14 Drugs which interact with phenobarbitone on a metabolic level

Phenytoin	Chlorpromazine
Warfarin	Phenylbutazone
Bishydroxycoumarin	Pethidine
Lignocaine	Cyclophosphamide
Digitoxin	Griseofulvin
Fenoprofen	Cortisol
DDT	

lists some of the drugs that interact with phenobarbitone at a metabolic level. Of particular interest is the interaction of phenobarbitone and phenytoin which are both used in the treatment of epilepsy. Treatment of patients already given phenytoin with phenobarbitone reduced the steady-state serum concentration of phenytoin markedly (Figure 7.16). Withdrawal of phenobarbitone treatment

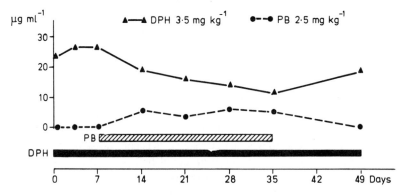

Figure 7.16 Effect of phenobarbitone pre-treatment on the steady-state serum concentration of phenytoin in man. (Taken from Cucinelli, S.A. (1972) In *Anti-epileptic drugs* (D.M. Woodbury, J.K. Penry and R.P Schmidt), Raven Press. Used with permission.)

returned serum concentrations of phenytoin to control levels. Control of seizures by phenytoin can thus be greatly influenced by the presence of phenobarbitone, itself a drug used to control seizure. The complex interactions theoretically available make the use of phenytoin and phenobarbitone in combination a somewhat unpredictable and therefore dangerous therapy.

The interaction of phenobarbitone with digitoxin (a drug with low therapeutic index) is also of major concern to the clinician. Digitoxin is a cardiac glycoside used in the treatment of heart failure, but with major side-effects at slightly above clinical doses (toxicity includes anorexia, CNS disturbances, atrial fibrillation and tachycardia). Steady-state concentrations of digitoxin fell to about a half following treatment with phenobarbitone, with a marked fall in plasma half-life of digitoxin from about 8 to 4 days. Polar metabolites of digitoxin increased in urine following phenobarbitone treatment. It thus appears that phenobarbitone increased the metabolism of digitoxin, thereby reducing its serum concentration and effectiveness. Increasing the dose of digitoxin to counter this effect will lead to excess, toxic concentrations of digitoxin being present in serum when phenobarbitone is withdrawn (Figure 7.17). A very similar effect is seen with warfarin (this has been discussed in chapter 3). The use of phenobarbitone to increase drug-metabolising capacity in liver diseases has been attempted. For instance patients with liver disease metabolise phenylbutazone very slowly (plasma $t_{1/2}$ of about 100 h) and this can be shortened to about 50–55 h by treatment with phenobarbitone. Patients suffering from unconjugated hyperbilirubinaemia (caused by a relative deficiency of UDP–glucuronosyltransferase in the liver, whether the mild Gilbert's disease or the more severe Crigler-Najjar syndrome) can be treated with phenobarbitone to relieve the symptoms. Dramatic reductions in serum bilirubin levels can easily be achieved by this method which probably relies on the ability of

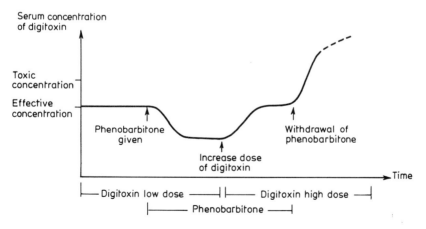

Figure 7.17 Changes in serum concentration of digitoxin following treatment with, and withdrawal of, phenobarbitone.

phenobarbitone to induce hepatic UDP–glucuronosyltransferase activity as there is a linear relationship between hepatic UDP–glucuronosyltransferase activity and bilirubin clearance. Other barbituates such as barbitone, hexobarbitone and amylobarbitone show similar effects to phenobarbitone and should, perhaps, be viewed as a group.

Of the other drugs that are considered to be inducers of drug metabolism, the majority are seen to induce their own metabolism. Tolerance to glutethimide, meprobamate and diazepam, for instance, develops partly due to the increased metabolism of the drug owing to autoinduction. Carbamazepine is a drug recently investigated in terms of induction of metabolism of itself, and of other exogenous and endogenous compounds. The clearance of antipyrine, measured by the saliva test, increased after two weeks treatment while carbamazepine half-life, measured in plasma, decreased from a control level of 32.3 h to 19.1 h during the same period. Increases in enzymes involved in endogenous metabolism were also found in this study, with 6β-hydroxylation of cortisol increased, and the level was also raised of leucocyte δ-aminolevulinic acid synthetase (the rate-limiting enzyme in the biosynthesis of haem). Carbamazepine has also been shown to induce the metabolism of phenytoin and warfarin.

Oral contraceptives containing oestrogens and/or progestins have been reported to inhibit hepatic drug metabolism, probably by competitive inhibition. Steroids are metabolised in the liver by the same enzyme systems as drugs and therefore such inhibitory interactions are not unlikely. Aminopyrine clearance is significantly lower in women taking an oral contraceptive pill but there is no effect on paracetamol clearance.

Another compound known to affect drug metabolism is ethanol which again shares a common breakdown enzyme with drugs and steroids. Ethanol may act acutely to inhibit drug metabolism but in the longer term as an inducer of cytochrome P4502E1. Co-administration of ethanol with certain drugs can, therefore, enhance the effect of the drug by leading to a slower clearance. This is part of the problem associated with the enhanced action of benzodiazepines when taken with ethanol. The habitual drinker, however, may have an enhanced drug metabolising capacity – the cytochrome P4502E1 induction caused by ethanol is a defence mechanism of the body as this isoenzyme is the one that metabolises ethanol (also known as the microsomal ethanol oxidising system – see chapter 1). Cytochrome P4502E1 can also metabolise paracetamol, isoniazid and carcinogenic amines. The interaction with paracetamol is thought to lead to an enhanced toxicity of the analgesic by increasing the formation of the toxic metabolite of the drug.

It can be seen from these examples that drug–drug interactions involving induction or inhibition of drug metabolism can be of great importance in determining the action and toxicity of drugs.

Induction and inhibition are, however, important in another respect and that is the interaction of environmental factors with hepatic drug metabolism. One major group of compounds, widespread in our environment, which have a major effect on hepatic drug metabolism are the polycyclic hydrocarbons (e.g. benzo[*a*]pyrene). These are found in cigarette smoke and in any food cooked over open heat (e.g. charcoal-broiled meat). Much work has been done on the effects of polycyclic hydrocarbons on drug metabolism and the relationship to the intake of tobacco smoke and charcoal-broiled meat.

The clearance of antipyrine and paracetamol is greatly increased by smoking (Figure 7.18). It is seen that there is a graded response to the number of cigarettes smoked. The effect of cigarette smoking on the plasma concentrations of phenacetin is even more dramatic (Figure 7.19). The area under the concentration curve is seen to be much less in smokers, indicating that the bioavailability of phenacetin is lower, but half-life is similar in both groups.

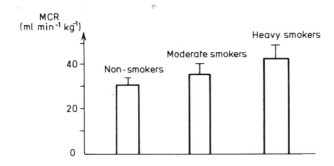

Figure 7.18 Relationship between daily cigarette consumption and clearance of antipyrine. MCR = mean clearance rate. (Taken from Vestal, R.E. *et al.*(1975) *Clin. Pharm. Ther.*, **18** 425–32.)

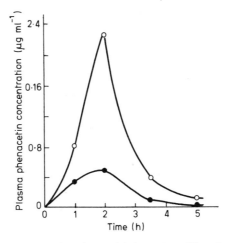

Figure 7.19 Mean plasma concentration of phenacitin in smokers (●), and non-smokers (○) as a function of time following oral adminstration of a 900 mg dose. (Taken from Pantuck, E. *et al.* (1972) *Science*, **175** 1248–50. Used with the permission of the author and the American Association for the Advancement of Science. © 1972 AAAS.)

Animal studies have shown that benzo[a]pyrene – major constituent of tobacco smoke – induces mixed-function oxidase activity in the small intestine and the increased first-pass effect caused by such induction may be the explanation of the reduced bioavailability without increased hepatic metabolism seen in man. Benzo[a]pyrene is known to induce cytochrome P4501A1 and 1A2 in man and it is these isoenzymes that perform the enhanced metabolism seen in smokers. Other drugs, however, are unaffected by smoking with respect to their metabolism. In drug therapy it is therefore important to know the smoking habits of the patients particularly if the drug to be used is metabolised by cytochrome P4501A1 or 1A2.

Looking at polycyclic hydrocarbon inducers in food, we find that any meat cooked over open heat (i.e. any browning of food) causes build-up of such compounds. These have been shown to be potent inducers of drug metabolism in a very similar manner to cigarette smoking and, indeed, the same compounds are responsible for the effects (i.e. benzo[a]pyrene induction of cytochrome P4501A1 and 1A2). Plasma levels of phenacetin are markedly reduced in subjects on a charcoal-broiled meat diet – the subjects in this case acting as their own controls so cutting down problems from inter-individual variations (Table 7.15). As with tobacco smoking the area under the curve is significantly reduced (Figure 7.20) indicating a lack of bioavailability of phenacetin in subjects eating charcoal-broiled meat probably because the inducers have increased enzyme activity in the small intestine so stopping uptake of the drug. It is seen that at least 75% of phenacetin never enters the plasma in subjects on a charcoal-broiled meat diet. This has obvious clinical relevance for treatment with this drug; a patient may need four times the dose to achieve the same effect simply because of eating charcoal-broiled meat.

If antipyrine and theophylline plasma half-life and clearance are examined in subjects on a charcoal-broiled meat diet a different picture emerges. For both antipyrine and theophylline, plasma half-life is decreased and total clearance

Table 7.15 The effect of a diet containing charcoal-broiled meat on the plasma concentration of phenacetin in man ·

Time after administration (h)	Plasma phenacetin concentration (ng ml^{-1})	
	Control diet	Charcoal diet
1	1328 ± 481[†]	319 ± 90
2	925 ± 166	163 ± 32
3	313 ± 60	74 ± 17
4	149 ± 27	34 ± 9
5	66 ± 14	15 ± 4

[†]mean ± (standard deviation)

(Data from Pantuck, E. et al. (1972) Science, **175** 1248–50. Used with permission of the author and the American Association for the Advancement of Science. © 1972 AAAS.)

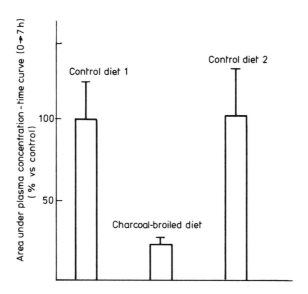

Figure 7.20 Effect of feeding a charcoal-broiled meat diet on the area-under-curve for phenacetin. (Taken from Pantuck, E. *et al* (1982) *Science*, **175** 1248–50. Used with the permission of the author and the American Association for the Advancement of Science. © 1972 AAAS.)

increased. As antipyrine and theophylline are both predominantly cleared by hepatic metabolism, it seems reasonable to suggest that the effect of charcoal-broiled meat, in this instance, is on the liver and that we are seeing induction of hepatic mixed-function oxidases by the polycyclic hydrocarbons in the diet. This is similar to the effect of tobacco smoke seen earlier.

Induction and inhibition of drug metabolism whether by other drugs, environmental or dietary chemicals can be important factors in the action of drugs. Changes in metabolism caused by such factors should be taken into account when treating patients.

7.5 Summary

Using as a theoretical basis the mathematical interpretation of drug concentrations in the body and drug elimination from the body (i.e. pharmacokinetics), we can measure various parameters of the drugs used in modern medicine. These parameters (such as half-life, clearance, etc.) can be related to the duration and intensity of action of a drug to give a meaningful measure of a drug's usefulness and possible toxicity.

The methods used in measuring these parameters have been discussed and examples of how these methods can be used, have been given. The clinical relevance of the examples chosen has been explained where known.

It is hoped that this chapter has given some insight into the usefulness of pharmacokinetics and drug metabolic measurements in man but that at the same time it has also pointed out the weaknesses of the methods and, perhaps, stimulated some thought as to how these techniques could be improved or better used.

Further reading

Books and symposia

Curry, S.H. and Whelpton, R. (1983) *Manual of laboratory pharmacokinetics,* J. Wiley & Sons, Chichester.

Dost, F.H., (1968) *Grundlagen der Pharmakokinetic,* Thieme, Stuttgart.

Gibaldi, M. and Perrier, D., (1980) *Pharmacokinetics,* Dekker, New York.

Gibaldi, M. (1984) *Biopharmaceutics and clinical pharmacology,* Lea and Febiger, Philadelphia.

Gillette, J. R. and Mitchell, J.R., (eds), (1977) *Concepts in biochemical pharmacology, Part 3, handbook of experimental pharmacology, Vol. 28,* Springer-Verlag, Berlin, pp. 1–34, 35, 85, 169–212, 234–58, 272–314, 359–82, 383–461.

Hladky, S.B. (1990) *Pharmacokinetics,* Manchester University Press, Manchester.

Rowland, M. and Tozer, T.M. (1989) *Clinical pharmacokinetics: concepts and applications.* 2nd Edition., Lea and Febiger, Philadelphia.

Reviews and original articles

Alvan, G. (1992) Genetic polymorphisms in drug metabolism. *J. Internal, Med.,* **231** 571–3.

Alvan, G. (1991) Clinical consequences of polymorphic drug oxidation. *Fund. Clin. Pharmacol.,* **5** 209–28.

Alvares, A.P., *et al* (1979) Regulation of drug metabolism in man by environmental factors, *Drug Metab. Rev.,* **9** 185–206.

Berry., M.N. *et al* (1992) Techniques for pharmacological and toxicological studies with isolated hepatocyte preparations. *Life Sci.,* **51,** 1–16.

Berthou, F. *et al.*(1989) Comparison of caffeine metabolism by slices, microsomes and hepatocyte cultures from adult human liver. *Xenobiotica,* **19** 410–17.

Bock, K.W. *et al.* (1987) Paracetamol as a test drug to determine glucuronide formation in man. *Eur. J. Clin Pharmacol.,* **31** 677–83.

Brosen, K. (1990) Recent developments in hepatic drug oxidations. Implications for clinical pharmacokinetics. *Clin. Pharmacokinet.,* **18** 220–39.

Butler, M.A. *et al* (1989) Human cytochrome P450PA(P4501A2), the phenacetin O-deethylase, is primarily responsible for the hepatic 3-demethylation of caffeine and N-oxidation of carcinogenic arylamines. *PNAS,* **86** 7696–7700.

Critchley, J.A.J.H. *et al.* (1986) Inter-subject and ethnic differences in paracetamol metabolism. *Brit. J. Clin. Pharm.,* **22** 649–57.

Dayer, P. *et al.* (1989) Dextramethorphan O-demethylation in liver microsomes as a prototype reaction to monitor cytochrome P450dbl activity. *Clin. Pharmacol. Ther.,* **45** 34–40.

Dollery, C.T., *et al* (1979) Contribution of environmental factors to variability in human drug metabolism. *Drug Metab. Rev.,* **9** 207–20.

Eichelbaum, M. and Gross, A.S. (1990) The genetic polymorphism of debrisoquine/sparteine metabolism – clinical aspects. *Pharmacol. Ther.,* **46,** 377–94.

Fabre, G. *et al.* (1990) Human hepatocytes as a key model to improve preclinical drug development. *Eur. J. Drug Metab. Pharmacokinet.,* **15** 165–71.

George, J. and Farrell, G.C. (1991) Role of human hepatic cytochromes P450 in drug metabolism and toxicity. *Aust. NZ J. Med.,* **21** 356–62.

Gonzalez, F.J. and Meyer, U.A. (1991) Molecular genetics of the debrisoquine/sparteine polymorphism. *Clin. Pharmacol. Ther.,* **50** 233–8.

Guttendorf, R.J. and Wedlund, P.J. (1992) Genetic aspects of drug disposition and therapeutics. *J. Clin. Pharmacol.*, **32** 107–17.

Howden, C.W. *et al.* (1989) Drug metabolism in liver disease. *Pharmacol. Ther.*, **40** 439–74.

Idle, J.R. and Smith, R.L., (1979) Polymorphisms of oxidation at carbon centres of drugs and their clinical significance. *Drug Metab. Rev.*, **9** 301–18.

Ingleman-Sundberg, M. *et al.* (1990) Drug metabolising enzymes: genetics, regulation and toxicology. *Proceedings of the VIIIth International Symposium on Microsomes and Drug Oxidations*, Stockholm.

Israili, Z.H., (1979) Correlation of pharmacological effects with plasma levels of antihypertensive drugs in man. *Ann. Rev. Pharm. Tox.*, **19**, 25–52.

Jusko, W.J., (1979) Influence of cigarette smoking on drug metabolism in man. *Drug Metab. Rev.*, **9** 221–36.

Kalow, W. and Tang, B.K. (1991) Caffeine as a metabolic probe: exploration of the enzyme-inducing effect of cigarette smoking. *Clin. Pharmacol. Ther.*, **49** 44–8.

Kraul, H. *et al.* (1991) Comparison of *in vitro* and *in vivo* biotransformation in patients with liver disease of differing severity. *Eur. J. Clin. Pharmacol.*, **41** 475–80.

Kroemer, H.K. and Klotz, U. (1992) Glucuronidation of drugs. *Clin. Pharmacokinet.*, **23** 292–310.

Ladona, M.G. *et al.* (1991) Differential foetal development of the *O*- and *N*- demethylation of codeine and dextromethorphan in man. *Brit. J. Clin Pharmacol.*, **32** 295–302.

Lavrijsen, K. *et al.* (1992) Comparative metabolism of flunarizine in rats, dogs and man: an *in vitro* study with subcellular liver fractions and isolated hepatocytes. *Xenobiotica*, **22** 815–36.

Loft, S. and Poulsen, H.E. (1990) Prediction of xenobiotic metabolism by non-invasive methods. *Pharmacol. Toxicol.*, **67** 101–8.

Lou, Y.C. (1990) Differences in drug metabolism polymorphism between Orientals and Caucasians. *Drug Metab. Rev.*, **22** 451–75.

Lucas, D. *et al.* (1990) Ethanol-inducible cytochrome P450: assessment of substrates specific chemical probes in rat liver microsomes. *Alcoholism Clin. Expt. Res.*, **14** 590–4.

Moshage, H. and Yap, S.H. (1992) Primary cultures of human hepatocytes: a unique system for studies in toxicology, virology, parasitology and liver pathophysiology in man. *J. Hepatol.*, **15** 404–13.

Mucklow, J.C., (1980) Environment, diet and drug metabolism. *Topics in Therap.*, **6** 103–110.

Osborne, N.J. *et al.* (1991) Interethnic differences in drug glucuronidation: a comparison of paracetamol metabolism in Caucasian and Chinese. *Brit. J. Clin. Pharmacol.*, **32** 765–7.

Paine, A.J. (1990) The maintenance of cytochrome P450 in rat hepatocyte cultures. Some applications of liver cell cultures to the study of drug metabolism, toxicity and the induction of the P450 system. *Chemico-Biol. Interact.*, **74** 1–31.

Park, B.K. (1981) Assessment of urinary 6β-hydroxycortisol as an *in vivo* index of mixed-function oxygenase activity. *Brit. J. Clin. Pharm.*, **12** 97–102.

Park, B.K., (1982) Assessment of drug metabolism capacity of the liver. *Brit. J. Clin. Pharm.*, **14** 631–51.

Perrier, G.D. and Gibaldi, M. (1974) Clearance and biologic half-life as indices of intrinsic hepatic metabolism. *J. Pharm. Exptl. Ther.*, **191** 17–24.

Price-Evans, D.A. (1989) *N*-Acetyltransferase. *Pharmacol. Ther.*, **42** 157–234.

Rawlins, M.D. (1980) *Methods for studying drug metabolism in man.* In *Topics in Therap.* (H.F.Woods), **6** 86–94.

Relling, M.V. (1989) Polymorphic drug metabolism. *Clin. Pharmacol.*, **8** 852–63.

Srivastava, P. *et al.* (1991) Effect of *Plasmodium berghei* infection and chloroquine on the hepatic drug metabolising system of mice. *Int. J. Parasitol.*, **4** 463–6.

Vessell, E.S. (1977) Genetic and environmental factors affecting drug disposition in man. *Clin. Pharm. Ther.*, **22** 659–79.

Vessell, E.S. (1978), Disease as one of the many variables affecting drug disposition and response: alterations of drug disposition and response: alterations of drug dispositions in liver disease. *Drug Metab. Rev.*, **8** 265–92.

Vessell, E.S. (1979), The antipyrine test in clinical pharmacology. Conceptions and misconceptions. *Clin. Pharm. Ther.* **26** 275–86.

Vestal, R.E. (1989) Aging and determinants of hepatic drug clearance. *Hepatology*, **9** 331–4.

Watkins, P.B. *et al.* (1989) Erythromycin breath test as an assay of glucocorticoid-inducible liver cytochrome P450. *J. Clin. Invest.*, **83** 688.

Wilkinson, G.R. and Shand, D.G., (1975) A physiological approach to hepatic drug clearance. *Clin. Pharm. Ther.*, **18** 377–90.

Wilkinson, G.R. *et al.* (1989) Genetic polymorphism of *S*-mephenytoin hydroxylation. *Pharmacol. Ther.*, **43** 53–76.

Wrighton, S.A. and Stevens,, J.C. (1992) The human hepatic cytochromes P450 involved in drug metabolism. *Crit. Rev. Toxicol.*, **22** 1–21.

Yasumore, T. *et al.* (1990) Polymorphism in hydroxylation of mephenytoin and hexobarbital stereoisomers in relation to hepatic P450 human-2. *Clin. Pharmacol. Ther.*, **47** 313–22.

8 Techniques and experiments illustrating drug metabolism

8.1 Introduction

This chapter is designed to illustrate experimentally some of the concepts discussed in this book, and the experiments described herein are derived from undergraduate practicals that have been running in the authors' laboratories for several years. The design of adequate experiments illustrating drug metabolism is not an easy task. For example, practical classes can suffer from time constraints in that the experiments usually have to be completed in one day. In addition, experimental design must also take account of practical constraints such as availability of reagents or analytical instrumentation. Accordingly, we have described a series of experiments that are flexible and can be tailored to suit either the size of a practical class, the time available or access to specific instrumentation.

This chapter is sub-divided into the following four sections:

- *In vitro* assays for drug-metabolising enzymes.

- Factors affecting drug metabolism including cofactor requirements, species differences, tissue differences, sex differences and temperature of incubation.

- Induction of drug metabolism and a correlation of *in vitro* drug action with *in vitro* hepatic drug-metabolising activity.

- Excretion of paracetamol in man.

The first section provides a spectrum of methods and analytical techniques, that depending on availability, can be used to illustrate the experiments described in detail in the other three sections. In certain experiments, particular assays of drug metabolism are described, but it must be emphasised that alternative assays can be used and these are usually indicated in each experiment.

8.2 *In vitro* assays for drug-metabolising enzymes

8.2.1 Preparation of tissue homogenates

One of the most widely used methods to study *in vitro* drug metabolism is the use of tissue homogenates, particularly liver homogenates. It should be noted that in the preparation of tissue homogenates, all apparatus and solutions should be cooled and stored on ice (or 4°C) prior to the start of the experiment. In addition, to minimise degradation of tissue enzymes, it is important that the tissue does not exceed 4°C during any stage of preparation and isolation.

The animals are killed in an appropriately humane manner (for example cervical dislocation), remembering that no chemical or drug should be used as this may influence the activity or content of the drug-metabolising enzymes. Thus sacrificing animals by treatment with ether, chloroform or barbiturates should be avoided, unless absolutely necessary.

The tissue(s) to be used are rapidly excised and immediately placed in ice-cold 0.25 M sucrose to wash off excess blood and to cool the tissue. The tissue is then blotted dry, weighed and added to four times its weight of 0.25 M sucrose, i.e. a 20% (w/v) homogenate. The tissue is finely chopped with scissors and homogenised such that no large pieces of tissue are evident. The amount of homogenisation required depends on the tissue being used, some tissues being more difficult to disrupt and homogenise than others. The recommended homogeniser is the Potter–Elvehjem type consisting of a teflon pestle and a glass homogeniser tube. Normally four passes of the homogeniser are sufficient to disrupt the tissue and the homogeniser tube should be immersed in an ice bucket and excessive 'frothing' should be avoided, a sure sign that protein (enzyme) denaturation is occurring.

Having obtained a tissue homogenate as above, the homogenate is centrifuged in a refrigerated centrifuge to isolate subcellular fractions. Two main subcellular fractions are routinely used in the study of drug metabolism, namely the post-mitochondrial supernatant and the endoplasmic reticulum (microsomal) fraction. The choice of subcellular fraction used depends on several factors including time constraints in tissue preparation or the availability of a refrigerated ultracentrifuge.

For preparation of the post-mitochondrial supernatant, the tissue homogenate is centrifuged at 12 500 g for 15 min to pellet intact cells, cell debris, nuclei and mitochondria. The resultant supernatant (the post-mitochondrial supernatant) is *carefully* decanted and contains the microsomal plus soluble (cell sap) fractions of the cell. Clearly this method of preparation is rapid and is useful when tissue homogenates are required quickly.

Microsomal tissue fractions can be prepared from the post-mitochondrial supernatant by one of two centrifugation techniques, one involving the use of an ultracentrifuge and the other involving a calcium precipitation of the microsomes at a lower g force.

Ultracentrifugation method. Aliquots (approximately 10–12 ml) of the post-mitochondrial supernatant are transferred to ultracentrifuge tubes and centrifuged at 100 000 g for 45 min in a refrigerated ultracentrifuge. After centrifugation, the supernatant (cell sap fraction) is decanted and discarded and the microsomal pellet rinsed with 3×5 ml of 0.25 M sucrose, transferred to a small homogenisation vessel, and gently resuspended in 5 ml of 0.1 M Tris buffer, pH 7.4. This procedure yields the final microsomal suspension.

Calcium precipitation method. This method is based on the calcium dependent aggregation of endoplasmic reticulum fragments and subsequent 'low speed' centrifugation of the aggregated microsomal particles. The advantages of this method are that it is less time-consuming and does not require an ultracentrifuge. Aliquots (approximately 10–12 ml) of post-mitochondrial supernatant are mixed with 88 mM $CaCl_2$, such that 0.1 ml, 88 mM $CaCl_2$ is added per ml of supernatant (final $CaCl_2$ concentration is 8 mM) and left to stand on ice for 5 min, with occasional gentle swirling. The mixture is then centrifuged at 27 000 g for 15 min, the supernatant discarded and the pellet resuspended by homogenisation in 5 ml of 0.1 M Tris buffer, pH 7.4, yielding the microsomal suspension.

If time permits, the microsomal fractions prepared by both of the above methods may be further washed by resuspending the microsomal pellet in 0.1 M Tris buffer, pH 7.4, containing 0.15 M KCl to remove either adventitous protein or excess $CaCl_2$. The microsomal pellet is then precipitated as above and resuspended in 5 ml 0.1 M Tris buffer, pH 7.4. It is not mandatory to resuspend the final microsomal preparations in Tris buffer and other buffers such as phosphate may be used. It should be noted that the yield of microsomal protein per g liver is usually around 20 mg/g liver.

The final post-mitochondrial supernatant prepared as above can then be used to study drug metabolism. It is preferable to use the tissue fractions fresh on the day of preparation, but in some cases this may not be possible. Accordingly, the tissue fractions may be stored frozen (–20 to –80°C) for several weeks without appreciable loss of activity if glycerol (20% v/v) is added to the final preparation.

An abbreviated version of preparation of subcellular homogenates is given in Table 8.1, and is extensively discussed by Lake (1987).

Table 8.1 Preparation of subcellular tissue fractions

1. Kill animal and remove tissue as rapidly as possible.
2. Blot tissue dry and weigh.
3. Make a 20% w/v homogenate in 0.25 M sucrose.
4. To prepare a post-mitochondrial supernatant, centrifuge the homogenate at 12 500 g for 15 min, decant, reserve the supernatant and discard the pellet.
5. To prepare microsomal fractions by the ultracentrifugation method, centrifuge the post-mitochondrial supernatant at 100 000 g for 45 min, discard the supernatant and resuspend the microsomal pellet in 5 ml of 0.1 M Tris buffer, pH 7.4.
6. To prepare microsomal fractions by the calcium chloride precipitation method, take an aliquot of the post-mitochondrial supernatant, add calcium chloride (8 mM final), swirl occasionally for 5 min and centrifuge at 27 000 g for 15 min.

Reagents required

- 0.25 M Sucrose (256.8 g to 3l H_2O)

- 88 mM $CaCl_2$: (1.93 g to 100 ml H_2O)

Other materials

- Experimental animals
- Surgical instruments
- Potter–Elvehjem homogenisers (50 ml and 10 ml)
- Appropriate refrigerated centrifuge, rotor, tubes.

8.2.2 Induction of hepatic drug metabolising enzymes

As described in earlier chapters, the activity or specific content of the hepatic drug metabolising enzymes may be induced by pretreatment of experimental animals with drugs and other xenobiotics, the most commonly used being phenobarbitone or β-naphthoflavone.

Phenobarbitone induction. Experimental animals are given three daily intraperitoneal injections of 80 mg/kg (sodium salt, dissolved in saline), and subcellular fractions prepared on the fourth day as described above. Control animals should receive an equivalent volume of saline. Alternatively, sodium phenobarbitone may be administered in the drinking water as a 0.1% (w/v) solution over a period of 5 days, normal drinking water being returned to the animals overnight before sacrifice.

β-Naphthoflavone induction. Animals are given an intraperitoneal injection of 80 mg/kg β-naphthoflavone (dissolved in corn oil) once daily for 3 days, prior to sacrifice. Control animals are given corn oil (equivalent volume to the test group) as an intraperitoneal injection according to the same schedule.

If an experiment is designed to investigate the influence of xenobiotic induction on hepatic (or other tissue) drug biotransformation, other inducing agents may be used. These additional inducers include isosafrole (Ryan *et al.*, 1980), pregnenolone-16 α-carbonitrile (Elshourbagy and Guzelian, 1980), ethanol (Ohnishi and Lieber, 1977) and clofibrate (Gibson and Lake, 1991). The required doses and pretreatment schedules are given in the cited references. In addition, much practical information on induction protocols for several enzyme inducers are extensively documented by Waterman and Johnson (1991).

8.2.3 Protein determination

When comparing tissue fractions for their ability to catalyse drug biotransformation, a measure of the tissue protein is required. Amongst several methods, protein is readily determined by the colorimetric method of Lowry *et al.* (1951), with reference to a standard curve of bovine serum albumin. The coloured complex is thought to arise as a result of a complex between the alkaline copper–phenol reagent used and tyrosine and tryptophan residues of the protein. For each tissue sample, determine the protein present (in duplicate at least, and

Table 8.2 Determination of tissue protein content by the Lowry method

Tissue sample

1. Dilute the tissue sample 1:100 with 0.5 M NaOH.
2. Take 0.2, 0.4, 0.6, 0.8 and 1.0 ml of the diluted tissue sample and make up to a final volume of 1 ml with 0.5 M NaOH. Prepare a blank containing 1.0 ml of 0.5 M NaOH instead of the tissue sample.
3. Add 5 ml of copper reagent to all samples (including the blank), mix thoroughly by vortexing or inversion, and allow to stand for 10 min.
4. Add 0.5 ml of 1N Folin reagent, mix immediately and completely and stand for 30 min.
5. Read absorbance at 750 nm on a spectrophotometer, after zeroing the instrument on the blank.
6. The tissue protein content can then be directly interpolated from the standard curve below.

Bovine serum albumin standard curve

1. Make a stock solution of bovine serum albumin (100 μg/ml) in 0.5 M NaOH.
2. Take 0, 0.2, 0.4, 0.6, 0.8, and 1.0 ml of the above stock solution (equivalent to 0, 20, 40, 60, 80 and 100 μg protein/ml respectively) and make up to a final volume of 1 ml with 0.5 M NaOH.
3. Process the standard curve as described in A above starting from 3 and continuing to 5.
4. Construct the standard curve by plotting absorbance against μg bovine serum albumin per assay.

Notes

1. Prepare the stock bovine serum albumin and copper reagent fresh on day of use.
2. If the tissue protein content absorbance values read higher than the standard curve range, further dilute the tissue sample to 1:500 and repeat the determination.
3. If a spectrophotometer is not available to read at 750 nm, absorbances can also be read at 540 nm.
4. If tissue samples have been stored in glycerol, an appropriate correction must be made in the blank, as glycerol gives a positive reaction with the copper reagent.

in several dilutions) and a standard curve (in duplicate at least) as described in Table 8.2.

Reagents required

- 2% (w/v) Sodium carbonate in 0.1 M NaOH.
- 1% (w/v) Copper sulfate (hydrated) in water.
- 2% (w/v) Sodium potassium tartrate in water.
- Copper reagent is prepared fresh by mixing the above sodium carbonate, copper sulfate and sodium potassium tartrate solutions, in the ratios of 100:1:1 by volume, respectively.
- Bovine serum albumin, 100μg/ml in 0.5 M NaOH.

Other materials

- Vortex mixer
- Spectrophotometer capable of reading absorbances at either 700 nm or 540 nm.

8.2.4 Cofactor solutions

Reduced nicotinamide adenine dinucleotide phosphate (NADPH) is a necessary cofactor for many drug biotransformation reactions and serves as a source of reducing equivalents in the reaction (particularly hydroxylation and demethylation reactions). When studying drug metabolism reactions, NADPH can be added directly to the incubation mixture, but suffers from the drawback that it is relatively expensive to use on a large scale. However, if NADPH is used, a final concentration of 1 mM in the incubation mixture is usually sufficient to support drug metabolism.

An alternative method is frequently used to generate NADPH and this involves the use of an auxiliary enzymatic reaction as follows

$$\text{Isocitrate} + \text{NADP}^+ \xrightarrow[\substack{\text{Isocitrate} \\ \text{dehydrogenase}}]{\text{Mg}^{2+}} \alpha\text{-Ketoglutarate} + \text{NADPH H}^+ + \text{CO}_2$$

Accordingly, an NADPH generating system is easily made up as shown in Table 8.3. An alternative NADPH generating system may be used taking advantage of the following reaction

$$\text{Glucose-6-phosphate} + \text{NADP}^+ \xrightarrow[\substack{\text{phosphate} \\ \text{dehydrogenase}}]{\text{Glucose-6-}} \text{6-Phospho-gluconolactone} + \text{NADPH H}^+$$

Table 8.3 Preparation of an NADPH-generating cofactor solution

The following components are mixed:

0.1 M Tris buffer, pH 7.4	8.5 ml
0.15 M MgCl$_2$	1.0 ml
0.5 M Nicotinamide	1.0 ml
Trisodium isocitrate	40 mg
Isocitrate dehydrogenase	2 Units
NADP$^+$	8 mg

Notes
1. The above components should be thoroughly mixed and dissolved just prior to use.
2. It is particularly important that this mixture is not left to stand for more than a few minutes, otherwise the generated NADPH will break down. Accordingly, it is recommended to make up the above solution, and add the NADP$^+$ immediately prior to use.
3. The nicotinamide is included to prevent the destruction of pyridine nucleotide by tissue nucleosidases.
4. For drug metabolism reactions, 1 ml of the above cofactor solution is usually required per assay. Therefore the above solution is sufficient for 10 assays.

When this regenerating system is used, the isocitrate and isocitrate dehydrogenase (Table 8.3) is substituted by glucose-6-phosphate (4 μmol/ml in final mixture) and glucose-6-phosphate dehydrogenase (20 units/ml in final mixture). It should be noted that when the post-mitochondrial supernatant is used as a source of tissue enzymes, the glucose-6-phosphate dehydrogenase may be omitted from the cofactor solution, as this fraction already contains the necessary enzyme. A more detailed discussion of the cofactor requirements and cofactor solution preparation is to be found in chapters 26 and 27 of *Fundamentals of Drug Metabolism and Drug Disposition* (B.N. La Du, H.C. Mandel and E.L. Way, eds, Williams and Wilkins, Baltimore, 1972), and Lake (1987).

Reagents required

- 0.15 M $MgCl_2$ (15.25 g of hexahydrate to 500 ml H_2O)

- 0.5 M Nicotinamide (30.5 g to 500 ml H_2O)

- NADPH, NADP+, isocitrate, isocitrate dehydrogenase, glucose-6-phosphate and glucose-6-phosphate dehydrogenase as supplied.

8.2.5 Spectral determination of cytochrome P450

Cytochrome P450 is a haemoprotein and use is made of the fact that when the haem iron is reduced and complexed with carbon monoxide, a characteristic absorption spectrum results. The reduced, carbon monoxide difference spectrum of cytochrome P450 absorbs maximally at around 450 nm (hence the name) and the extinction coefficient for the wavelength couple 450–490 nm has been accurately determined to be 91 mM^{-1} cm^{-1}, thus allowing quantitative determination of this haemoprotein.

Because of the turbidity of tissue homogenates containing cytochrome P450, spectrophotometric determination of the haemoprotein must be carried out in a split beam instrument, i.e. one containing both a sample and reference compartment to offset the high turbidity. The spectrophotometric assay is described in Table 8.4. The cytochrome P450 content is calculated as in the following example.

Absorbance difference (450–490 nm) = 0.22

Extinction coefficient (450–490 nm) = 91 mM^{-1} cm^{-1}

Therefore using Beer's Law and assuming a cuvette path length of 1 cm, the cytochrome P450 concentration is given by

$$\frac{0.22 \times 1000}{91} \quad \text{nmol/ml diluted sample}$$
$$= 2.4 \quad \text{nmol/ml diluted sample}$$

Table 8.4 Spectrophotometric determination of cytochrome P450

---

1. Tissue samples are diluted in 0.1 M Tris buffer, pH 7.4 containing 20% (v/v) glycerol to approximately 2 mg/ml.
2. 2 ml of the diluted sample are then added to both matched sample and reference cuvettes and a baseline recorded between 400 and 500 nm.
3. A few grains of solid sodium dithionite are added to both sample and reference cuvettes with gentle stirring and the sample cuvette *only* is gently bubbled with carbon monoxide for approximately 1 min.
4. The spectrum is then re-scanned from 400 to 500 nm.

Notes
1. Glycerol is included in the buffer to minimise conversion to the inactive cytochrome P420.
2. Use only a few grains of dithionite as excess reductant will destroy the haemoprotein.
3. Gas the sample with carbon monoxide as soon after dithionite addition as possible, as the reduced ferrous form of cytochrome P450 is relatively unstable.
4. When gassing with carbon monoxide, the gas flow rate should be approximately 1 bubble per second. Excessively high flow rates will result in frothing and protein denaturation.
5. If a prominent peak is observed at 420 nm after gassing with carbon monoxide, this is indicative of the presence of inactive cytochrome P420, and is to be avoided.

The *specific* content of cytochrome P450 in the original tissue sample is then calculated knowing the dilution factor used and the protein content of the original sample. For example, if the dilution was 1:10 and the original tissue protein was 26 mg/ml, then the cytochrome P450 specific content is given by

$$\frac{2.4 \times 10}{26} \text{ nmol/mg protein}$$
$$= 0.92 \quad \text{nmol/mg protein}$$

This value will vary depending on the tissue examined, animal pretreatment with inducers and the species, strain, age and sex of the animal used. As a general rule of thumb, for uninduced (control), male adult rats this value will usually fall in the range 0.4 to 1.0 nmol cytochrome P450/mg microsomal protein derived from hepatic tissue.

It should be noted that the tissue content of cytochrome b_5 can also be analysed using the same sample. If both cytochrome P450 and cytochrome b_5 concentration are required from the same sample, the cytochrome b_5 must be determined first as in the method given below.

Reagents

• 0.1M Tris buffer, pH 7.4 containing 20% (v/v) glycerol

• Solid sodium dithionite

• Carbon monoxide

Other materials

• Two matched glass or quartz cuvettes (3 ml capacity)

- Split-beam recording spectrophotometer

- Tissue homogenate

8.2.6 Spectral determination of cytochrome b_5

This is achieved by determining the difference absorbance spectrum of NADH-reduced versus oxidised cytochrome b_5. The reduced, ferrous form of cytochrome b_5 has an absorbance maximum at 424 nm in difference spectrum and the extinction coefficient for the wavelength couple 424–490 nm is 112 mM^{-1} cm^{-1}. NADH is used as the reductant because of the presence of the flavoprotein enzyme NADH–cytochrome b_5 reductase in tissue preparations, an enzyme that relatively specifically and quantitatively reduces cytochrome b_5. The spectral determination of cytochrome b_5 is summarised in Table 8.5.

Table 8.5 Spectrophotometric determination of cytochrome b_5

1. Tissue samples are diluted to approximately 2 mg protein/ml as for cytochrome P450 determination and split between a sample and reference cuvette as in Table 8.4.
2. A baseline is recorded between 400 and 500 nm.
3. 25 µl of a 2% (w/v) NADH solution is added to the sample cuvette *only*, the cuvette contents gently stirred and the spectrum re-recorded between 400 and 500 nm.
4. The absorbance difference between 424 and 490 nm (relative to the baseline) is then determined and the cytochrome b_5 concentration determined as described in the text.

Note
When the cytochrome b_5 has been determined as above, the same sample may be analysed for cytochrome P450 by proceeding from step 3 in Table 8.4.

The tissue cytochrome b_5 content is then calculated as in the following example:

$$\text{Absorbance difference (424–490 nm)} = 0.11,$$

$$\text{Extinction coefficient (424–490 nm)} = 112 \text{ mM}^{-1} \text{ cm}^{-1}$$

Applying Beer's Law for a 1 cm cuvette, the cytochrome b_5 concentration is given by

$$\frac{0.11 \times 1000}{112} \text{ nmol/ml diluted sample}$$
$$= 0.98 \qquad \text{nmol/ml diluted sample}$$

In a similar manner to the example given for the cytochrome P450 calculation above, the *specific* content of cytochrome b_5 is given by (assuming a 1:10 dilution and an original tissue protein concentration of 26 mg/ml)

$$\frac{0.98 \times 10}{26} \quad \text{nmol/mg protein}$$

$$= 0.38 \quad \text{nmol/mg protein}$$

Again, as for cytochrome P450, the value of the specific content is dependent on various factors. In general, for hepatic microsomal fractions derived from adult, male rats (non-induced), the specific content of cytochrome b_5 is in the region of 0.2 to 0.5 nmol/mg protein, i.e. approximately one half of the cytochrome P450 specific content in the same tissue.

Reagents

• Freshly prepared 2% (w/v) NADH (10 mg to 0.5 ml H_2O – sufficient for 20 assays)

Other materials

• Two matched glass or quartz cuvettes (3 ml capacity)

• Split-beam recording spectrophotometer

• Tissue homogenate

8.2.7 Spectral determination of substrate binding to hepatic microsomal cytochrome P450

As described in chapter 2, many drugs and xenobiotics can bind to cytochrome P450, resulting in characteristic perturbations of the absorbance of the haem iron. The absorbance changes can be utilised to quantitatively describe drug binding to the haemoprotein, resulting in the determination of the apparent spectral dissociation constant (K_s) and maximum spectral change elicited by the drug (ΔA_{max}). These two parameters are formally similar to the K_m and V_{max} values described by Michaelis-Menton kinetics for enzyme-catalysed reactions. In the broadest sense, K_s is a measure of drug affinity for cytochrome P450 and ΔA_{max} is the maximum spectral change. These two spectral parameters are therefore of use in comparing drug interaction with various forms of cytochrome P450 or in comparing the interactions of different drugs with the same form of cytochrome P450.

The method for determining hexobarbitone-induced spectral changes of cytochrome P450 is given in Table 8.6 and results of a typical experiment are given in Figure 8.1. As can be seen from this latter figure, increasing concentrations of hexobarbitone result in increasing spectral changes as judged by the difference in absorbance between 390 and 420 nm (ΔA 390–420). The shape of the 'titration' is hyperbolic in nature (Figure 8.2a), indicating saturation of cytochrome P450 at high substrate concentrations. When the data are analysed

Table 8.6 Quantitative spectral interaction of hexobarbitone with cytochrome P450

1. Rat liver microsomes are diluted to 2 mg protein/ml in 0.1 M Tris buffer, pH 7.4.
2. 2 ml samples of the diluted microsomes are placed in both a sample and a reference cuvette of a split beam recording spectrophotometer, and a baseline recorded between 350 and 500 nm.
3. Aliquots of a stock solution of 50 mM sodium hexobarbitone are then added to the sample cuvette *only* as follows: 1.7 μl (micro syringe) of the stock hexobarbitone is added to the sample cuvette and gently, but thoroughly, stirred. The spectrum is re-scanned from 350 to 500 nm.
4. Further additions of 1.7, 7.0 and 30 μl of hexobarbitone are added to the sample cuvette and the spectrum re-recorded between 350 and 500 nm after each addition.

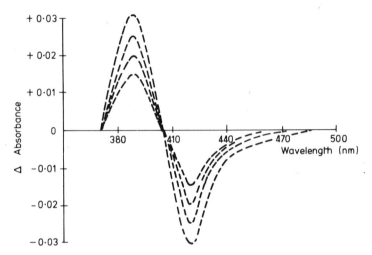

Figure 8.1 Spectral interaction of hexobarbitone and rat liver microsomes.

by the double-reciprocal plot procedure (Lineweaver–Burke plot), a straight line is usually obtained (Figure 8.2b). The K_s and ΔA_{max} parameters are derived from the Lineweaver-Burke plot from the axis intercepts as shown in Figure 8.2b. In this example

$$-\frac{1}{K_s} = -21.2, \text{ hence } K_s = 0.047 \text{ mM}$$

and

$$\frac{1}{\Delta A_{max}} = 16, \text{ hence } \Delta A_{max} = 0.063$$

It should be noted that hexobarbitone usually gives a type I spectral change with an absorbance maximum and minimum at approximately 390 nm and 420 nm respectively, with an isosbestic point around 407 nm. Other type I substrates may be used including those described in Table 2.4, which also includes type II and reverse type I substrates. Although the spectra of type II and reverse type I substrates are different from that described for hexobarbital above, the methodology and data analysis are the same.

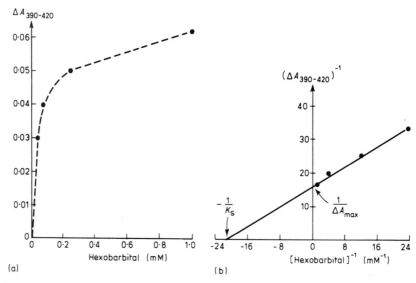

Figure 8.2 Determination of K_s and ΔA_{max} for the interaction of hexobarbitone with rat liver microsomal cytochrome P450. (a) Titration curve, (b) Lineweaver–Burke plot.

For a more detailed analysis of the interaction of drugs and xenobiotics with cytochrome P450, the reader is referred to the review by Schenkman *et al.* (1981) and the original paper of Schenkman *et al.* (1967), the latter containing many valuable experimental details for a variety of drugs and xenobiotics.

Reagents

- 0.1 M Tris buffer, pH 7.4
- 50 mM Sodium hexobarbital: (13 mg to 1 ml)

Other materials

- Two matched glass or quartz cuvettes (3 ml capacity)
- Split-beam recording spectrophotometer
- Hepatic microsomes

8.2.8 NADPH–cytochrome c (P450) reductase

NADPH–cytochrome c (P450) reductase is a flavoprotein enzyme localised in the microsomal fraction of the liver that transfers the necessary reducing equivalents from NADPH to cytochrome P450 during certain drug metabolism reactions as

NADPH $\longrightarrow$ NADPH–cytochrome c (P450) reductase $\longrightarrow$ cytochrome P450

As the reduction of cytochrome P450 is relatively difficult to assay directly, a simplified determination of enzyme activity is widely used, utilising exogenous cytochrome c (oxidised, ferric form) as an artificial electron acceptor. Accordingly, the reduction of cytochrome c by NADPH–cytochrome c (P450) reductase mirrors the reduction of cytochrome P450.

The principle of the method is that oxidised (ferric) cytochrome c has a characteristic absorption spectrum as does the reduced (ferrous) form. However, the reduced form has a characteristic absorption band at 550 nm, a band that is absent in the oxidised form. Therefore the enzyme activity can be conveniently assayed by measuring the increase in absorbance at 550 nm as a function of time. The detailed method for determination of this enzyme activity is given in Table 8.7.

Table 8.7 Spectrophotometric determination of NADPH–cytochrome c (P450) reductase activity in hepatic microsomal fractions

1. Mix 250 μl cytochrome c (ferric form, 5 mg/ml), 2.15 ml of 0.1 M Tris buffer, pH 7.4 and 0.1 ml of a liver microsomal preparation (10 mg protein/ml) in a 3 ml spectrophotometer cuvette.
2. Place the cuvette in the spectrophotometer and initiate the reaction by the addition of 25 μl of a 2% NADPH solution. Mix well and as rapidly as possible.
3. Record the absorbance change at 550 nm as a function of time for the linear period of the reaction.

Note

For tissue samples that have a high turbidity, this can be offset by using a split-beam spectrophotometer and proceeding as in (1) above but with cytochrome c, buffer and microsomes in both a sample and a reference cuvette. The reaction is initiated by the addition of NADPH as in (2) above, the NADPH being added to the sample cuvette *only*.

Calculation of enzyme activity

Protein concentration in cuvette	= 0.4 mg/ml
Extinction coefficient for reduced (ferrous) cytochrome c at 550 nm	= 19.6 mM^{-1} cm^{-1}
Absorbance change (550 nm) per min (linear portion)	= 0.784

Therefore using Beer's Law and assuming a cuvette pathlength of 1 cm, then the specific activity of NADPH–cytochrome c (P450) reductase is given by

$$\text{Specific activity} = \frac{0.784}{19.6 \times 0.4}$$

$$= 0.1 \text{ μmol cytochrome reduced/min/mg protein}$$

Reagents

- Freshly prepared 2% (w/v) NADPH (10 mg to 0.5 ml H$_2$O – sufficient for 40 assays)

- 5 mg/ml Cytochrome c (50 mg to 10 ml H_2O – sufficient for 40 assays) – prepare fresh or store frozen

- 0.1 M Tris buffer, pH 7.4

Other materials

- Two glass or quartz cuvettes (3 ml capacity)

- Recording spectrophotometer to read at 550 nm

- Liver microsomal preparation (10 mg protein/ml).

8.2.9 Assay of aniline 4-hydroxylase activity

Many drugs are hydroxylated in the liver by the cytochrome P450-dependent, mixed-function oxidase system, and the 4-hydroxylation of aniline is a convenient, reproducible assessment of this reaction as

$$C_6H_5\text{-}NH_2 \xrightarrow[\text{NADPH, O}_2]{\text{Microsomes}} OH\text{-}C_6H_4\text{-}NH_2$$

aniline   4-aminophenol

The 4-aminophenol metabolite produced is chemically converted to a phenol-indophenol complex with an absorption maximum at 630 nm and is based on the method of Schenkman *et al.* (1967). It should be borne in mind that this assay only measures 4-aminophenol and therefore can give an underestimate of total aniline hydroxylation, which can also occur at the 2- and 3-positions. It has been suggested that haemoglobin can catalyse the 4-hydroxylation of aniline and it is therefore important to remove as much blood from the tissue (during preparation) as is possible. The detailed method is given in Tables 8.8 and 8.9.

Calculation of enzyme activity is as follows. The amount of metabolite formed can be calculated by direct reference to the standard curve and should be expressed as nmol product formed (4-aminophenol) per min per mg protein *or* per gm wet weight of tissue as appropriate

Absorbance of unknown sample	= 0.2
Incubation time	= 30 min
Protein content	= 2.5 mg/ml
Concentration of product from standard curve	= 2 nmol/ml
Hence amount of product in incubation (2 ml)	= 4 nmol

$$\text{Hence enzyme activity} = \frac{4}{\text{time} \times \text{total protein in 2 ml}} \text{ nmol/min/mg protein}$$

$$= \frac{4}{30 \times 5} \quad \text{nmol/min/mg protein}$$
$$= \ 0.027 \quad \text{nmol/min/mg protein}$$

Table 8.8 The 4-hydroxylation of aniline by rat liver homogenates

1. Mix 1 ml of cofactor solution (Table 8.3) with 0.5 ml of 10 mM aniline HCl solution in suitable flasks or test tubes at 37°C for 2 min in a water bath. A suitable blank is prepared by replacing aniline with 0.5 ml H_2O.
2. Initiate the enzyme reaction by adding 0.5 ml of microsomes or post-mitochondrial supernatant (containing 10 mg protein/ml) and continue incubation at 37°C for 30 min.
3. Stop the reaction with 1 ml, ice-cold 20% trichloroacetic acid and stand on ice for 5 min and transfer to centrifuge tubes.
4. Centrifuge to give a clear solution (5 min in a bench centrifuge at maximum speed is usually sufficient).
5. Take 1 ml of the supernatant fluid and add to 1 ml, 1% phenol in a separate test tube, mix well and add 1 ml sodium carbonate. Mix well.
6. Stand for 30 min at room temperature and read the absorbance at 630 nm, after zeroing the instrument on the blank.
7. Construct a standard curve using known concentrations of 4-aminophenol as in Table 8.9.

Notes
1. All incubations should preferably be done in triplicate or at least duplicate.
2. If the final solution to be read in (6) above is at all turbid or cloudy, clarify by centrifugation in a bench centrifuge.
3. Under the above conditions, the final aniline concentration in the incubation mixture is 2.5 mM (2.5 μmol/ml) and the protein concentration is 2.5 mg/ml.

Table 8.9 Standard curve for 4-aminophenol

1. Make a stock solution of 10 μM 4-aminophenol.
2. Take 0, 0.2, 0.4, 0.6, 0.8 and 1.0 ml of 10 μM 4-aminophenol stock solution and make up to a constant volume of 1 ml with 6% trichloroacetic acid.
3. Proceed as in Table 8.8 (step 5) replacing the supernatant fluid with the standard curve samples.
4. Construct a standard curve for 4-aminophenol by plotting the absorbance value at 630 nm against the known 4-aminophenol concentration.

Reagents

- Cofactor solution (Table 8.3)

- 10 mM Aniline HCl (93 mg to 100 ml H_2O – store in dark bottle)

- 6% (w/v) Trichloroacetic acid (60 g to 1 l H_2O)

- 20% (w/v) Trichloroacetic acid (200 g to 1 l H_2O)

- 1% (w/v) Phenol (20 g phenol and 40 g NaOH to 2 l H_2O)

- 1 M Na_2CO_3 (200 g anhydrous Na_2CO_3 to 2 l H_2O)

- 10 μM 4-Aminophenol (36.5 mg of 4-aminophenol made up to 10 ml with H_2O. Take 0.1 ml of this aminophenol solution, add to 15 g trichloroacetic acid and make up to 250 ml with H_2O).

Other materials

- 10 or 25 ml Ehrlenmeyer conical flasks *or* 10 ml test tubes for incubation

- Thermostatted, shaking water bath

- Liver microsomal or post-mitochondrial supernatant fraction

- Bench centrifuge and centrifuge tubes

- Spectrophotometer to read at 630 nm

- Vortex mixer *or* parafilm

8.2.10 Assay of aminopyrine N-demethylase activity

N-demethylation of drugs is a common metabolic pathway and usually proceeds by initial hydroxylation at the α-carbon atom and subsequent breakdown of the carbinolamine intermediate liberating formaldehyde (Figure 8.3a). Therefore if the formaldehyde produced could be measured, this would then yield an appropriate assay for the *N*-demethylase activity. Formaldehyde may be trapped in solution as the semicarbazone and measured by the colorimetric procedure of Nash (1953), based on the Hantzsch reaction (Figure 8.3b).

It should be noted that both aminopyrine and monomethyl-4-aminoantipyrine are metabolised by other pathways (including additional demethylation reactions) and therefore this particular assay does not reflect the overall metabolism of the substrate. The specific procedures for this *N*-demethylase assay are given in Tables 8.10 and 8.11.

The rate of product formation (i.e. enzyme activity) can be calculated by direct reference to the formaldehyde standard curve and is normally expressed as nmol formaldehyde formed/min/mg protein or per gram wet tissue weight as appropriate. The calculations of enzyme activity are as described before for aniline-4-hydroxylase.

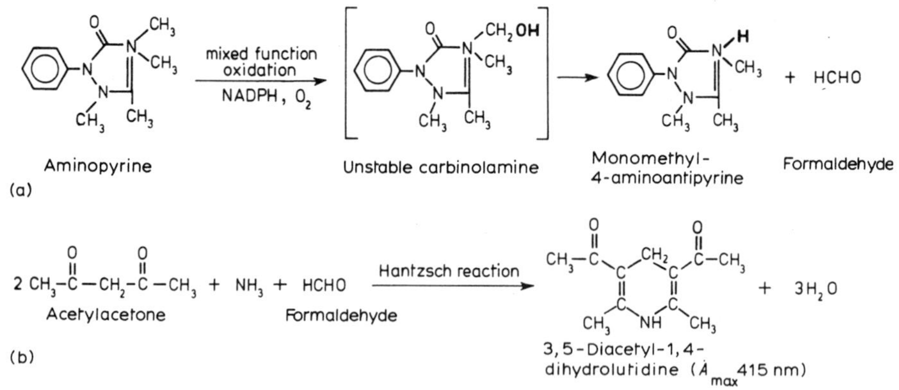

Figure 8.3 (a) Metabolic *N*-demethylation of aminopyrine and (b) colorimetric determination of formaldehyde,

Table 8.10 Assay for aminopyrine *N*-demethylase activity

1. Prepare a *modified* cofactor solution to include semicarbazide as follows. Replace the 1.0 ml of 0.15 M MgCl$_2$ in Table 8.3 by 1.0 ml of 0.15 M MgCl$_2$/0.1 M semicarbazide.
2. Mix 1 ml of modified cofactor solution and 0.5 ml, 20 mM aminopyrine and incubate in a shaking water bath at 37°C for 2 min. A suitable blank is prepared by replacing aminopyrine with 0.5 ml H$_2$O.
3. Initiate the enzyme reaction by adding 0.5 ml microsomes or postmitochondrial supernatant (containing 10 mg protein/ml) and continue the incubation for 30 min.
4. Terminate the incubation by the addition of 0.5 ml, 25% zinc sulfate, thoroughly mix and stand on ice for 5 min.
5. Add 0.5 ml, saturated barium hydroxide solution, mix again, stand for 5 min and centrifuge to a clear supernatant on a bench centrifuge (maximum speed for 5 min).
6. Take 1 ml of the clear supernatant (from (5)), add 2 ml Nash reagent and incubate at 60°C for 30 min. Cover tubes with marbles to prevent water loss and hence inaccuracy.
7. Cool the tubes and read the absorbance at 415 nm. If the tubes show any cloudiness, centrifuge briefly before reading. Zero the instrument on the blank.
8. Construct a standard curve for formaldehyde as in Table 8.11.

Notes
1. Under the above conditions, the final protein and aminopyrine concentrations in the incubation medium are 2.5 mg/ml and 5 mM (5 μmol/ml) respectively.
2. All incubations should be done in triplicate or duplicate.
3. This assay can be used for other substrates that undergo *N*-demethylation including ethylmorphine, benzphetamine and *p*-chloro-*N*, *N*-dimethylaniline.

Table 8.11 Standard curve for formaldehyde

1. Prepare a stock solution of 0.1 mM formaldehyde.
2. Take 0, 0.2, 0.4, 0.6, 0.8 and 1.0 ml of stock, 0.1 mM formaldehyde solution and make up to 1 ml with distilled water.
3. Proceed as in Table 8.10, from step 6, replacing the supernatant fluid with the standard curve samples.
4. Construct a standard curve for formaldehyde by plotting the absorbance values at 415 nm versus the known formaldehyde concentration.

Note
Prepare all tubes in triplicate or duplicate.

Reagents

- 0.15 M MgCl$_2$/0.1 M semicarbazide (15.25g MgCl$_2$.6H$_2$O and 3.75g semicarbazide to 500 ml H$_2$O)

- *Modified* cofactor solution (Table 8.10)

- 20 mM aminopyrine (1.16 g to 250 ml H$_2$O – store in a dark bottle)

- 25% (w/v) ZnSO$_4$ (125 g to 500 ml H$_2$O)

- Saturated barium hydroxide solution. Excess Ba(OH)$_2$ is added to boiling water and stirred for at least 2 h. Cool the mixture and filter to remove excess solute.

- Nash reagent. 30 g ammonium acetate and 0.4 ml acetylacetone made up to 100 ml with H_2O

- 0.1 mM formaldehyde. Take 0.75 ml of stock 40% formaldehyde solution and make up to 100 ml with H_2O. Take 0.25 ml of this dilution and make up to 250 ml with H_2O. Prepare fresh formaldehyde solution and keep in a tightly stoppered bottle.

Other materials

- Rat liver microsomal suspension or post-mitochondrial supernatant

- Thermostatted, shaking water bath

- Marbles

- Spectrophotometer to read at 415 nm

- 10 or 25 ml Ehrlenmeyer conical flasks *or* 10 ml test tubes for incubation

- Bench centrifuge

- Vortex mixer or parafilm

- Centrifuge tubes.

8.2.11 Assay of 4-nitroanisole O-demethylase activity

In a similar manner to the *N*-demethylation of xenobiotics, many drugs can undergo *O*-demethylation reactions, catalysed by the microsomal, cytochrome P450-dependent, mixed-function oxidase system. A useful substrate to monitor *O*-demethylation reactions is 4-nitroanisole which is converted to 4-nitrophenol as

$$NO_2\text{-}C_6H_4\text{-}O\text{-}CH_3 \xrightarrow[\text{NADPH, } O_2]{\text{Microsomes}} NO_2\text{-}C_6H_4\text{-}OH + HCHO$$

The 4-nitrophenol thus produced, forms an intense yellow colour at pH 10, with an absorbance maximum at 400 nm. Hence the activity of the enzyme system can be followed spectrophotometrically as described in detail in Tables 8.12 and 8.13.

Calculate the amount of product formed by reference to the 4-nitrophenol standard curve and express the activity as nmol product formed/min/mg protein or per gram wet tissue weight as appropriate. Calculation is similar to that for aniline-4-hydroxylase activity above.

Reagents

- Cofactor solution (see Table 8.3)

Table 8.12 Assay for 4-nitroanisole *O*-demethylase activity

1. Mix 1 ml cofactor solution (Table 8.3) and 1 ml of microsomes or postmitochondrial supernatant (containing 10 mg protein/ml) and incubate at 37°C for 2 min in a shaking water bath.
2. Initiate the reaction with 10 μl (micro syringe) of 500 mM 4-nitroanisole solution and continue incubation for 15 min.
3. Blank incubations should be prepared as above, but by substituting a tissue homogenate previously heated to 70–100°C for 10 min to denature the enzymes. This is necessary as the 4-nitroanisole has some yellow colour of its own.
4. Terminate the enzyme reaction by the addition of 1 ml, ice-cold, 20% trichloroacetic acid solution and allow to stand on ice for 5 min.
5. Centrifuge the mixture to obtain a clear supernatant (bench centrifuge, maximum speed for 5 min).
6. Take 1 ml of the supernatant and add 10 M NaOH until the pH is approximately 10–11. Add distilled water to give a final volume of 1.5 ml, mix well, and read the absorbance at 400 nm.
7. Construct a standard curve for 4-nitrophenol as in Table 8.13.

Notes
1. Under the above conditions, the final protein and 4-nitroanisole concentrations in the incubation medium are 5 mg/ml and 2.5 mM (2.5 μmol/ml) respectively.
2. Carry out all incubations in duplicate or triplicate.

Table 8.13 Standard curve for 4-nitrophenol

1. Prepare a stock 0.1 mM solution of 4-nitrophenol.
2. Take 0, 0.2, 0.4, 0.6, 0.8 and 1.0 ml of stock 0.1 mM 4-nitrophenol solution and make up to a constant volume of 1 ml with appropriate volumes of 6% trichloroacetic acid.
3. Proceed as in Table 8.12 from step 6, replacing the supernatant with the standard curve samples.
4. Construct a standard curve for 4-nitrophenol by plotting the absorbance values at 400 nm against the known 4-nitrophenol concentration.

Note
Prepare tubes in triplicate or duplicate.

- 500 mM 4-nitroanisole (765 mg to 10 ml of acetone. Keep the solution in a dark, air-tight bottle)

- 20% (w/v) trichloroacetic acid (200 g to 1 l H_2O)

- 6% (w/v) trichloroacetic acid (60 g to 1 l H_2O)

- 10 M NaOH (400 g to 1 l H_2O)

- 0.1 mM 4-nitrophenol (3.5 mg of 4-nitrophenol and 15 g trichloroacetic acid made up to 250 ml with H_2O)

Other materials

- Rat liver microsomes *or* post-mitochondrial supernatant

- Thermostatted, shaking water bath

- Spectrophotometer to read at 400 nm

- 10 or 25 ml Ehrlenmeyer conical flasks *or* 10 ml test tubes for incubation
- Centrifuge tubes and bench centrifuge
- Vortex mixer or parafilm.

8.2.12 Resorufin O-dealkylase assays

A series of alkyl-substituted resorufins has been extensively used in recent years as substrates for cytochrome P450-dependent, *O*-dealkylation activity. There are several reasons for the popularity of these assays including sensitivity of the fluorimetric analysis and the fact that different resorufin substrates are metabolised preferentially by different cytochrome P450 isoforms, e.g. ethoxyresorufin by cytochrome P4501A1 and pentoxyresorufin by cytochrome P4502B1 (Burke and Mayer, 1983). The experimental details are not covered here because they are discussed in extensive detail by Lake (1987).

8.2.13 Assay for glucuronosyl transferase activity

The glucuronosyl transferase family of enzymes are important in phase II drug conjugation reactions and many examples are known where glucuronic acid is conjugated with the hydroxyl, carboxyl or amino groups of the substrate. A useful compound to assess glucuronosyl transferase activity is 2-aminophenol, because this phenol readily forms an *O*-linked glucuronide conjugate in the presence of microsomal fractions and UDP–glucuronic acid.

The assay for glucuronidation of 2-aminophenol is based on the colorimetric diazotisation method for free primary amino groups, originally developed by Bratton and Marshall (1939) for the estimation of sulfonamides. The principle of the analytical method is based on the observation that when an aqueous solution of sodium nitrite is added to a cold, acidified solution of an aromatic amine, a diazonium salt is formed. Excess nitrite is removed by the addition of ammonium sulfamate and the diazonium salt is finally reacted with a complex aromatic amine (*N*-naphthylethylene diamine), to produce a brightly coloured azo compound that can be analysed spectrophotometrically. This method, therefore, detects the amino group of the 2-aminophenyl glucuronide. The method is relatively specific because excess substrate (2-aminophenol) is destroyed under the assay conditions (at pH 2.7) and therefore does not take part in the diazotisation reaction.

As the glucuronosyl transferases usually exhibit enzyme latency in the microsomal membrane, the assay is carried out in the presence of a detergent (usually Triton X-100) to offset the latency. Ascorbic acid is included as an anti-oxidant. Because the cofactor requirements for glucuronosyl transferase activity are different to those for cytochrome P450-dependent, mixed-function oxidase activity described earlier in this section, the following cofactor solution is required:

- 0.1 M Tris buffer, pH 8.0, 8.0 ml

- 0.15 M MgCl$_2$ 1.0 ml

- 1% (w/v) Triton X-100, 0.5ml

- 0.02 M ascorbic acid, 1.0 ml

- UDP–glucuronic acid, 10 mg

This is sufficient for ten assays. The assay procedure is given in Table 8.14 and the standard curve in Table 8.15. Calculate the amount of product formed by reference to the standard curve (Table 8.15) and express the activity as nmol product formed/min/mg protein or per gram wet tissue weight as appropriate.

Table 8.14 Assay for glucuronosyl transferase activity

1. Mix 1 ml cofactor solution with 0.5 ml of 1 mM 2-aminophenol and initiate the reaction with either 0.5 ml microsomal or post-mitochondrial fraction (containing 10 mg protein/ml) at 37°C in a shaking water bath.
2. A suitable blank is prepared by adding 0.5 ml H$_2$O instead of 2-aminophenol.
3. Continue the incubation for 30 min.
4. Stop the reaction with 1 ml, ice-cold 20% trichloroacetic acid in 0.1 M phosphate buffer, pH 2.7, stand on ice for 5 min and clarify the supernatant by centrifugation (bench centrifuge).
5. To 1 ml of the supernatant fluid, add 0.5 ml (fresh) 0.1% sodium nitrite, mix well and stand for 2 min.
6. Add 0.5 ml, 0.5% ammonium sulfamate, mix well and stand for 3 min.
7. Add 0.5 ml, 0.1% N-naphthylethylene diamine, mix well and allow to stand at room temperature in the dark for 60 min.
8. Read the absorbance at 540 nm against the substrate blank.
9. Prepare a standard curve (aniline) as described in Table 8.15.

Notes
1. Under the above conditions, the protein and 2-aminophenol concentrations in the incubation mixture are 2.5 mg/ml and 0.25 mM (0.25 μmol/ml) respectively.
2. Prepare incubations in triplicate or duplicate.
3. 2-aminophenol is one of the many substrates used to monitor glucuronosyl transferase activity. Many other substrates may be used (both endogenous and exogenous substrates) and the reader is referred to the articles by Burchell (1974) and Falany and Tephly (1983) for more detailed descriptions.

Table 8.15 Standard curve for 2-aminophenyl glucuronide

1. Prepare a stock solution of 0.1 mM aniline in 6% trichloroacetic acid. Aniline is used in the standard curve because it produces a chromophore of similar properties as 2-aminophenol glucuronide (not routinely available).
2. Take 0, 0.2, 0.4, 0.6, 0.8 and 1.0 ml of 0.1 mM aniline stock solution and make up to a constant volume of 1 ml with appropriate volumes of 6% trichloroacetic acid in 0.1 M phosphate buffer, pH 2.7.
3. To each tube of the standard curve, add 0.5 ml (fresh) 0.1% sodium nitrite, mix well and stand for 2 min.
4. Proceed as in Table 8.15, from step 6.
5. Construct a standard curve for aniline by plotting the absorbance values at 540 nm against the aniline concentration.

Note
Prepare the standard curve in triplicate or duplicate.

Reagents

- 1 mM 2-aminophenol (11 mg to 100 ml H_2O)
- 20% (w/v) trichloroacetic acid (200 g to 1 l H_2O)
- 6% (w/v) trichloroacetic acid (60 g to 1 l H_2O)
- 0.15 M $MgCl_2$ (15.25 g $MgCl_2$ (hexahydrate) to 500 ml H_2O)
- 1% (w/v) Triton X-100 (100 mg to 10 ml H_2O)
- 0.02 M ascorbic acid (180 mg to 50 ml H_2O)
- 20% (w/v) trichloroacetic acid (200 g to 1 l of 0.1 M phosphate buffer, pH 2.7)
- 6% (w/v) trichloroacetic acid (60 g to 1 l of 0.1 M phosphate buffer, pH 2.7)
- 0.1% (w/v) sodium nitrite (100 mg to 100 ml – make up just prior to use)
- 0.5% (w/v) ammonium sulfamate (500 mg to 100 ml)
- 0.1% (w/v) N-naphthlethylene diamine (100 mg to 100 ml)
- 0.1 mM aniline in 6% (w/v) trichloroacetic acid (13 mg aniline (HCl salt) plus 6 g trichloroacetic acid to 100 ml)

Other materials

- Rat liver microsomes *or* post-mitochondrial supernatant
- Thermostatted shaking water bath
- Spectrophotometer to read at 540 nm.
- 10 or 25 ml Ehrlenmeyer conical flasks *or* 10 ml test tubes for incubation.
- Centrifuge tubes and bench centrifuge.
- Vortex mixer or parafilm.

8.2.14 Assay for glutathione-S-transferase activity

The glutathione-S-transferases are a family of isoenzymes that catalyse the conjugation of the endogenous tripeptide glutathione (gamma-glutamylcys-teinylglycine) with a large number of structurally diverse, electrophilic xenobiotics or their metabolites. As discussed earlier, the glutathione-S-trans-ferases consist of two sub-units each of which is inducible by many drugs or xenobiotics, and although some exceptions are known (see chapter 7), their prime function is in the detoxication of biologically reactive electrophiles.

A convenient spectrophotometric method has been developed for the analysis of glutathione-S-transferase activity based on the enzyme catalysed condensa-tion of glutathione with the model substrate 2,4-dinitro-1-chlorobenzene (Figure 8.4). The product formed (2,4-dinitrophenyl-glutathione) absorbs light at 340

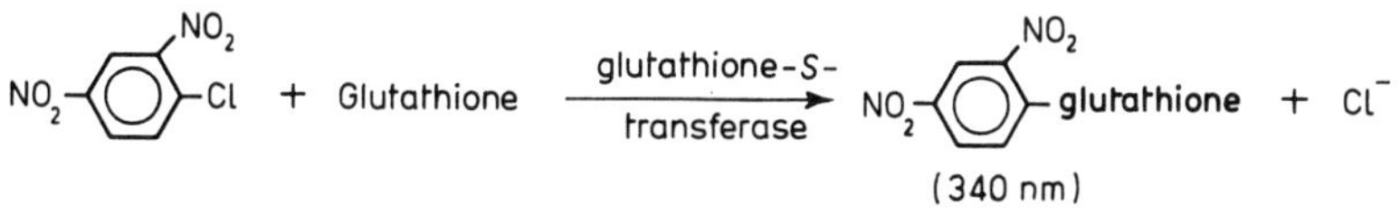

Figure 8.4 Conjugation of 1-chloro-2, 4-dinitrobenzene and glutathione as catalysed by glutathione-*S*-transferase.

nm and the extinction coefficient of this product is known to be 9.6 mM^{-1} cm^{-1}, thus facilitating the analysis of enzyme activity based on product formation. It should be pointed out that the glutathione-*S*-transferase isoenzymes have similar but overlapping substrate specificities for the electrophilic substrate to be conjugated. Therefore one substrate which is readily reactive with a particular isoenzyme may not be a substrate for another isoenzyme. With this limitation in mind, dinitrochlorobenzene is a good substrate for most of the glutathione-*S*-transferase isoenzymes, but it still must be remembered that the observed activity is a composite result of the activity of each isoenzyme present in the tissue preparation.

Table 8.16 Assay for glutathione-*S*-transferase activity

1. To each of 2 × 3 ml spectrophotometer cuvettes, add 0.1 ml of 30 mM glutathione, 0.1 ml of 30 mM dinitrochlorobenzene and 2.2 ml of 100 mM potassium phosphate buffer, pH 6.5
2. Place the cuvettes in the sample and reference compartment of a split beam recording spectrophotometer.
3. Initiate the reaction by adding 0.6 ml of a post-mitochondrial supernatant (or 100 000 *g* supernatant) from liver (10 mg/ml) and balance the reference cuvette volume by adding 0.6 ml of the appropriate buffer or medium (i.e. the medium the tissue homogenate was prepared in). Mix both cuvettes thoroughly. Carry out this step as rapidly as possible.
4. Record the increase in absorbance at 340 nm with time over a 5 min period.

Notes
1. A split-beam recording spectrophotometer is not essential and the assay may be carried out in a single cuvette instrument, remembering to subtract the enzyme blank from the test value. In addition a recording spectrophotometer is not essential in this case, record absorbance changes timed with a clock.
2. Depending on the activity of the tissue under study, the linearity period of the reaction may vary. If the linear period is short, then use less of the enzyme preparation (for example 0.1 ml). If the reaction is slow, then extend the observation period.
3. Many other substrates (in addition to dinitrochlorobenzene) may be used and the reader is referred to the original article by Habig *et al.* (1974) for additional substrates and for a detailed discussion of the glutathione-*S*-transferase assay procedure.

Conditions for the assay are given in Table 8.16 and a sample calculation of enzyme activity is as follows:

Protein concentration in cuvette	= 2 mg/ml
Extinction coefficient for glutathione adduct	= 9.6 mM^{-1}cm^{-1}
Absorbance change (340 nm) per min (linear portion)	= 0.4

Therefore using Beer's Law and assuming a cuvette path length of 1 cm, the specific activity of the glutathione-S-transferase is given by

$$\text{specific activity} \quad = \frac{0.4}{9.6 \times 2} \quad \text{mmol product formed/min/mg protein.}$$
$$= \quad 0.2 \quad \text{mmol product formed/min/mg protein.}$$

Reagents

- 30 mM dinitrochlorobenzene (62 mg to 10 ml ethanol)

- 30 mM glutathione (16 mg to 2 ml H_2O. This is sufficient for ten assays.)

- 100 mM potassium phosphate buffer, pH 6.5

Other materials

- Post-mitochondrial supernatant or 100 000 $\times$ g supernatant from rat liver

- Split-beam recording spectrophotometer to read at 340 nm

- 3 ml quartz cuvettes

8.2.15 *Additional* in vitro *assays for drug metabolism*

The above *in vitro* assays have been chosen and described in detail because they are easy to perform, give reproducible results, are rapid to perform and involve the use of a relatively widely available analytical end point, i.e. a spectrophotometer. However, many other analytical techniques may be used to assay the activity of drug metabolising enzymes including fluorimetry and radiochemical methods for example. Unfortunately these latter techniques are either time-consuming or require more expensive or less readily available instrumentation. On the other hand, fluorimetry and radiochemical methods are generally more sensitive than spectrophotometry, and dependent on the substrate investigated, may provide more incisive information about a particular metabolic pathway. Some of these assays are outlined in Tables 8.17 and 8.18 and a reference is also given to the detailed methodology and analytical technique required.

8.3 Factors affecting drug metabolism

8.3.1 *Experiment 1. Cofactor requirements of drug metabolism*

The cytochrome P450-dependent oxidation of xenobiotics in hepatic microsomes uses an electron transport pathway to deliver reducing equivalents from

Table 8.17 Additional assays for *in vitro* phase I drug metabolism

Enzyme involved	Metabolic pathway	Substrate	Analytical technique	Reference
Cytochrome P450	Ring hydroxylation	Coumarin	Fluorimetry	Jacobson *et al.* (1974)
Cytochrome P450	*O*-deethylation	7-Ethoxycoumarin	Fluorimetry	Jacobson *et al.* (1974)
Cytochrome P450	*O*-deethylation	Ethoxyresorufin	Fluorimetry	Burke and Mayer (1975)
Cytochrome P450	Ring hydroxylation	Benzo[*a*]pyrene	Fluorimetry	Nebert and Gelboin (1968)
Cytochrome P450	Alkyl hydroxylation	Lauric acid	TLC/radiochemical	Parker and Orton (1980)
Cytochrome P450	Alkyl hydroxylation	Lauric acid	HPLC/radiochemical	Gibson *et al.* (1991)
Cytochrome P450 and NADPH-cytochrome P450 reductase	Azoreductase	Amaranth	Spectrophotometry	Mallet *et al.* (1982)
Cytochrome P450	Epoxidation	Aldrin	GLC	Wolff *et al.* (1979)
Cytochrome P450	Ring hydroxylation	Testosterone or androstenedione	HPLC	Wood *et al.* (1983) and Tredger *et al.* (1984)
Cytochrome P450	Ring and *N*-hydroxylation	2-Acetylaminofluorene	HPLC	Åstrom *et al.* (1982)
Cytochrome P450	*N*-Hydroxylation	2-Acetylaminofluorene	TLC	Lotikar *et al.* (1974)
Cytochrome P450	*N*-Oxidation	*N*, *N*-Dimethylaniline	Spectrophotometric	Ziegler and Pettit (1964)
Cytochrome P450	Ring and benzylic hydroxylation	Warfarin	HPLC	Kaminsky *et al.* (1983)
Cytochrome P450	Deethylation	Phenacetin	Radiochemical	Guengerich and Martin (1980)
Cytochrome P450	Ring and side-chain oxidation	Propranolol	HPLC	Bargar *et al.* (1983)
Epoxide hydrase	Epoxide hydration	Styrene oxide	Radiochemical	Oesch *et al.* (1971)
Epoxide hydrase	Epoxide hydration	Benzo[*a*]pyrene-4, 5-oxide	Radiochemical	Schmassmann *et al.* (1976)
Epoxide hydrase	Epoxide hydration	Various epoxides	Spectrophotometric	Guengerich and Mason (1980)

Note. Additional information on *in vitro*, phase I drug metabolism assays (and purification of the enzymes) can be found in Guengerich, F.P. (1982) Microsomal enzymes involved in toxicology – analysis and separation. In *Principles and methods of toxicology* (A.W. Hayes), Raven press, New York, pp. 609–634.

Table 8.18 Additional assays of *in vitro* phase II drug metabolism

Enzyme involved	Metabolic pathway	Substrate	Analytical technique	Reference
UDP–glucurono-syltransferase	Glucuronidation	Morphine	Radiochemical	Sanchez and Tephly (1974)
UDP–glucurono-syltransferase	Glucuronidation	4-Nitrophenol	Colorimetric	Tukey *et al.* (1978)
UDP–glucurono-syltransferase	Glucuronidation	4-Methylumbel-liferone	Fluorimetric	Aitio (1974)
Gluthathione-*S*-transferase	Glutathione conjugation	Various	Spectrophotometric	Habig *et al.* (1974)

NADPH to the terminal electron acceptor, cytochrome P450. Two electrons are required in this reaction, the first of which must be supplied by NADPH via NADPH–cytochrome P450 reductase. The second electron can be supplied either from NADPH as above or from NADH via NADH–cytochrome b_5 reductase and cytochrome b_5 as described in detail in chapter 2.

According to the above scheme, NADH alone only poorly supports drug metabolism reactions, but if the second electron transfer is rate-limiting, then the addition of NADH to an NADPH-driven reaction will increase the rate of product formation. Accordingly, the following experiment is designed to show the validity of this scheme for the hepatic oxidative metabolism of drugs. It should be noted that some substrates show an increase in metabolism in the presence of NADH added to NADPH-fortified liver homogenates (termed NADH synergism), whereas other substrates do not. Aniline is a classical substrate for displaying NADH synergism, whereas the aminopyrine response is variable. Accordingly, the following experiment is designed to investigate NADH synergism for the metabolism of both aniline and aminopyrine. This experiment can easily be completed in one day (8 h).

Solutions (sufficient for two groups, each using one substrate).

- 0.25 M sucrose (85.6 g to 1 l H_2O)

- 88 mM $CaCl_2$ (if using $CaCl_2$ precipitated microsomes) (1.93 g to 100 ml H_2O)

- 5 mM NADPH (21 mg to 5 ml H_2O. Make up immediately prior to use and store on ice)

- 5 mM NADH (18 mg to 5 ml. Make up immediately prior to use and store on ice)

- 0.3 M Tris buffer, pH 7.4, 1 l

- 50 mM aniline (465 mg of hydrochloride salt to 100 ml H_2O)

- 100 mM aminopyrine (272 mg to 10 ml H_2O)

- 0.15 M $MgCl_2$ (15.25 g of the hexahydrate to 500 ml H_2O)

- 0.5 M nicotinamide (3.05 g to 50 ml H_2O)

- Solutions for protein assay, aniline hydroxylase assay and aminopyrine N-demethylase assay

Note that NADPH and/or NADH replaces the cofactor solution in this instance.

Apparatus (for two groups, using one substrate each)

- Test tubes, 120 × 15 mm, 200

- Bench centrifuge tubes, 50 ml, 20

- Ultracentrifuge tubes (if needed for microsome preparation)

- Beakers, 25, 50 and 250 ml, as required, 20

- Homogenisation vessels, 15 ml and 50 ml, one of each

- Cuvettes (disposable), 3 ml,

- Cuvettes (disposable), 1 ml, 50

- Balance (up to 30 g), one

- Timers, two

- Ice buckets, five

- Automatic pipettes: 10–100 μl, 200–1000 μl, 1–5 ml; two of each

- Shaking water bath, sufficient to take 28 tubes

- Refrigerated centrifuge, one, capable of 27 000 × g

- Ultracentrifuge, one, capable of 100 000 × g. Only required if microsomes are prepared by ultracentrifugation.

- Spectrophotometer, one, UV-visible

Method

All apparatus and solutions needed for the tissue preparation should be precooled on ice before the start of the experiment. It is important that the tissue does not exceed +4°C during preparation. Experimental animals are killed and hepatic microsomal fractions prepared as in section 8.2.1 either by the $CaCl_2$ aggregation method or by ultracentrifugation. Ten male rats (100–200 g body weight) are sufficient for this experiment. Determine the microsomal protein content (section 8.2.3) and dilute to 10 mg protein/ml.

Set up test tubes (in duplicate for both substrates) as described in Table 8.19. Tube 1 is a blank containing no NADPH or NADH and should be performed in addition to the substrate blank as described under the appropriate substrate. Tube

Table 8.19 Incubations to investigate the cofactor requirements of drug metabolism

Tube number	0.15 M MgCl$_2$ (ml)	0.5 M Nicotinamide (ml)	5 mM NADPH (ml)	0.3 M Tris buffer pH 7.4 (ml)	Microsomes 10 mg/ml, (ml)	5 mM NADH (ml)	H$_2$O (ml)
1	0.1	0.1	0	0.5	0.5	0	0.7
2	0.1	0.1	0	0.5	0.5	0.2	0.5
3	0.1	0.1	0.2	0.5	0.5	0	0.5
4	0.1	0.1	0.2	0.5	0.5	0.05	0.45
5	0.1	0.1	0.2	0.5	0.5	0.10	0.4
6	0.1	0.1	0.2	0.5	0.2	0.20	0.3
7	0.1	0.1	0.2	0.5	0.5	0.40	0.1

Note that after substrate addition, the final incubation volume is 2 ml.

2 contains only NADH as cofactor and tube 3 only NADPH. Tubes 4–7 contain differing proportions of NADH and NADPH. Tubes 2 and 3 will show the requirement for NADH and NADPH respectively when compared to the experimental blank (tube 1). Tubes 4–7 will show if any NADH synergism is evident.

The tubes are placed in a shaking water bath at 37°C for 2 min and the reaction started by adding 0.1 ml of either 50 mM aniline *or* 0.1 ml of 100 mM aminopyrine. Continue incubating at 37°C for 30 min for both substrates and stop the reaction and assay for aniline hydroxylase activity or aminopyrine *N*-demethylase activity as indicated in Tables 8.8 and 8.10 respectively.

Express both enzyme activities as nmol product formed/min/mg protein and tabulate your data to show the cofactor requirements. With reference to your results, you should be able to answer the following questions.

1. Is NADH or NADPH required for microsomal drug metabolism?

2. Can NADH alone as cofactor support drug metabolism? If so, how does this fit in with the accepted theory of oxidative metabolism.

3. Was NADH synergism observed with either substrate? If not, why?

4. If NADH synergism was observed, was there any difference in the degree of synergism seen at different rations of NADH/NADPH?

8.3.2 Experiment 2. Factors affecting drug metabolism

Many factors can affect the rate of metabolism of drugs by the liver including the species, sex and age of the animal, its genetic make-up and state of health. There are also major effects of hormonal, nutritional and environmental factors. These aspects of drug metabolism are discussed in more detail in chapters 4 and 5. The ability of different tissues to metabolise drugs is also of interest, particularly in terms of tissue selective toxicity and in cases where hepatic metabolism may be low as in liver disease. From a biochemical viewpoint, the temperature and pH of the incubation medium being used in the assay can also be of importance in determining the enzyme activity measured.

Outline

In this experiment, a number of the variables mentioned above are tested for their effect on drug metabolism using some of the assays described in section 8.2. In order to keep the experiment within one day (8 h), it is necessary to restrict the number of parameters investigated to around four per group and for each group to use two substrates. The groups given in Table 8.20 can be used as a single experiment to illustrate the effects of species, tissue, sex and temperature on drug metabolism. The large number of tissue samples used means that metabolism by post-mitochondrial supernatants must be measured unless access to a number of ultracentrifuges is available or the class is relatively small.

Table 8.20 Outline of experiments to illustrate some factors influencing drug metabolism

Animal	Groups
Male rat	Liver preparations incubated at 0, 20, 30, 37, 45 and 60°C
Male rat	Preparations from liver, kidney, brain and lung incubated at 37°C
Female rat	Liver preparations incubated at 37°C
Male frog	Liver preparations incubated at 0, 20, 30, 37, 45 and 60°C

Method

1. Prepare post-mitochondrial supernatants from male and female rats and the male frog for the tissues indicated in Table 8.20, following the method in section 8.2.1.

2. Determine the protein content of each tissue preparation as in section 8.2.3.

3. Split the class into appropriate groups and assign each group a particular experiment (Table 8.20). For each group determine the drug metabolising activity (in duplicate) for two substrates, and ensure that all groups investigate the same two substrates.

4. Express drug metabolising activity as both activity/mg protein and activity/g original wet tissue weight.

5. Collate the results from all groups and use them to answer the following questions.

- Are the effects of the various factors investigated the same for both substrates? If not, why?

- How do the temperature curves for enzyme activity compare between the male rat liver and male frog liver? If they are different, why?

- Do the male and female rat metabolise the two chosen substrates to the same extent. If not, why?

- In the male rat, place the ability of each tissue to metabolise both substrates in descending order. If the enzyme activity is expressed as per mg protein or per g original wet tissue weight, does this make any difference to the order of activity.

- Discuss the importance of the various factors studied in the regulation of drug metabolism.

- Discuss the relevance of the various factors studied in the clinical use of drugs.

Solutions

- 0.25 M sucrose (256.8 g to 3 l H_2O)

- 88 mM $CaCl_2$ if using $CaCl_2$-precipitated microsomes (1.93 g to 100 ml H_2O)

- Appropriate amounts of the solutions required for assay of the metabolism of two substrates, as in section 8.2.

Apparatus (sufficient for ten students/group)

- Test-tubes, 120×15 mm, 400

- Centrifuge tubes, 50 ml, 100

- Ultracentrifuge tubes (if required)

- 100 beakers, 25, 50 and 250 ml, as required

- Homogenisation vessels, 50 ml, minimum three

- Homogenisation vessels, 15 ml, minimum three

- Cuvettes (disposable), 3 ml, 100

- Cuvettes (disposable), 1 ml

- Balance, up to 30 g, one

- Timers, ten

- Ice-buckets, ten

- Automatic pipettes, $10–100$ μl, $200–1000$ μl and $1–5$ ml, ten of each, although a smaller number can be shared if necessary

- Thermostatted, shaking water baths, five

- Refrigerated centrifuge, up to $27\ 000 \times g$, one

- Refrigerated ultracentrifuge (if required), as many as are available to cut down on tissue processing time

- Spectrophotometer, UV–visible, one

8.4 Induction and inhibition of drug metabolism and a correlation of *in vivo* drug action with *in vitro* hepatic drug metabolising activity

8.4.1 Introduction

The duration and intensity of action of many drugs is critically influenced by the rate of their metabolism. As discussed previously in chapter 3, the rate of drug metabolism can be substantially altered (either increased or decreased) by the prior treatment of animals with various compounds, some of which may be structurally unrelated to the drug metabolised.

The present two experiments are designed to demonstrate the effects of a compound that stimulates (induces) the liver drug metabolising enzymes (phenobarbitone) or inhibits (destroys) these enzymes (CCl_4) on

- The *in vivo* duration of action of the hypnotic drug pentobarbitone

- The drug metabolising activity of the 12 500 g liver supernatant as measured by the *in vitro* N-demethylation of aminopyrine

- The levels of cytochrome P450 in the hepatic microsomal fraction

It is then possible to compare the duration of action of a drug *in vivo* with both the activities of the drug metabolising enzymes *in vitro* and the levels of cytochrome P450. Note that the following two experiments can easily be completed in one day provided that the class is large enough (around 20) and the class is split into groups. However, if the class is small (around six to ten) then the following two experiments may have to be attempted on separate days.

8.4.2 Experiment 1: The duration of action of the hypnotic drug pentobarbitone

Pentobarbitone is a hypnotic drug whose duration of action can be measured in rats by the sleeping time (i.e. the time from when the animal falls asleep to when it regains its 'righting reflex'). Therefore, because pentobarbitone is metabolised by the hepatic microsomal cytochrome P450 enzyme system (Figure 8.5), its duration of action can be altered by inducing agents or by inhibitors.

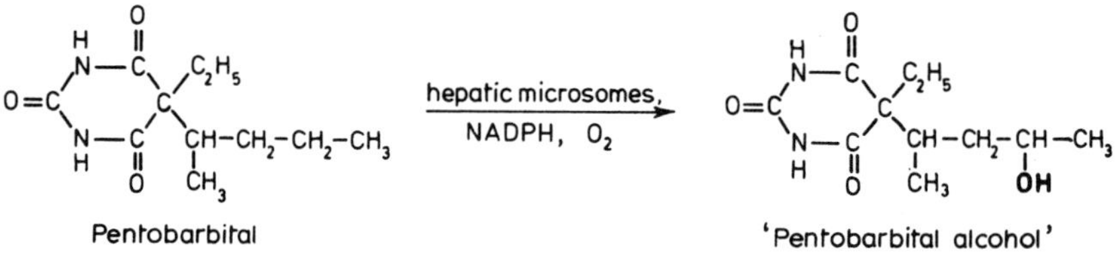

Pentobarbital   'Pentobarbital alcohol'

Figure 8.5 The cytochrome P450-dependent metabolism (side-chain hydroxylation) of pentobarbitone.

Animal pretreatment

Male rats, initially weighing 80–100g and fed a standard laboratory diet are used in groups of ten per treatment. It is important that the rat body weights are as close together as possible at the start of the pretreatment, in view of the well documented age differences in drug metabolism and drug response. Ten rats are injected intraperitoneally once daily for 3 days prior to the experiment with either sodium phenobarbitone, 80 mg/kg (in saline) or an equivalent volume of saline, the latter saline treated group serving as vehicle controls. In addition, a third group of ten rats are injected on the third day only with a single, intraperitoneal injection of carbon tetrachloride, 1.25 ml/kg (in corn oil). Although a corn oil vehicle control group of rats should ideally be used, previous experience indicates that the corn oil control is not significantly different from the saline control and hence the latter group serves as a control group for both pretreatments. If the above protocol is followed, then all groups of rats will be ready for the start of the experiment on the fourth day, i.e. 24 h after the last injection.

Method

Three groups of rats (ten in each group) are now available to study the influence of pretreatment on the *in vivo* duration of action of pentobarbitone. It is advisable to start this experiment in the morning so that when the sleeping times are being monitored, the tissue homogenates are being simultaneously prepared for use in the afternoon.

Every rat, in all three groups, is then given an intraperitoneal injection of pentobarbitone at a dose of 30 mg/kg. The rats can be separately caged or appropriately marked to monitor individual sleeping times. Note the times at which each rat is

(a) injected

(b) falls asleep as measured by its loss of the righting reflex

(c) wakes up as measured by regaining of the righting reflex, twice within a
    period of 10 s

The righting reflex is easily monitored by gently placing the rat on its back – if the righting reflex is still present, the animal will 'right' itself. If the reflex has been abolished, the animal will attempt to get up but is unable to do so. Clearly from the above discussion, the 'sleeping time' is the difference between (b) and (c).

It should be noted that, dependent on the rat strain used, the drug response may vary. In our experience for the stated dose in male Wistar rats, the control group will sleep for around 1 h, the CCl_4 treated group for around 3 h and the phenobarbitone treated group for much less than an hour.

Treatment of data

The mean sleeping time, ± S.E. and S.D. for each group of rats should be calculated and compared statistically with the control group to determine if the pretreatment has had a statistically significant effect in either increasing or decreasing the sleeping time.

8.4.3 Experiment 2: Influence of pretreatment on the in vitro N-*demethylation of aminopyrine and microsomal cytochrome P450 content*

The purpose of this experiment is to determine the ability of rat liver to N-demethylate aminopyrine, to determine the hepatic microsomal cytochrome

P450 content and to investigate the influence of pretreatment with either pheno-barbital or CCl_4 on these two parameters. Because the animal pretreatment involves the same two compounds used to assess the influence on the sleeping times in the previous experiment, then the two experiments can be finally compared to determine if modulation of *in vitro* drug metabolising activity is reflected in any change in drug action *in vivo*.

Animal pretreatment

In order to compare the results of this experiment with the previous one the pretreatment schedules are identical to that described for the sleeping times, with the only exception that smaller groups of animals are used. This is largely to minimise the numbers of animals used and because of constraints of available centrifuge space and time of preparation of individual tissue homogenates. Accordingly, it is recommended to use only five animals per group, with the same three groups of control, phenobarbitone treated and CCl_4 treated rats. The treatment should start on the same day as the sleeping time experiment.

Method

The rats are killed, the livers removed, blotted dry and weighed and a 12 500 g supernatant made from each individual liver in all groups, as described in section 8.2.1. Remove 12 ml of each of the 12 500 g supernatant preparations and determine the protein content of each sample, as in section 8.2.3. This prepara-tion is then used for the aminopyrine N-demethylase determination, as described in section 8.2.10. The remainder of the 12 500 g supernatant is then centrifuged at 100 000 g to prepare microsomal fractions. Alternatively, microsomal fractions may be prepared by the $CaCl_2$-aggregation method. Determine the protein content and cytochrome P450 content of each of the microsomal preparations.

Treatment of data

1. Calculate the aminopyrine N-demethylase specific activity of each sample, expressing your results as both activity per mg 12 500 g supernatant protein and activity per g wet liver weight. For each pretreatment group, calculate the mean specific activity for aminopyrine N-demethylation, the S.E. and S.D. Statistically compare the influence of both phenobarbital and CCl_4 pretreatments on drug metabolism activity as compared to the control (saline treated) group of rats.

2. Calculate the cytochrome P450 specific content of each microsomal prepara-tion, expressed as nmol cytochrome P450 per mg microsomal protein. For each pretreatment group, determine the mean ($\pm$ S.E. and S.D.) cytochrome P450 content and statistically test if the pretreatment has influenced the results obtained, by comparison to the control group.

3. Finally, compare the results of experiments 1 and 2 to determine if

modulation of *in vitro* drug metabolising enzyme activity is mirrored by appropriate changes in the *in vivo* sleeping times.

Solutions

The following solutions and materials are required, assuming that both experiments are completed in the one day.

- Phenobarbitone (20 mg/ml)

- Pentobarbitone (6 mg/ml)

- CCl_4 (undiluted)

- Corn oil (undiluted)

- Saline (0.9%, w/v, NaCl) (900 mg to 100 ml H_2O)

- 0.25 M sucrose (85.6 g to 1 l H_2O)

- 88 mM $CaCl_2$ (if using $CaCl_2$ precipitated microsomes) (1.93 g to 100 ml H_2O)

- Sufficient solutions for protein determination, aminopyrine-*N*-demethylation and cytochrome P450 determination

Apparatus and other materials

45 male rats, 80–100 g body weight

All other materials are as given in the list of apparatus for section 8.3.2

8.5 Urinary excretion of paracetamol in man

Paracetamol (acetaminophen) in normal therapeutic doses is generally considered one of the safest of all minor analgesics, although it should be pointed out that large overdoses of paracetamol may produce hepatic necrosis in man and other animals. After administration, paracetamol is eliminated from the body by the apparent, first order processes of metabolism, and to a small extent, excretion, the principal metabolites in man being the glucuronide and sulfate conjugates (Figure 8.6).

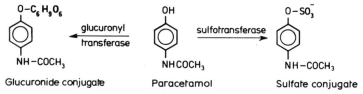

Figure 8.6 The *in vivo* metabolism of paracetamol.

The elimination of paracetamol may be rationalised mathematically according to the method of Cummings *et al.* (1967). Using this approach, it has been shown that a plot of the log rate of excretion of 'total drug' will ultimately become a straight line of slope equal to

$$\frac{K_E}{2.303}$$

where K_E is the elimination rate constant. Thus in this experiment, the log excretion rate of 'total drug' (mg/h) is plotted at the mid-point of each time interval of urine collection. As discussed in chapter 7, the elimination rate constant (K_E) is estimated from the slope of the above plot and the half-life ($t_{1/2}$) of paracetamol can be calculated from

$$t_{1/2} = \frac{0.693}{K_E}$$

Human subjects

In normal, healthy individuals, the dose of paracetamol used in this experiment is entirely without side effects and is a dose taken routinely as an analgesic for headaches. However, it must be emphasised that the drug should **not** be taken by people who:

- have a history of hepatic or kidney disease of any type
- habitually take paracetamol
- exhibit allergic or hypersensitivity reactions to this drug
- are under current therapy with other drugs
- are generally in poor health

If the subject is in *any doubt* at all about whether or not to take paracetamol, they should seek professional medical advice before participating in the experiment. Furthermore, if the experiment is being conducted as a class practical, it is the *organiser's* responsibility to ensure that the experimental protocol is in agreement with the local ethical and safety guidelines laid down by the appropriate institutional body.

Preliminary notes

1. This experiment can be conducted in pairs, one member of each pair taking the drug. This protocol then gives the advantage that the excretion of paracetamol can be compared from subject to subject.

2. In view of the fact that urine samples have to be collected over a 6 h period, it is convenient for the subject to take the drug and collect urine samples the day prior to being analysed. The urine samples can be stored overnight at 4°C without appreciable decomposition and analysed the following day.

Paracetamol administration and collection of urine

1. In order to maintain a reasonable urine flow, the subject should initially drink about 200 ml of water. After 30 min, the bladder should be voided into a suitable container – this sample represents the blank urine.

2. Paracetamol (500 mg) is ingested with 200 ml of water and a clock started – this is time zero.

3. After 1 h, the bladder is voided again, the volume of urine measured, the sample is annotated and an additional 100 ml of water taken.

4. The same procedure as in (3) is repeated every hour for 2, 3, 4, 5 and 6 h.

5. The 'total drug' in each urine sample is measured (in duplicate) as below.

Analytical method

The urine samples will be analysed for 'total paracetamol' by treatment of urine samples with acid. In this method, paracetamol and its sulfate and glucuronide conjugates present in urine are hydrolysed in the presence of acid to 4-aminophenol. This compound is subsequently coupled with phenol in the presence of hypobromite to form an indophenol dye whose concentration is determined spectrophotometrically with reference to a standard curve as follows:

(1) The standard curve is obtained by initially preparing a stock solution of paracetamol (1 mg/ml) in water. Dilutions of this stock are made with water giving standard paracetamol solutions of 50, 100, 200, 400, 600 and 800 μg/ml.

(2) Pipette (in duplicate) 1 ml of blank urine into a test-tube followed by 4 ml of 4 M HCl and 1 ml of each standard paracetamol solution. Mix thoroughly. A suitable blank is prepared (in duplicate) in which 1 ml of water is added instead of the standard paracetamol solution.

(3) Cover the tubes with marbles and place in a boiling water bath (in a fume cupboard) for 1 h.

(4) Cool the tubes and accurately make the volume up to 10 ml with water. Mix thoroughly.

(5) Pipette 1 ml from the 10 ml hydrolysed urine sample into a separate test-tube and add 10 ml of the 'colour forming solution'. Mix gently and allow to stand for 40 min.

(6) Measure the absorbance of each solution at 620 nm in a spectrophotometer, zeroing the instrument on the drug-free, blank urine sample.

(7) Starting from (2) above, treat each collected urine sample (in duplicate, preferably at the same time) in a similar manner, substituting the timed urine

sample for the blank urine. In addition, replace the 1 ml standard paracetamol solution with 1 ml of water.

Treatment of results

1. Plot a calibration curve of absorbance at 620 nm versus the known concentration of paracetamol (in μg/ml).

2. The 'total drug' in each urine sample is then determined from the calibration
curve and hence the amount per hour, knowing the volume of each urine
sample.

3. A graph of the log rate of excretion (mg/h) is plotted against the mid-point of
each time interval.

4. From the plot in (3), estimate the elimination rate constant (K_E) and the half-
life ($t_{1/2}$) for paracetamol excretion.

5. Compare the class results and note any substantial differences in the kinetic
parameters for paracetamol excretion from subject to subject. If a substantial
variation in K_E or $t_{1/2}$ is noted, suggest a reason(s) why this should be so.

Simple qualitative tests on urine to determine the nature of the metabolites

These following tests should be carried out on all the urine samples,
including the blank.

(a) Naphthoresorcinol test for glucuronide conjugates

Urine (0.5 ml), solid naphthoresorcinol (approx. 2 mg) and concentrated
HCl (1 ml) are boiled (fume cupboard) for 3 min, then cooled. Ethyl acetate
(3 ml) is added and the mixture shaken. A purple coloration in the organic
layer indicates the presence of glucuronic acid or a glucuronide. Compare
with a control of normal urine. This is a sensitive test. (N.B. This test cannot be
used for biliary metabolites owing to the large amounts of bilirubin glucuronide
present).

Further information on the glucuronide may be obtained by carrying out
Benedict's test on the urine. Glucoronides of carboxyl groups (ester
glucuronides) and *N*-glucoronides will give a positive test as they are hydrolysed
by the alkaline conditions of the test. Glucoronides of hydroxyl groups (ether
glucuronides) will not react as this glycosidic linkage is stable to alkali.

(b) Barium chloride test for sulfate conjugates

Adjust a urine sample (0.5 ml) to pH 4–6 and add 2 ml of a 2% $BaCl_2$
solution. Centrifuge the $BaSO_4$ precipitate formed from the inorganic sulfate present. Add 2 drops of concentrated HCl to the supernatant and boil (fume
cupboard) for 3 min. The formation of a further precipitate or turbidity
suggests the presence of a sulfate conjugate. Compare with a control of normal
urine. This test is rather insensitive.

(c) Ferric chloride test for phenols

To a urine sample (0.5 ml) adjusted to pH 7 add 2% $FeCl_3$ solution dropwise. The first few drops produce a precipitate of ferric phosphate which may be centrifuged if necessary. Further dropwise addition of $FeCl_3$ may produce a purple or green coloration if a phenol is present. The sensitivity of this test varies for different phenols and many do not produce a colour at all.

Solutions (sufficient for ten pairs/group)

- 1 mg/ml paracetamol, (100 mg to 100 ml H_2O)

- 4 M HCl, 2 l

- 0.2 M NaOH (32 g to 4 l – for colour forming reagent)

- 1% (w/v) phenol (5 g to 500 ml – for colour forming reagent) Make up fresh 2 M sodium carbonate – bromine solution. Dissolve 53 g anhydrous sodium carbonate in water and dilute to 500 ml. Add 75 ml of bromine-saturated water solution to 500 ml of the sodium carbonate solution. Used in colour forming reagent. Make up fresh.

- Colour forming reagent: Mix 4 l of 0.2 M NaOH, 500 ml of 1% phenol and 500 ml of the carbonate–bromine reagent. Make up fresh.

- Solid naphthoresorcinol

- Concentrated HCl, 200 ml

- Ethyl acetate, 600 ml

- 2% (w/v) $BaCl_2$ (8 g to 400 ml)

- 2% (w/v) $FeCl_3$ (2 g to 100 ml)

Apparatus and other materials

- Urine samples

- Measuring cylinders, 50, 100, 250 ml, ten of each

- Filter funnels, ten of each

- Beakers, 50, 100, 250 ml, ten of each

- Plastic storage bottles, 100 ml, 100 of each

- Paracetamol, 10 × 500 mg capsules

- Clocks, ten

- Test tubes, 120 × 15 mm, 400

- Marbles, 400

- UV–vis spectrophotometer (reading to 620 nm)
- Bench centrifuge, ten
- pH paper or pH meter

8.6 Practice problem

Propranolol, a β-adrenergic blocking drug, was administered both orally (80 mg) and intravenously (10 mg) on separate occasions to a patient (weight,70kg) and the following plasma levels of propranol obtained.

Time after administration (h)	Plasma level (ng/ml) Oral	i.v.
0.5	-	52.5
1	80.7	46.0
2	95.2	33.5
3	100.0	25.0
4	83.6	18.3
5	69.5	13.6
6	57.7	10.2
7	48.0	7.5
8	40.0	5.6

(a) From the i.v. data determine the half-life ($t_{1/2}$), the rate constant of elimination, K_E and the volume of distribution of propranolol. Comment on your results.

(b) From the oral data, determine the $t_{1/2}$ and K_E of propranolol.

(c) Determine the areas under the curve (AUC) for propranolol following both oral and i.v. administration. (The AUC is a measure of the availability of the drug, i.e. the amount of the drug that reaches the systemic circulation. The AUC may be determined by various methods such as weighing the areas or by the trapezoidal rule.) You must correct for the different amounts of drug given by the two routes. In this problem, the amount of orally administered drug reaching the systemic circulation is

$$\frac{\text{AUC (oral)}}{\text{AUC (i.v.)}} \times \frac{10}{80} \times 100\%$$

Suggest possible reasons for the different results obtained from both routes of administration.

Further reading and references

A. Aitio. (1974) *Int. J. Biochem.*, **5** 325–30.

A. Åstrom and J.W. de Pierre. (1982) 2-Acetylaminofluorene induces forms of cytochrome P-450 active in its own metabolism, *Carcinogenesis*, **3** 711–3.

E.M. Bargar, U.K. Walle, S.A. Bai and T.Walle. (1983) Quantitative metabolic fate of propranolol in the dog, rat and hamster using radiotracer, high pressure liquid chromatography and gas chromatography/mass spectrometry techniques, *Drug Metab. Dispn.*, **11** 266–72.

A.C. Bratton and E.K. Marshall. (1939) A new coupling component for sulphanilamide determination, *J. Biol. Chem.*, **128** 537–50.

B. Burchell (1974) Substrate specificity of UDP-glucuronyltransferase, purified to apparent homogeneity from phenobarbital-treated rat liver, *Biochem. J.*, **173** 749–57.

M.D. Burke and R.T. Mayer. (1975) Inherent specificities of purified cytochromes P-450 and P-448 towards biphenyl hydroxylation and ethoxyresorufin deethylation, *Drug Metab. Dispn.*, **3** 245–50.

M.D. Burke and R.T. Mayer. (1983) *Chemico–Biological Interactions*, **45** 243–51.

Cummings, Martin and Park. (1967) *Brit. J.Pharmacol. Chemother.*, **29** 136.

N.A. Elshourbagy and P.S. Guzelian. (1980) Separation, purification and characterisation of a novel form of hepatic cytochrome P-450 from rats treated with pregnenolone-16α-carbonitrile, *J. Biol. Chem.*, **255** 1279–85.

C.N. Falany and T.R. Tephly. (1983) Separation, purification and characterisation of three isoenzymes of UDP-glucuronyltransferase from rat liver microsomes, *Arch. Biochem. Biophys.*, **227** 248–58.

G.G. Gibson and B.G. Lake. (1991) Induction protocols for the cytochrome P4504 family in animals and primary hepatocyte culture. In *Methods in Enzymology*, **206** 353–64.

F.P. Guengerich and H. Martin. (1980) Purification of cytochrome P-450, NADPH cytochrome P-450 reductase and epoxide hydrase from a single preparation of rat liver microsomes, *Arch. Biochem. Biophys.*, **205** 365–79.

F.P. Guengerich and P.S. Mason. (1980) Alcohol dehydrogenase-coupled spectrophotometric assay of epoxide hydratase activity, *Anal. Biochem.*, **104** 445–51.

W.H. Habig, M.J. Pabst and W.B. Jakoby. (1974) Glutathione-*S*-transferase, the first enzymatic step in mercapturic acid formation, *J. Biol. Chem.*, **249** 7130–9.

M. Jacobson, W. Levin, P.J. Poppers, A.W. Wood and A.H. Conney. (1974) Comparison of the *O*-dealkylation of 7-ethoxycoumarin and hydroxylation of benzo(*a*)pyrene in human placenta, *Clin. Pharmacol. Ther.*, **16** 701–10.

G.C. Kahn, A.R. Boobis, S. Murray, M.J. Brodie and D.S. Davies. (1982) *Brit. J. Clin. Pharmacol.*, **13** 637.

L.S. Kaminsky, F.P. Guengerich, G.A. Dannan and S.D. Aust. (1983) Comparisons of warfarin metabolism by liver microsomes of rats treated with a series of polybrominated biphenyl congeners and by the component purified cytochrome P-450 isoenzymes, *Arch. Biochem. Biophys.*, **225** 398–404.

B.G. Lake. (1987) Preparation and characterisation of microsomal fractions for studies on xenobiotic metabolism. In *Biochemical toxicology, a practical approach* (K. Snell and B. Mullock), IRL press, Oxford, pp 182–215.

P.D. Lotlikar, L. Luha and K. Zaleski. (1974) Reconstituted hamster liver microsomal enzyme system for *N*-hydroxylation of the carcinogen, 2-acetyl-aminofluorene, *Biochem. Biophys. Res. Commun.*, **59** 1349–55.

O.H. Lowry, N.J. Rosebrough, A.L. Farr and R.J. Randall. (1951) Protein measurement with the Folin phenol reagent, *J. Biol. Chem.*, **193** 265–75.

A.K. Mallett, L.J. King and R. Walker. (1982) A continuous spectrophotometric determination of hepatic microsomal azoreductase activity and its dependence on cytochrome P-450, *Biochem. J.*, **201** 589–95.

T. Nash. (1953) The colorimetric estimation of formaldehyde by means of the Hantzsch reaction, *J. Biol. Chem.*, **55** 416–22.

D.W. Nebert and H.V. Gelboin. (1968) Substrate-inducible microsomal aryl hydrocarbon hydroxylase in mammalian cell culture. I. Assay and properties of the induced enzyme, *J. Biol. Chem.*, **243** 6242–9.

F. Oesch, D.M. Jerina and J. Daly. (1971) A radiometric assay for hepatic hydratase activity with (³H)-styrene oxide, *Biochim. Biophys. Acta*, **227** 685–91.

K. Ohnishi and C.S. Lieber. (1977) Reconstitution of the microsomal ethanol-oxidising system. Qualitative and quantitative changes of cytochrome P-450 after chronic ethanol consumption, *J. Biol. Chem.*, **252** 7124–31.

G.L. Parker and T.C. Orton. (1980) Induction by oxyisobutyrates of hepatic and kidney microsomal cytochrome P-450 with specificity towards hydroxylation of fatty acids. In *Biochemistry, biophysics and regulation of cytochrome P-450*, (J.A. Gustafsson, J. Carlstedt-Duke, A. Mode and J. Rafter), Elsevier, Amsterdam 373–7.

D.E. Ryan, P.E. Thomas and W. Levin. (1980) Hepatic microsomal cytochrome P-450 from rats treated with isosafrole. Purification and characterisation of four enzymic forms, *J. Biol. Chem.*, **255** 7941–55.

E. Sanchez and T.R. Tephly. (1974) Morphine metabolism. Evidence for separate enzymes in the glucuronidation of morphine and para-nitrophenol by rat hepatic microsomes, *Drug Metab. Dispn.*, **2** 247–53.

J.B. Schenkman, H. Remmer and R.W. Estabrook. (1967) Spectral studies of drug interactions with hepatic microsomal cytochrome P-450 *Mol. Pharamcol.*, **3** 113-23.

J.B. Schenkman, S.G. Sligar and D.L. Cinti. (1981) Substrate interaction with cytochrome P-450, *Pharmacol. Ther.*, **12** 43–71.

H.U. Schmassmann, H.R. Glatt and F. Oesch. (1976) A rapid assay for epoxide hydratase activity with benzo(*a*)pyrene 4,5-oxide as substrate, *Anal. Biochem.*, **74** 94–104.

K. Snell and B. Mullock (eds). (1987) *Biochemical toxicology, a practical approach*, IRL Press, Oxford.

J.M. Tredger, H.M. Smith and R. Williams. (1984) Effects of ethanol and enzyme-inducing agents on the monooxygenation of testosterone and xenobiotics in rat liver microsomes, *J. Pharmacol. Exp. Ther.*, **229** 292–8.

R.H. Tukey, R.E. Billings and T.R. Tephly. (1978) Separation of oestrone UDP-glucuronyltransferase and para-nitrophenol UDP-glucuronyltransferase activities, *Biochem. J.*, **171** 659-63.

V. Ullrich and P. Weber. (1972) The *O*-dealkylation of 7-ethoxycoumarin by liver microsomes, *Hoppe-Seyler's Z. Physiol. Chem.*, **353** 1171–7.

M. Waterman and E.F. Johnson, (eds). (1991) *Methods in enzymology: cytochrome P450*, Academic Press, San Diego.

T. Wolff, E. Demi and H. Wanters. (1979) Aldrin epoxidation, a highly sensitive indicator for cytochrome P-450-dependent monooxygenase activity, *Drug Metab. Dispn.*, **7** 301–5.

A.W. Wood, D.E. Ryan, P.E. Thomas and W. Levin. (1983) Regio- and stereoselective metabolism of two C_{19} steroids by five highly purified and reconstituted rat hepatic cytochrome P-450 isoenzymes, *J. Biol. Chem.*, **258** 8839–47.

C.S. Yang, F.S. Strickhart and L.P. Kicha. (1978) Analysis of the aryl hydrocarbon hydroxylase assay, *Biochem. Pharmacol.*, **27** 2321–6.

R.N. Wixtrom and B.D. Hamock. (1988) Continuous spectrophotometric assays for cytosolic epoxide hydrolase. *Analytical Biochemistry*, **174** 291–9.

D. Zakim and D.A. Vessey (eds). (1985) *Biochemical pharmacology and toxicology, Volume 1. Methodological aspects of drug metabolising enzymes*, Wiley, New York.

D.M. Ziegler and H. Pettit. (1964) Formation of an intermediate *N*-oxide in the oxidative demethylation of *N, N*-dimethylaniline catalysed by liver microsomes, *Biochem. Biophys. Res. Commun.*, **15** 188–93.

Index